CASE STUDIES

Stahl's Essential Psychopharmacology
Volume 6

This sixth volume in Stahl's Case Studies series presents a selection of clinical case studies in forensic psychopharmacology. Focusing on critical syndromes and clinical presentations found in the severely mentally ill who have become justice involved and/or required care in a state or forensic hospital facility, these cases illustrate questions that are routinely asked in psychopharmacological consultations. Following a consistent, user-friendly layout, each case features icons, tips, and questions about diagnosis and management as it progresses over time, a pre-case self-assessment question, followed by the correct answers at the end of the case. Formatted in alignment with the American Board of Psychiatry and Neurology's maintenance of psychiatry specialty certification, cases address multifaceted issues in an understandable way. Covering a wide-ranging and representative selection of clinical scenarios, each case is followed through the complete clinical encounter, from start to resolution, acknowledging the complications, issues, decisions, twists, and turns along the way.

Carolina A. Klein is the Associate Medical Director and Lead Psychiatrist in Advancement & Innovation at California Department of State Hospitals in Sacramento, California.

Stephen M. Stahl is Adjunct Professor of Psychiatry at the University of California, San Diego; Clinical Professor of Psychiatry and Neuroscience at the University of California, Riverside; and Honorary Visiting Senior Fellow in Psychiatry at the University of Cambridge.

CASE STUDIES: Stahl's Essential Psychopharmacology

Forensic Psychiatry
Volume 6
Edited by
Carolina A. Klein
California Department of State Hospitals, Sacramento
Stephen M. Stahl
University of California, San Diego and Riverside

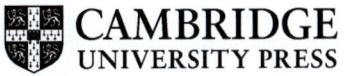

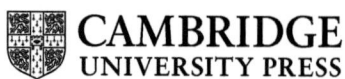
CAMBRIDGE
UNIVERSITY PRESS

Shaftesbury Road, Cambridge CB2 8EA, United Kingdom

One Liberty Plaza, 20th Floor, New York, NY 10006, USA

477 Williamstown Road, Port Melbourne, VIC 3207, Australia

314–321, 3rd Floor, Plot 3, Splendor Forum, Jasola District Centre, New Delhi – 110025, India

103 Penang Road, #05–06/07, Visioncrest Commercial, Singapore 238467

Cambridge University Press is part of Cambridge University Press & Assessment, a department of the University of Cambridge.

We share the University's mission to contribute to society through the pursuit of education, learning, and research at the highest international levels of excellence.

www.cambridge.org
Information on this title: www.cambridge.org/9781009335867
DOI: 10.1017/9781009335874

© Cambridge University Press & Assessment 2026

This publication is in copyright. Subject to statutory exception and to the provisions of relevant collective licensing agreements, no reproduction of any part may take place without the written permission of Cambridge University Press & Assessment.

When citing this work, please include a reference to the DOI 10.1017/9781009335874

First published 2026

Printed in the United Kingdom by CPI Group Ltd, Croydon CR0 4YY

A catalogue record for this publication is available from the British Library

Library of Congress Cataloging-in-Publication Data
Names: Klein, Carolina A. editor | Stahl, Stephen M., 1951– editor
Title: Case studies : Stahl's essential psychopharmacology : forensic psychiatry,
  volume 6 / edited by Carolina A. Klein, Stephen M. Stahl.
Description: Cambridge ; New York, NY : Cambridge University Press, 2025. |
  Includes bibliographical references and index.
Identifiers: LCCN 2025014286 | ISBN 9781009335867 paperback | ISBN 9781009335874 ebook
Subjects: LCSH: Forensic psychiatry – Case studies | Psychopharmacology – Case studies
Classification: LCC RA1151 .C315 2025
LC record available at https://lccn.loc.gov/2025014286

ISBN 978-1-009-33586-7 Paperback

Cambridge University Press & Assessment has no responsibility for the persistence or accuracy of URLs for external or third-party internet websites referred to in this publication and does not guarantee that any content on such websites is, or will remain, accurate or appropriate.

Every effort has been made in preparing this book to provide accurate and up-to-date information that is in accord with accepted standards and practice at the time of publication. Although case histories are drawn from actual cases, every effort has been made to disguise the identities of the individuals involved. Nevertheless, the authors, editors, and publishers can make no warranties that the information contained herein is totally free from error, not least because clinical standards are constantly changing through research and regulation. The authors, editors, and publishers therefore disclaim all liability for direct or consequential damages resulting from the use of material contained in this book. Readers are strongly advised to pay careful attention to information provided by the manufacturer of any drugs or equipment that they plan to use.

For EU product safety concerns, contact us at Calle de José Abascal, 56, 1°,
28003 Madrid, Spain, or email eugpsr@cambridge.org

Contents

List of Contributors vii
List of icons ix
List of Abbreviations xi

Section I. Aggression and Violence in the Forensic Setting

1. Psychotic aggression: the magic combo 3
   Jongseung Baek and Seth Judd

2. Impulsive affective aggression: Action in a second 17
   Maanasi Chandarana

3. Predatory violence: The wolf in sheep's clothing 29
   Maanasi Chandarana

Section II. Self-Injurious Behaviors (SIB) or Non-suicidal self-injury (NSSI)

4. Self-injurious behavior (SIB) and violence: Inward and outward 43
   Jennifer O'Day

5. Non-suicidal self-injury (NSSI): Death by a thousand cuts 51
   Maanasi Chandarana

6. Prolonged fasting: Starved for care 65
   Amanie Salem and Carolina A. Klein

7. Severe suicidality: To die at any cost 73
   Amanie Salem and Carolina A. Klein

Section III. Critical Associated Syndromes of Severe Mental Illness (SMI)

8. Who's who? Misidentification syndromes in severe mental illness (SMI) 85
   Carolina A. Klein and Amanie Salem

9. Primary polydipsia: Unquenchable thirsts 97
   Shrey Patel and Seth Judd

10. Catatonia: Turning into stone 117
    Amanie Salem and Carolina A. Klein

11. Negative syndrome: Nothing and nobody 131
    Michael McGee and Rocco Marotta

12. Post-psychotic depression: Too good to be true, so it's blue 139
    Maanasi Chandarana

SECTION IV. Iatrogenic Syndromes and Drug-Associated Side Effects

13. Neuroleptic malignant syndrome: Altered and rigid — 161
    Ajay Nair, Carolina A. Klein, and Amanie Salem

14. Constipation and capacity: The full stop — 171
    Seth Judd and Kim-Long Hua-Rupp

Section V. Complex Comorbidities

15. TBI and CTE: Bruised brains — 189
    Carolina Klein and Hunter Neely

16. Addictions: Everyone, everywhere, everything — 201
    Long Hoang and Seth Judd

17. Personality disorders: Fixing the foundation — 219
    Emilia Laing and Seth Judd

18. Schizo-obsessive disorder: Repeatedly compelling — 235
    Ajay Nair, Amanie Salem, and Carolina A. Klein

19. Anxiety disorders: Constant worries — 247
    Maanasi Chandarana

20. COVID-19: The new player in town and here to stay — 271
    Maanasi Chandarana

21. Neurological disorders: Near and Fa(h)r — 289
    Maanasi Chandarana

Section VI. Specialty Forensic Populations

22. Incompetent to stand trial (IST) Murphy Conservatorship (MurCON): Conserved or convicted? — 309
    Maanasi Chandarana

23. Sexually violent predators (SVPs): Interrupting the circuit — 329
    Rachel Powers and Carolina A. Klein

24. Pregnancy: Treating for two — 343
    Imran Hassan and Gillian Friedman

25. Schizo-obsessive compulsive disorder (SCZ-OCD), addictions, paraphilia: The collision — 349
    Hunter Neely

Case Studies: Index — 363
Index of drug names — 375

Contributors

Jongseung Baek, DO, Florida Healthcare Psychiatry Residency Program, University of Florida HCA

Maanasi Chandarana, DO, California Department of State Hospitals

Imran Hassan, MD, California Department of State Hospitals

Long Hoang, DO, California Department of State Hospitals; Psychiatry Residency Training Program, St. Joseph's Medical Center, Dignity Health

Kim-Long Hua-Rupp, MD, California Department of State Hospitals; St. Joseph's Medical Center, Dignity Health

Seth Judd, DO, California Department of State Hospitals; College of Osteopathic Medicine, Touro University California

Carolina A. Klein, MD, California Department of State Hospitals; The Maia Institute

Emilia Laing, DO, Sutter Roseville Internal Medicine Residency Program

Rocco Marotta, MD Ph.D., Center for the Treatment and Study of Neuropsychiatric Disorders; Yale University School of Medicine; CUNY School of Medicine

Michael McGee, MD, WellMind, Inc.; Optima Healing and Recovery

Ajay Nair, MD, NYU Grossman School of Medicine, Bellevue Hospital

Hunter Neely, MD, California Department of State Hospitals

Jennifer O'Day, MD, California Department of State Hospitals; Clinical Faculty, University of California Riverside School of Medicine

Shrey Patel, MD, California Department of State Hospitals; Psychiatry Residency Training Program, St. Joseph's Medical Center, Dignity Health

Rachel Powers, PsyD, California Department of State Hospitals

Amanie Salem, MD, California Department of State Hospitals

List of icons

?	Pre- and post-test self-assessment question; question
📋	Patient evaluation on intake; patient evaluation on initial visit
🧠	Psychiatric history
ABC	Social and personal history
🩺	Medical history
🏠	Family history
℞	Medication history
💊	Current medications/history

List of icons

	Psychotherapy history; psychotherapy moment
	Mechanism of action moment
	Attending physician's mental notes
	Further investigation
	Case outcome; use of outcome measures
	Case debrief
	Take-home points
	Performance in practice: confessions of a psychopharmacologist
	Tips and pearls
	Two-minute tutorial

Abbreviations

ACE	angiotensin-converting enzyme	CSF	cerebrospinal fluid
ACEi	angiotensin-converting enzyme inhibitor	CTE	chronic traumatic encephalopathy
ADHD	Attention-Deficit/Hyperactivity Disorder	D_2	dopamine-2
		DBS	deep brain stimulation
AIDS	Acquired Immunodeficiency Syndrome	DBT	dialectical behavioral therapy
		dmPFC	dorsomedial prefrontal cortex
ANC	absolute neutrophil count	DSM-5-TR	*Diagnostic and Statistical Manual of Mental Disorders* (5th ed., text rev.)
ARB	angiotensin receptor blocker		
ASPD	antisocial personality disorder	ECT	electroconvulsive therapy
AUD	alcohol use disorder	EKG	electrocardiogram
BDNF	brain-derived neurotrophic factor	EPS	extrapyramidal symptoms
BFCRS	Bush–Francis Catatonia Rating Scale	ESR	erythrocyte sedimentation rate
BID	twice daily	FEP	first-episode psychosis
BMI	body mass index	FGA	first-generation antipsychotic
BNP	brain natriuretic peptide		
BPD	borderline personality disorder	FSD	functional somatic disorders
CAH	command auditory hallucinations	GABA	gamma aminobutyric acid
cAMP	cyclic adenosine monophosphate	GAD	generalized anxiety disorder
CBC	complete blood count	GED	general educational development
CBT	cognitive behavioral therapy	GERD	gastroesophageal reflux disease
CDSS	Calgary Depression Scale for Schizophrenia	GI	gastrointestinal
cGMP	cyclic guanosine monophosphate	GnRH	gonadotropin-releasing hormone
CRT	cognitive rehabilitation treatment	GnRHa	gonadotropin-releasing hormone agonist

xi

List of Abbreviations

HCR-20	Historical Clinical Risk Management 20	PDGFB	Platelet Derived Growth Factor, subunit B
HDL	high-density lipoprotein	PPD	purified protein derivative
HPA	hypothalamic–pituitary axis	PRN	pro re nata (as needed)
		PTH	parathyroid hormone
IBGC	Idiopathic Basal Ganglia Calcification	PTSD	post-traumatic stress disorder
ICD-10	International Classification of Diseases 10	qHS	every night at bedtime
		rTMS	repetitive transcranial magnetic stimulation
IM	intramuscular		
IMO	involuntary medication order	SCZ-OCD	schizo-obsessive compulsive disorder
IST	incompetent to stand trial	SGAs	second-generation antipsychotics
IV	intravenous		
LDL	low-density lipoprotein	SI	suicidal indeation
LPS	Lanterman Petris Short	SIADH	Syndrome of Inappropriate Antidiuretic Hormone Secretion
MDD	major depressive disorder		
MI	myocardial infarction	SIB	self-injurious behaviors
MMSE	Mini-Mental State Examination	SLC20A2	Solute Carrier Family 20, member 2
MoCA	Montreal Cognitive Assessment	SLE	systemic lupus erythematosus
mRNA	messenger RNA	SMI	severe mental illness
MSE	mental status examination	SNRI	serotonin–norepinephrine reuptake inhibitor
MurCON	Murphy Conservatorship	SSRI	selective serotonin reuptake inhibitor
NBIA	neurodegeneration with brain iron accumulation	SUD	substance use disorder
NGRI	not guilty by reason of insanity	SVP	sexually violent predator
		TBI	traumatic brain injury
NMDA	N-methyl-D-aspartate	TCA	tricyclic antidepressants
NMDA-R	N-methyl-D-aspartate receptor	TID	three times daily
		TMS	transcranial magnetic stimulation
NMS	neuroleptic malignant syndrome		
NSSI	non-suicidal self-injury	TRS	treatment-resistant schizophrenia
OCD	obsessive–compulsive disorder	TSH	thyroid stimulating hormone
OCS	obsessive–compulsive symptoms	TTE	transthoracic echocardiogram
OSA	obstructive sleep apnea	(WASI-I)	Wechsler Abbreviated Scale of Intelligence
PANSS	Positive and Negative Symptom Scale	XPR1	Xenotropic and Polytropic Retrovirus Receptor
PCP	phencyclidine		

SECTION I
Aggression and Violence in the Forensic Setting

1
Psychotic aggression: the magic combo

The Psychopharmacological Dilemma: Finding biological treatment modalities for reducing psychotic aggression

Jongseung Baek and Seth Judd

Pretest self-assessment question
Which of the following classes of medication should not be considered for long-term adjunct therapy for treatment-resistant schizophrenia (TRS)?

A. Benzodiazepines
B. Mood stabilizers
C. Anticonvulsants
D. Electroconvulsive therapy (ECT)
E. Antidepressants

Patient evaluation on intake
- A male in his late 40s with a long history of schizophrenia, alcohol use disorder (AUD), benzodiazepine use disorder, and cannabis use disorder was transferred to a forensic state hospital for management of psychotic and aggressive behaviors toward himself and others
- The patient showed multiple violent behaviors at the time of hospital admission:
  - He attempted to kick the leg of a staff member who was taking his vitals
  - After sleeping, he went to the restroom and attempted to push his peer
  - He tried to chase after another staff member but was verbally redirected
  - Lastly, he volitionally jumped off his bed backward. He hit the back of his head on the door, sustaining a 3 cm laceration. He reported he was "okay" but refused to talk further
- He declined to answer questions.
- Mental status examination (MSE):
  - General: in hospital attire, fairly kempt
  - Motor: neutral
  - Speech: occasional selective mutism
  - Mood/Affect: "Okay" / neutral and blunted
  - Thought process: linear
  - Thought content: He has urges to assault others in response to auditory hallucination. He denies suicidal and homicidal thoughts

- Insight: limited as noted by his request for addictive substances
- Cognition: below-average intelligence with poor judgment
• It was decided to continue the current regimen of clozapine 300 mg every evening and haloperidol decanoate 250 mg IM every 2 weeks and provide as-needed medications (PRNs) appropriately and judiciously (to avoid drug-seeking behavior)

Psychiatric history

• The patient was diagnosed and treated for schizophrenia in his late teens
  - His primary psychiatric symptoms include auditory hallucinations that command him to harm himself and others
  - His symptoms began a few months after his sibling's suicide
  - He has been on various psychotropic treatment regimens
• He was placed on a state conservatorship shortly after his initial hospitalization
• He has been hospitalized in different levels of mental health facilities
• He previously asked for PRN medicines when he was not outwardly agitated
  - He reported that he wants PRN medicines for the "high"
  - He also reports enjoying being in restraints because it makes him feel "high"
• He previously received ECT but with minimal improvement
• He reported worsening of psychotic symptoms during times of heightened stress

Social and personal history

• He was born in an intact family
• He has three siblings – of whom two are alive
• His mother is deceased and his father is still alive
• He graduated from high school and had sparse employments due to his mental illness
• He has no known history of trauma or abuse
• He has been homeless in between psychiatric placements
• He has a history of multiple substance abuse including benzodiazepines, alcohol, and cannabis
• He has extensive nonviolent and violent criminal history

Medical history

• He had a seizure while taking clozapine 600 mg/day without divalproex
• He developed hypothyroidism and renal insufficiency from lithium toxicity

PATIENT FILE

- Other medical conditions include right retinal detachment, bilateral glaucoma, hypertension, hyperlipidemia, iron deficiency anemia, and stress urinary incontinence

Family history
- He has no family history of mental illnesses

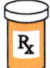

Medication history
- The patient has been on numerous psychotropic medications, including antipsychotics, mood stabilizers, benzodiazepines, and antidepressants
- The following medication amount is the maximum dose per day, unless otherwise stated:
  - Antipsychotics: aripiprazole 15 mg, clozapine 600 mg, fluphenazine 45 mg, haloperidol 350 mg every 2 weeks, olanzapine 50 mg, quetiapine 1200 mg, risperidone 10 mg, ziprasidone 200 mg
  - Antidepressants: bupropion 400 mg, citalopram 40 mg, escitalopram 20 mg, fluoxetine 80 mg, mirtazapine 15 mg, sertraline 100 mg
  - Anticonvulsant/mood stabilizer divalproex 1500 mg, lamotrigine 250 mg, lithium 1200 mg, and valproic acid 1250 mg
- Patient was also prescribed propranolol (60 mg) for akathisia, clonazepam (4 mg) and lorazepam (2 mg) for impulse control
- Adverse reactions: divalproex – pancreatitis; lithium – renal insufficiency

Current medications
- Clozapine 300 mg once every night
- Haloperidol decanoate 250 mg intramuscular (IM) twice monthly
- Hydroxyzine 50 mg three times a day
- Haloperidol 5 mg every 2 hours as needed, but no more than 3 doses per 24 hours
- Levothryroxine 100 ug every day
- Tamsulosin 0.8 mg every night
- Ferrous sulfate 325 mg once every noon
- Metformin once every day
- Multivitamin w/folic acid once every morning
- Lactulose 20 mg every 4 hours as needed for constipation
- Polyethylene glycol 3350 pack once every night

PATIENT FILE

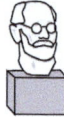

Psychotherapy history
- Due to the presence of ongoing psychotic symptoms and aggressive behaviors, he has been unable to participate in meaningful therapy beyond learning stress management skills (listening to music, taking hot shower, playing the guitar, sitting in his rocking chair, utilizing weighted blanket and essential oils – lavender). He briefly attended sensory modulation therapy

Mechanism of action moment
- Clozapine: atypical antipsychotic
- Target receptors/effect
    - D4 antagonism: high clozapine affinity; however, effect is unknown
    - D_2 antagonist: reduce positive symptoms of psychosis and stabilize affective symptoms
    - $5\text{-}HT_{2A}$ antagonist: enhance dopamine release thus reducing motor side effects and possibly improving cognitive and affective symptoms
    - For some patients, $5\text{-}HT_{2C}$ and $5\text{-}HT_{1A}$ receptor interaction may contribute to efficacy for cognitive and affective symptoms

Attending physician's mental notes
- This patient has tried a variety of antipsychotics with suboptimal results
- His prior history shows frequent decompensation with increased violent tendencies and actions
- There are multiple factors that may be associated with patient's violent behavior
    - Patient reports command auditory hallucinations, which suggests that he was in the state of psychosis when he was acting violently
    - Recent study has shown that patients who experience command auditory hallucinations (CAH) to harm others were twice as likely to be violent as those without CAH
    - This aspect could be controlled by appropriate pharmacotherapy
    - Clozapine and olanzapine are effective in treating aggression stemming from schizophrenia
    - Patient reported urge to inflict self-injury and violence toward others
    - Urge entails impulsivity in the context of strong emotion
    - Impulsivity has been shown to be contributing factor to increased violent behavior
    - This aspect could be addressed through further destressing techniques
- Benzodiazepine PRN for aggression should be avoided, if possible, to prevent reinforcement of drug-seeking behavior

PATIENT FILE

Further investigation
- Is there anything else you would like to know about this patient? What additional information is needed to change or adjust the treatment plan?
  - Clozapine level should be monitored to determine whether it is in therapeutic range. Initially, the patient's clozapine level was 865 mcg/L
  - Dosage was increased to 400 mg to reach maximum therapeutic level of 1000 mcg/L per hospital guidelines
  - For patients on the schizophrenia spectrum and who have failed multiple trials of antipsychotic medications, including clozapine, ECT should be considered. Medical records indicate that he has a history of ECT treatments, but these were discontinued due to lack of response

Case outcome (3 months): use of outcome measures
- The patient continues to exhibit violent behaviors. During the first 2 months, he engaged in over 30 aggressive behaviors per month
- He reports that he is "suffering" from hearing the voices, which he characterizes as "strong" and difficult to resist
- His psychiatric medications were adjusted (clozapine 400 mg every night and haloperidol decanoate 200 mg IM every 2 weeks)
- He is adherent to antipsychotic medications based on plasma level
  - Last clozapine level was 1000 mcg/L which is at the maximum therapeutic level per hospital policy
- The Mini-Mental State Examination was administered and he obtained 21/30 which is suggestive of mild cognitive impairment. However …
  - His impaired vision partially explains the lower score – he had difficulty completing the part of the examination that requires visual acuity
  - He was also drowsy during the session as he had just received a PRN medication

Attending physician's mental notes: first interim progress report
- The patient is taking the highest dose of clozapine, confirmed by plasma level, with modest benefit
- Following adjunct therapy must be considered
  - Previous research has shown small benefit when clozapine is augmented with secondary antipsychotics; however, recent meta-analysis showed no benefit with risperidone (most-used augmentation)

PATIENT FILE

- Although previous meta-analysis research has shown small benefit when clozapine is augmented with a mood stabilizer such as lamotrigine, the difference was no longer statistically significant after removing an outlier
- Out of the available antidepressants, only citalopram has been shown to have improvement in a small study
- ECT adjunct has efficacy rates ranging from 40% to 70% in TRS
- Repetitive transcranial magnetic stimulation (rTMS) has shown evidence of treating auditory hallucination and potential negative symptoms; however, it is not yet FDA approved for treating schizophrenia
- Lastly, deep brain stimulation (DBS) is supported by case studies
• Records indicate the patient had trials of adjunct secondary antipsychotics, mood stabilizers, antidepressants, and ECT without much improvement

Further investigation
• Which adjunct therapy should be considered? What additional information do you need to choose adjunct therapy?
   - Although previous ECT trials showed subpar responses, they were performed under suboptimal clozapine treatment. With optimal clozapine therapy, ECT treatments could improve his psychotic symptoms
   - Other "failed" adjunct therapy could be reconsidered if the concurrent clozapine level was not at the maximum therapeutic level

Case outcome: interim follow-up progress report 6 months
• Patient began receiving three ECT treatments per week
   - ECT team was unable to elicit a seizure until energy level increased to 100%. Changes in the general anesthetic were also made to lower seizure threshold in order to produce a seizure. Methohexital dose was reduced, and ketamine was added, but patient did not tolerate the ketamine well. Anesthesiologist then switched from methohexital to etomidate, a pro-seizure anesthetic. IV caffeine was also added and titrated up to 540 mg
• Patient has been responding positively with ECT treatment, showing a decrease in aggressive behaviors from over 30 incidents over 90 days pre-ECT, to fewer than 5 aggressions per month for the past 3 months
• He reports that he is "doing better" and denies auditory hallucination and thoughts of harming self and others
• His main complaint is his worsening vision from retinal detachment

PATIENT FILE

- Given his improvement, ECT frequency was reduced. However, shortly afterward the frequency of the patient's psychotic behaviors increased. The patient then went back to receiving ECT three times a week
- During recent ECT treatments, ECT nurses and anesthesiologist noted that it was becoming increasingly difficult to obtain intravenous (IV) access
    - Larger-gauge needles on more peripheral veins were used but patient reports pain when receiving caffeine IV
- Clozapine level was rechecked. At 400 mg, the level was 1480 mcg. Patient did not show any signs of clozapine toxicity, such as seizures, arrhythmia, cardiotoxicity, or neutropenia. Dose was reduced to 350 mg and follow-up level was in therapeutic range

Attending physician's mental notes
- The patient's high seizure threshold required additional pharmacological adjustment to standard ECT protocol
    - Anesthetic
        - Methohexital, a barbiturate, is the most commonly used anesthetic agent for ECT. It is characterized by fast emergence time; however, it is seizure-threshold neutral
        - Ketamine can lower seizure threshold, increase seizure duration, and lead to better-quality seizure compared to barbiturates
            - It was chosen initially over etomidate as it reduces transient cognitive dysfunction from ECT
        - Etomidate decreases seizure threshold and increases seizure duration
            - Acute hemodynamic response to ECT becomes more prominent
            - There is concern about adrenal function depression in long-term use
    - Caffeine IV
        - Caffeine was titrated to prolong seizure response during ECT
- Although patient is tolerating ECT, IV access issues need to be addressed for patient comfort and successful ECT treatments. The following strategy can be used to resolve this issue:
    - Local anesthetic agent could be used
    - More skilled personnel could assist in getting IV access
    - Veinviewer infrared scanner could be used to find deeper vein

- Although patient's increase in violence coincided with ECT tapering, other causes should be investigated to confirm the source of increased aggression
  - Measure clozapine and norclozapine levels to confirm medication compliance
  - Ophthalmology referral and surgery to reduce stress factor associated with decreased vision

Further investigation
- Is there an upper limit of how many ECT treatments can be given in one patient? When would you stop ECT treatment for this patient?
  - There is no upper limit to number of ECT treatments
  - As long as it is indicated and well tolerated, ECT can be continued

Case debrief
- Our patient has a long psychiatric history with diagnosis of schizophrenia and substance use disorder. He has an extensive psychotropic medication history including numerous failed trials of antipsychotic and other psychotropic medications
- Although he was on clozapine at the time of his initial visit, he was not at the maximum therapeutic dosage
- Even after maximum therapeutic level was reached, patient still suffered from CAH and violent behavior
- ECT trial led to a decrease in violent behavior

Take-home points
- Individuals with schizophrenia have a greater risk of engaging in violent behaviors
- Between 10% and 60% of patients with schizophrenia experience treatment resistance
- Clozapine is first-line therapy for TRS
- There is an association between schizophrenia and substance use disorder. The treatment team should evaluate whether aggressive behavior is a part of drug-seeking behavior
- Benzodiazepine does not play a role in anti-psychosis; therefore, it should be only used for acute agitation
- Antidepressants, anticonvulsants, mood stabilizers, and ECT can be used as adjunct therapy. However, ECT is preferred as it has highest rates of efficacy

PATIENT FILE

Performance in practice: confessions of a psychopharmacologist

What could have been done better to prevent deterioration of his symptoms?

- Early critical period in psychosis is important for secondary prevention of impairments and disabilities
- The patient received first dose of clozapine at the state forensic hospital 10 years after his initial diagnosis and psychiatric hospitalization. He may have benefited from an earlier clozapine trial

What could have been done in the outpatient setting to prevent relapses?

- Frequent bloodwork and follow-up to determine medical adherence. Routine drug screens to monitor substance use
- Adding long-acting antipsychotic medications (e.g., haloperidol) to increase compliance

What additional adjunct therapy can be used for this patient if symptoms relapse?

- Impulsivity is also associated with the risk of violence. Increasing cognitive capacities and reducing negative symptoms can help patients more adequately engage with psychotherapy to modulate impulsivity and violent behaviors
- Minocycline: double-blinded clinical study (n = 52) showed improvement in total symptoms, negative symptoms, and cognition with adjunct minocycline (100 mg po BID) compared to placebo
- Memantine: double-blinded clinical study (n = 52) showed improvement in total symptoms, negative symptoms, and composite memory score with adjunct memantine (titrated to 20 mg p.o. QD), compared to placebo
- Famotidine: double-blinded clinical study (n = 30) showed improvement in Positive and Negative Syndrome Scale (PANSS) with adjunct famotidine (titrated to 100 mg p.o. QD), compared to placebo

Tips and pearls

- It is important to gather prior medication history to understand the rationale behind dosage and medication changes to choose an appropriate treatment plan
- Psychiatrists should first try maximizing medicine as much as a patient tolerates, before considering medicine to be ineffective
- TRS definition – Kane Criteria
  - No relief ≥ 3 treatments, ≥ 6 weeks length, ≥ antipsychotics
  - Persistent poor functioning
  - Failure to respond to prospective high-dose first-generation antipsychotic (FGA) trial

PATIENT FILE

- Based on long-term studies, there is clozapine response in up to 60% of TRS, compared to < 5% with non-clozapine antipsychotics
- Clozapine can reduce violence, aggression, and substance abuse
- Clozapine receptor-mediated side effects
  - Sedation: caused by clozapine and norclozapine H1 antagonist activity
  - Hypersalivation:
    - Clozapine partial agonist in M1 and norclozapine's full agonist in M1
    - Clozapine's full antagonist in M3 and norclozapine's partial agonist at M3
    - Clozapine's impairment of swallowing reflex
  - Orthostatic hypotension and tachycardia: antimuscarinic activity
  - GI hypomotility / constipation:
    - Caused by clozapine and norclozapine activity on colonic M3 receptor
  - Weight gain
    - Due to increase in appetite mediated by clozapine H1 antagonism
  - Myoclonus and seizure
    - Possible explanation: D_2, H1, A1 receptor blockade
- Clozapine-induced myocarditis
  - Reported incidents vary from 0.06% to 3.88%, with mortality ranging from 10% to 30%
  - Highest risk within first month of therapy
  - Postulated to be caused by following: IgE-mediated hypersensitivity, inflammatory response from hypercatecholaminergic state, myocardial oxidative stress, reduced antioxidants, apoptosis
  - Management: withdrawal of drug, diuretics, angiotensin-converting enzyme (ACE) inhibitor, digoxin, beta-blocker
- Clozapine-induced neutropenia/agranulocytosis
  - 3% and 0.8% respectively, with the highest risk between 4 and 20 weeks; 85–90% of cases occur within 1 year
  - There are two proposed pathologic mechanisms: (1) immune-mediated response against haptenized neutrophil; (2) metabolite toxicity
  - Clinical presentation: fever, mouth ulcer, sore throat, but can be asymptomatic. Absolute neutrophil count less than 0.5×10^9/L
  - Management: weekly complete blood count (CBC) for the first 18 weeks, then every 2 weeks until week 52. Discontinue clozapine if agranulocytosis develops
- Smoking increases clozapine metabolism through induction of CYP1A2. This may explain possible discrepancies between reported medicine compliance and lab work

PATIENT FILE

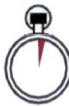

Two-minute tutorial
- Violent behavior in schizophrenia
  - Patients with schizophrenia have increased risk of violent behavior that leads to arrest or conviction compared to the general population
- Clozapine is a first-line treatment for TRS
  - Severe adverse reactions include: myocarditis, seizure, and agranulocytosis
    - Assess clinical symptoms (flu-like symptoms) and laboratory results (CBC, clozapine/norclozapine level)
    - Management: discontinue clozapine. Depending on severity, it can be reinitiated at lower dose with close monitoring if benefit outweighs adverse reaction
  - Other side effects include: sedation, hypersalivation, orthostatic hypotension, gastrointestinal (GI) hypomobility, weight gain
    - Constipation may cause ileus and possible mortality. Laxative prophylaxis reduces this risk
- ECT adjunct therapy should be used if patient doesn't respond with optimal clozapine plasma level
  - On average, initial ECT trial consist of 6 to 12 treatments; usually performed two to three times a week for 2–4 weeks. There is no set number
  - Continue if patient tolerates well and has good clinical outcome
  - There is no maximum number of treatments
- ECT treatment can be adjusted with different pharmacological agents to be safe and effective, and help manage clinical complexities such as an elevated seizure threshold

Post-test question
Which of the following classes of medication should not be considered for long-term adjunct therapy for TRS?

A. Benzodiazepines
B. Mood stabilizers
C. Anticonvulsants
D. Electroconvulsive therapy (ECT)
E. Antidepressants

Answer: A

References

1. Birchwood, M., Todd, P., & Jackson, C. (1998). Early intervention in psychosis: the critical period hypothesis. *British Journal of Psychiatry: Supplement*, 172(33), 53–59.
2. Correll, C. U. & Howes, O. D. (2021). Treatment-resistant schizophrenia: definition, predictors, and therapy options. *Journal of Clinical Psychiatry*, 82(5). https://doi.org/10.4088/JCP.MY20096AH1C.
3. Correll, C. U., Yu, X., Xiang, Y., Kane, J. M., & Masand, P. (2017). Biological treatment of acute agitation or aggression with schizophrenia or bipolar disorder in the inpatient setting. *Annals of Clinical Psychiatry: Official Journal of the American Academy of Clinical Psychiatrists*, 29(2), 92–107.
4. Dold, M., Li, C., Gillies, D., & Leucht, S. (2013). Benzodiazepine augmentation of antipsychotic drugs in schizophrenia: a meta-analysis and Cochrane review of randomized controlled trials. *European Neuropsychopharmacology*, 23(9), 1023–1033. https://doi.org/10.1016/j.euroneuro.2013.03.001.
5. Espinoza, R. T. & Kellner, C. H. (2022). Electroconvulsive therapy. *New England Journal of Medicine*, 386(7), 667–672. https://doi.org/10.1056/NEJMra2034954.
6. Faay, M. D. M. & Sommer, I. E. (2021). Risk and prevention of aggression in patients with psychotic disorders. *American Journal of Psychiatry*, 178(3), 218–220. https://doi.org/10.1176/appi.ajp.2020.21010035.
7. Fazel, S., Gulati, G., Linsell, L., Geddes, J. R., & Grann, M. (2009). Schizophrenia and violence: systematic review and meta-analysis. *PLoS Medicine*, 6(8), e1000120. https://doi.org/10.1371/journal.pmed.1000120.
8. Higgins, J. M., San, C., Lagnado, G., Chua, D., & Mihic, T. (2019). Incidence and management of clozapine-induced myocarditis in a large tertiary hospital. *Canadian Journal of Psychiatry. Revue Canadienne de Psychiatrie*, 64(8), 561–567. https://doi.org/10.1177/0706743718816058.
9. Hodgins, S., & Klein, S. (2017). New clinically relevant findings about violence by people with schizophrenia. *Canadian Journal of Psychiatry. Revue Canadienne de Psychiatrie*, 62(2), 86–93. https://doi.org/10.1177/0706743716648300.
10. Hoptman, M. J. (2015). Impulsivity and aggression in schizophrenia: a neural circuitry perspective with implications for treatment. *CNS Spectrums*, 20(3), 280–286. https://doi.org/10.1017/S1092852915000206.

11. Hoyer, C., Kranaster, L., Janke, C., & Sartorius, A. (2014). Impact of the anesthetic agents ketamine, etomidate, thiopental, and propofol on seizure parameters and seizure quality in electroconvulsive therapy: a retrospective study. *European Archives of Psychiatry and Clinical Neuroscience*, 264(3), 255–261. https://doi.org/10.1007/s00406-013-0420-5.
12. Kane, J. (1988). Clozapine for the treatment-resistant schizophrenic: a double-blind comparison with chlorpromazine. *Archives of General Psychiatry*, 45(9), 789. https://doi.org/10.1001/archpsyc.1988.01800330013001.
13. Kelly, D. L., Sullivan, K. M., McEvoy, J. P., et al. (2015). Adjunctive minocycline in clozapine-treated schizophrenia patients with persistent symptoms. *Journal of Clinical Psychopharmacology*, 35(4), 374–381. https://doi.org/10.1097/JCP.0000000000000345.
14. Khokhar, J. Y., Dwiel, L. L., Henricks, A. M., Doucette, W. T., & Green, A. I. (2018). The link between schizophrenia and substance use disorder: a unifying hypothesis. *Schizophrenia Research*, 194, 78–85. https://doi.org/10.1016/j.schres.2017.04.016.
15. McNiel, D. E., Eisner, J. P., & Binder, R. L. (2000). The relationship between command hallucinations and violence. *Psychiatric Services*, 51(10), 1288–1292. https://doi.org/10.1176/appi.ps.51.10.1288.
16. Meskanen, K., Ekelund, H., Laitinen, J., et al. (2013). A randomized clinical trial of histamine 2 receptor antagonism in treatment-resistant schizophrenia. *Journal of Clinical Psychopharmacology*, 33(4), 472–478. https://doi.org/10.1097/JCP.0b013e3182970490.
17. Mijovic, A. & MacCabe, J. H. (2020). Clozapine-induced agranulocytosis. *Annals of Hematology*, 99(11), 2477–2482. https://doi.org/10.1007/s00277-020-04215-y.
18. Mørup, M. F., Kymes, S. M., & Oudin Åström, D. (2020). A modelling approach to estimate the prevalence of treatment-resistant schizophrenia in the United States. *PloS One*, 15(6), e0234121. https://doi.org/10.1371/journal.pone.0234121.
19. Nucifora, F. C., Woznica, E., Lee, B. J., Cascella, N., & Sawa, A. (2019). Treatment resistant schizophrenia: clinical, biological, and therapeutic perspectives. *Neurobiology of Disease*, 131, 104257. https://doi.org/10.1016/j.nbd.2018.08.016.
20. Schoretsanitis, G., Kane, J. M., Ruan, C.-J., Spina, E., Hiemke, C., & de Leon, J. (2019). A comprehensive review of the clinical utility of and a combined analysis of the clozapine/norclozapine ratio in therapeutic drug monitoring for adult patients. *Expert Review of Clinical Pharmacology*, 12(7), 603–621. https://doi.org/10.1080/17512433.2019.1617695.

PATIENT FILE

21. Sinclair, D. J. M., Zhao, S., Qi, F., Nyakyoma, K., Kwong, J. S. W., & Adams, C. E. (2019). Electroconvulsive therapy for treatment-resistant schizophrenia. *Schizophrenia Bulletin*, 45(4), 730–732. https://doi.org/10.1093/schbul/sbz037.
22. Stahl, S. M. (2011). Antipsychotic agents. In: *Stahl's Essential Psychopharmacology: Prescriber's Guide*, 4th ed. New York: Cambridge University Press, pp. 133–138.
23. Tiihonen, J., Suokas, J. T., Suvisaari, J. M., Haukka, J., & Korhonen, P. (2012). Polypharmacy with antipsychotics, antidepressants, or benzodiazepines and mortality in schizophrenia. *Archives of General Psychiatry*, 69(5), 476–483. https://doi.org/10.1001/archgenpsychiatry.2011.1532.
24. Veerman, S. R. T., Schulte, P. F. J., Smith, J. D., & de Haan, L. (2016). Memantine augmentation in clozapine-refractory schizophrenia: a randomized, double-blind, placebo-controlled crossover study. *Psychological Medicine*, 46(9), 1909–1921. https://doi.org/10.1017/S0033291716000398.

PATIENT FILE

2

Impulsive affective aggression: Action in a second

The Psychopharmacological Dilemma: How is impulsive aggression treated?

Maanasi Chandarana

Pretest self-assessment question
What is the gold standard for treating impulsive aggression?
A. Lithium
B. Clozapine
C. Haloperidol
D. There is no gold standard for treating impulsive aggression
E. Combination therapy of treatment with antipsychotic and mood stabilizer medications

Answer: B

Patient evaluation on intake
The patient is a 33-year-old male with previous diagnoses of Borderline Intellectual Functioning, Unspecified Schizophrenia Spectrum and Other Psychotic Disorder, Unspecified Personality Disorder, and Stimulant – Methamphetamine-type Use Disorder. Due to his persistent violent behaviors, the patient is transferred from one forensic hospital to another forensic state hospital. The patient is admitted to the specialized unit consisting of increased programming, structure, and security measures, and reserved for the most unstable and violent patients. While hospitalized in the specialized unit, the patient became upset when his dinner was late and, resultantly, broke the television. He is documented by staff as easily frustrated and often engages in property destruction.

Psychiatric history
- Mental health history with onset in childhood
  - He reported delusional content including delusions of grandeur and persecutory delusions, auditory hallucinations, and visual hallucinations
  - He exhibited disorganized speech and behavior
  - He was described as prone to affective dysregulation and behavioral destabilization

PATIENT FILE

- He did not graduate from high school or obtain a general educational development (GED) certificate
- Behaviorally, the patient exhibited intrusive, impulsive, and unpredictable acts
  - The patient has a history of self-injurious, sexually inappropriate, and verbally threatening behavior and interpersonal conflict
    - The patient has a history of pica, ingesting foreign objects, and inserting objects into his mouth and anus
- The patient has an extensive history of violence with multiple arrests, charges, and in-custody offenses
- The patient has been hospitalized in forensic psychiatric facilities multiple times

Social and personal history
- The patient was raised by his biological mother until early childhood
- At 6 years of age, he was removed from his mother's home and placed in a group home
- Multiple encounters with law enforcement noted, with first documented arrest and incurred charge when he was 14 years of age
- He reported working as a bus boy and drug dealer
- He received Social Security benefits for his mental health diagnoses
- He was never married and denied having any children

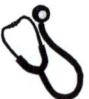
Medical history
- Hypothyroidism
- History of head trauma following a motor vehicle accident
- The patient is being evaluated by consultants for a comorbid seizure disorder

Family history
- There is no known familial history to report

Medication history
- The patient was prescribed multiple trials of medications including antipsychotics, mood stabilizers, benzodiazepines, and beta-blocker medication

Current history
- The patient presented to the evaluation as calm, polite, and cooperative
- He was dressed in hospital attire, and his grooming and hygiene were deemed fair
- His speech rate, rhythm, and volume were normal

- The patient did not demonstrate psychomotor agitation, retardation, and abnormal involuntary movements
- He reported that his mood was depressed, but he exhibited a broad affective range. He denied suicidal thoughts and said that he could not die. He denied experiencing homicidal ideations
- He stated that ghosts were following and sexually assaulting him, but he denied experiencing auditory hallucinations
- His thought process was linear, and goal-directed
- The patient was alert, and oriented to person, time, and place. His recent and remote memory, ability to abstract, and attention were deemed fair
- He demonstrated deficits in his fund of knowledge, cognition, insight, and judgment

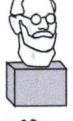

Psychotherapy history
- There is no known psychotherapy history to report

Mechanism of action moment
- Clozapine
  - Antagonizes D_2 receptors and serotonin 2A receptors
    - Blocking D_2 receptors reduces positive symptoms of psychosis and provides mood stabilization
    - Blocking serotonin 2A receptors enhances dopamine release in brain regions to minimize motor side effects and improve cognitive and affective symptoms
  - Interacts with $5-HT_{2C}$ and $5-HT_{1A}$ which may promote increased efficacy in treatment of cognitive and affective symptoms
- Divalproex
  - Stabilizes neuronal membrane by optimizing K+ efflux and Na+ influx
    - Decreases the glutamate : gamma-aminobutyric acid (GABA) ratio
      - Decreases glutamate by stimulating glutamine synthetase
      - Increases GABA by increasing GABA levels, GABA release, $GABA_B$ receptor density, and neuronal responsiveness to GABA; and decreases GABA catabolism and turnover
  - Dampens excitatory systems by decreasing aspartate release, cerebrospinal fluid (CSF) somatostatin, and N-methyl-D-aspartate- (NMDA-) mediated circuits
  - Increases dopamine turnover

PATIENT FILE

- Haloperidol decanoate
  - Blocks D_2 receptors:
    - Reduces positive symptoms and aggressive behaviors
    - In the nigrostriatal pathway, D_2 blockade improves tics and associated symptoms of Tourette's
- Lithium carbonate
  - Mechanism of action is complex and not well understood
  - Thought to recruit second messenger signaling pathway including that of cyclic adenosine monophosphate (cAMP) and cyclic guanosine monophosphate (cGMP)
  - Involved in genetic transcription and post-translational modification
    - Competes with other cations involved in signal transduction
  - Decreases the glutamine : GABA ratio
    - Prevents loss of phosphorylated cAMP Response Element Binding Protein
      - Inhibits glutamate activation of protein kinases
        - Provides neuroprotective effects

Attending physician's mental notes

- The patient has a history of experiencing psychotic symptoms, including auditory and visual hallucinations, as well as persecutory delusions and delusions of grandeur
- His cognitive deficits limit his ability to engage in prosocial behaviors and contribute to dysregulated, impulsive, and aggressive behaviors
- The patient demonstrates behaviors that deviate from sociocultural norms in the domains of cognition, affectivity, interpersonal functioning, and impulse control
- Medications prescribed by the referring facility appear to be targeting his symptoms of affective and behavioral dysregulation
  - Clozapine 450 mg p.o. qHS
  - Divalproex 2000 mg p.o. qHS
  - Haloperidol decanoate 200 mg IM every month
  - Lithium carbonate 1200 mg p.o. qHS

Further investigation

- The patient developed seizure activity and was referred to neurology
  - An MRI revealed two areas of left frontal gyral cortical atrophy without mass effect, gliosis, or edema
  - An EEG was negative for a seizure focus
  - A valproic acid level resulted as 123 ug/mL

PATIENT FILE

- Clozapine and divalproex were decreased in dosage by 50 mg, respectively
  - Following the changes in his medications, further seizure activity was not observed
  - In a follow-up appointment, it was not thought that clozapine was the causative agent or etiology of the patient's seizures, and it was thought that divalproex antiepileptic and seizure-prophylactic properties were beneficial
    - Clozapine and divalproex were both increased to further treat the patient's seizures and behaviors

Case outcome
- The patient's case is followed monthly
- Through his hospitalization, the patient engaged in multiple aggressive behaviors that resulted in his placement in seclusion and/or restraints, benefited from treatment with PRN medications, prompted increase in his prescribed medications to therapeutic dosing, and warranted his continued treatment on the specialized unit reserved for the most unstable and violent patients
- Clozapine, divalproex, and lithium were gradually increased. Haloperidol decanoate was gradually increased in dosing and frequency of administration
  - Clozapine increased to 850 mg p.o. qHS
    - Level of 1064 ng/mL
  - Divalproex increased to 4000 mg p.o. qHS
    - Level of 100.5 ug/mL
  - Lithium increased to 1350 mg p.o. qHS
    - Level of 0.89 mmol/L
  - Haloperidol decanoate increased to 300 mg IM q 2 weeks
    - Level of 13.2 ng/mL
- The patient's impulsivity improved with increased dosages of clozapine and divalproex with the most perceived therapeutic benefit associated with divalproex
- However, the patient exhibited persistent impulsive aggressive behaviors including verbal aggression / verbal threats, physical aggression, repetitive self-harm behaviors, placing nonfood objects in his rectum, eating nonfood items, and punching and kicking inanimate objects

Case debrief
- Our patient suffered from a psychotic disorder, comorbid with cognitive limitations, addiction, and personality disorders

PATIENT FILE

- Due to his persistent violent behaviors, the patient was transferred from one forensic hospital to the unit reserved for the most unstable and violent patients of another forensic state hospital
- Despite increased dosing of clozapine, divalproex, and lithium, and increased dosing and frequency of haloperidol decanoate, the patient exhibited impulsive aggressive behaviors which posited him as a danger to himself and others, and benefited from multiple psychopharmacological and nonpharmacological therapeutic interventions

Take-home points

- Aggression is defined as any act with the potential to harm self or others, whereas violence is a subcategory of aggression that results in harm to others
- Aggression can result from a mismatch of "top-down" and "bottom-up" neuroanatomical control systems due to system dysfunction
  - Top-down: Aggression is controlled by inhibitory neurotransmitters (serotonin) in the prefrontal and orbitofrontal cortices and the anterior cingulate cortex, as well as GABA
  - Bottom-up: Excitatory neurotransmitters (aspartate, glutamate) from the amygdala facilitate aggression
- Impulsive violence is represented in greater proportions in forensic settings when compared to other subtypes of violence
  - Comparative percentages attributed to impulsive, predatory, and psychotic violence are: impulsive (54%) > predatory (29%) > psychotic (17%)
  - Impulsive violence is triggered by provocative, threatening, or stressful stimuli; is accompanied by angered, fearful, and frustrated mood states; and presents with increased autonomic arousal
  - Predatory violence is planned behavior with a defined outcome; it is not necessarily a response to threatening or noxious stimuli; it is not accompanied by autonomic arousal
  - Psychotic violence is driven by positive symptoms of psychosis including persecutory delusions, delusions of grandeur, and command hallucinations
    - Symptoms include persecutory thoughts of threat control override, being poisoned, and generalized suspiciousness
- Classifying the subtype of violence aids with treatment management
  - Impulsive violence
    - Treatment includes cognitive remediation and pro-cognitive (top-down) and antipsychotic (bottom-up) medications
  - Predatory violence
    - Represents the most severe and least treatable of the subtypes of aggressive acts

PATIENT FILE

- No current treatment management and guidelines
  o Psychotic violence
    - Treatment of the underlying psychiatric condition (top-down and bottom-up), behavioral therapy (top-down), and use of pro-cognitive (top-down) and antipsychotic (bottom-up) medications

Performance in practice: confessions of a psychopharmacologist

What are clinical considerations when treating impulsive violence?

- Impulsive violence can be distinguished from predatory and psychotic violence in that impulsive violence *is* in response to a threatening stimulus, accompanied by autonomic arousal, and associated with anxious, irritable, and/or angry mood state; and *is not* accompanied by positive symptoms of psychosis, planning, and obtaining a specific outcome or goal
- The pharmacodynamic, anti-aggressive effect of clozapine is independent of the psychotropic medication's antipsychotic effect, at an average serum concentration of 171 ng/dL, and at therapeutic drug levels less than 350 ng/dL
- Clozapine's mitigating effect on aggression is more noticeable in individuals with cognitive dysfunction
- Other psychopharmacological augmentation strategies, including antipsychotic medications, valproic acid, central B-adrenergic blockade, and selective serotonin reuptake inhibition, have limited treatment effect if the patient's response to clozapine is suboptimal despite therapeutic dosing

Tips and pearls

- The various subtypes of violent behaviors are linked to different neurochemical and neuroanatomical deviations
  o Impulsive violence is associated with higher emotional sensitivity and disproportionate response to perceived threats; imbalance between cortical top-down inhibition and bottom-up impulsivity; and structural and functional deficits in the frontal and temporal lobes
    - Suboptimal functioning of the dorsolateral and ventromedial prefrontal cortex and the orbitofrontal cortex leads to inability to recognize consequences, apply learned information to reward and punishment, recognize social cues, and process stimuli as emotionally neutral (versus negative)

PATIENT FILE

- Dysfunction in the temporal lobe includes hyperactivity of the amygdala in impulsive aggression
- Neurobiologically, there is an imbalance between serotoninergic and dopaminergic pathways
  - In the prefrontal cortex, serotonin is decreased, and dopamine is increased
    - Dopamine hyperactivity in the striatum weakens inhibitory pathways modulating impulsivity
    - Serotonin hypoactivity in the anterior cingulate and orbitofrontal cortex decreases top-down control of the prefrontal cortex
  - Predatory violence
    - Associated with amygdala hypo-functioning and decreased fear conditioning
  - Psychotic violence
    - Accompanies neuronal and dopamine overactivity in the mesolimbic dopamine pathway
- Persistent violence in inpatient and forensic settings is mostly enacted by individuals diagnosed with schizophrenia spectrum disorders, intellectual disability, and cognitive disorders
  - Bottom-up processing is reinforced resulting in automatic or compulsive behaviors
    - In individuals with less cortical inhibition and input, opioid-mediated learned behaviors shift toward a dopamine-dependent anticipation and knowledge of a reward
    - With reinforcement, the dorsal striatum of the subcortical reward center is repeatedly flooded with dopamine, as opposed to the ventral striatum (learned goal-directed behavior) fueling impulsivity
    - Individuals will react automatically and repeatedly
- Identifying the subtype of violent behavior can guide and assist treatment
  - Impulsive violence: treat with clozapine to therapeutic level of 171 ng/mL
    - Impulsive violence is associated with poor executive functioning, and clozapine affects aggression despite cognitive impairments
  - Predatory violence: no standardized treatment guidelines
    - Individuals engaging in predatory violence may benefit from placement in carceral and forensic settings
  - Psychotic violence
    - First-line treatment with antipsychotic +/– mood-stabilizer medication to treat affective symptoms

PATIENT FILE

- For treatment-refractory cases, treat with clozapine and increase dose with corresponding trough level > than 350 ng/dL
- Adjunctive treatment includes potent D_2 antagonist antipsychotic or aripiprazole
- Third-line treatment includes short-term treatment with valproate (8-week treatment course), SSRI antidepressant medication, or central-acting B adrenergic antagonist

Two-minute tutorial

- Inpatient psychiatric facilities and forensic hospitals are dangerous work environments with patient assaults contributing to disabling employee injuries
- A minority of the forensic patient population are responsible for the majority of violent and aggressive behaviors – however, when enacted, these can cause serious harm
- Impulsive aggression is associated with interpersonal conflicts, receipt of staff instructions, or when denied a request
- Aggression treatment and management remains difficult
- Classifying the type and nature of aggressive patient behaviors enables the practitioner to identify potential treatment options
- In forensic settings, violence is more frequently categorized as impulsive (54%) versus predatory (29%) and psychotic (17%)
- Violence results from dysfunction of top-down and bottom-up neuroanatomic control systems
  - Deficits in top-down processing are due to decreased serotonin in the prefrontal and orbitofrontal cortices and reduced inhibition by the prefrontal cortex
  - Deficits in bottom-up processing are because of hyperactivity of the amygdala and dopamine in the striatum modulating and decreasing the inhibitory control of the prefrontal cortex
- Persistent impulsive violence is enacted most by individuals diagnosed with schizophrenia spectrum disorders, intellectual disability, and cognitive disorders
  - Repetitive reinforcement of bottom-up processing leads to automatic and compulsive behaviors by shifting dopamine from the learned behavior reward system in the ventral striatum to the anticipatory reward system in the dorsal striatum
- Current treatment options include targeting and restoring top-down control and reducing bottom-up impulsive and emotional drive
- In impulsive aggression, clozapine is an effective medication and reduces aggressive symptoms independent of the presence of comorbid psychotic symptoms and cognitive impairment

PATIENT FILE

Post-test question

Which of the following statements regarding the neurobiology and treatment of impulsive aggression are false?

A. Impulsive aggression is singularly due to prefrontal cortical lesions and resultant behavioral disinhibition
B. Impulsive aggression is attributed to deficits in bottom-up and top-down processing leading to failure of risk:reward stratification and inhibitory behavioral response
C. Adjunctive treatment strategies include antipsychotics, mood stabilizers, beta-blockers, and SSRIs augmentation
D. A and C
E. None of the above is true regarding the neurobiology and treatment of impulsive aggression
F. All of the above are true

Answer: D

References

1. Blair, R. J. (2016). The neurobiology of impulsive aggression. *Journal of Child and Adolescent Psychopharmacology*, 26(1), 4–9. https://doi.org/10.1089/cap.2015.0088.
2. Citrome, L. & Volavka, J. (2014). The psychopharmacology of violence: making sensible decisions. *CNS Spectrums*, 19(5), 411–418. https://doi.org/10.1017/S1092852914000054.
3. Meyer, J. M., Cummings, M. A., Proctor, G., & Stahl, S. M. (2016). Psychopharmacology of persistent violence and aggression. *Psychiatric Clinics of North America*, 39(4), 541–556. https://doi.org/10.1016/j.psc.2016.07.012.
4. Nassif, J. B. & Felthous, A. R. (2022). Mapping the neurocircuitry of impulsive aggression through the pharmacologic review of anti-impulsive aggressive agents. *Journal of Forensic Services*, January 10, 67(3), 844–853. https://doi.org/10.1111/1556-4029.15000.
5. Quanbeck, C. D., McDermott, B. E., Lam, J., Eisenstark, H., Sokolov, G., & Scott, C. L. (2007). Categorization of aggressive acts committed by chronically assaultive state hospital patients. *Psychiatric Services*, April, 58(4), 521–528. https://doi.org/10.1176/ps.2007.58.4.521.
6. Seo, D., Patrick, C. J., & Kennealy, P. J. (2008). Role of serotonin and dopamine system interactions in the neurobiology of impulsive aggression and its comorbidity with other clinical disorders. *Aggression and Violent Behavior*, June 10, 13(5), 383–395. https://doi.org/10.1016/j.avb.2008.06.003.

PATIENT FILE

7. Stahl, S. M. (2014). Deconstructing violence as a medical syndrome: mapping psychotic, impulsive, and predatory subtypes to malfunctioning brain circuits. *CNS Spectrums*, October, 19(5), 35–365. https://doi.org/10.1017/S1092852914000522.
8. Stahl, S. M. (2014). *Stahl's Essential Psychopharmacology: Prescriber's Guide*, 5th ed. New York: Cambridge University Press.

PATIENT FILE

3

Predatory violence: The wolf in sheep's clothing

The Psychopharmacological Dilemma: What treatment options are available for persistent predatory acts of violence?

Maanasi Chandarana

Pretest self-assessment question

What is the most common type of violence in forensic hospital settings?

A. There isn't a prevalent type of violence represented in forensic hospital settings
B. Predatory
C. Impulsive
D. Psychotic
E. All of the above

Answer: C

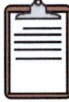

Patient evaluation on intake

The patient is a 39-year-old male with previous diagnoses of delusional disorder, neurocognitive disorder due to a traumatic brain injury, and substance use disorder (stimulant – methamphetamine type, cannabis use disorder). After he was adjudicated not guilty by reason of insanity (NGRI), he was court ordered, committed, and admitted to the state forensic hospital system. The patient's behaviors were notable for repeated aggressive acts directed toward peers and staff. His behaviors were retaliatory and non-self-defensive in nature and often occurred after an interpersonal disagreement or a perceived slight. During his brief hospitalization, he was prescribed as-needed medication (PRN) including oral haloperidol, lorazepam, and diphenhydramine with intramuscular (IM) back-ups; however, he was not prescribed scheduled medications. A week after he was told by a hospital staff member that he could not go to a musical event on campus, he punched, attempted to choke, and assaulted that staff member in a blind hallway during shift change. Three weeks after his admission, and to maintain the safety of the patients and staff, he was transferred to a maximum-security unit at another state forensic facility.

- The patient presented to the evaluation as calm, polite, and cooperative
- His grooming and hygiene were deemed fair

- His speech rate, rhythm, and volume were deemed normal and described as spontaneous and goal-directed
- The patient did not demonstrate psychomotor agitation, retardation, and abnormal involuntary movements
- He characterized his mood as "good," and demonstrated a stable affect. He denied suicidal thoughts and homicidal ideations
- He denied experiencing perceptual disturbances
- His thought process was linear, goal-directed, and organized
- The patient was alert, and oriented to person, time, and place. His memory, ability to abstract, fund of knowledge, attention, insight, and judgment were deemed fair
- His cognitive abilities were deemed akin to his baseline functioning

Psychiatric history

- Mental health history with onset in childhood
  - He reported that he lost consciousness following a motor vehicle accident when he was 5 years old, subsequently developing partial seizures, and perceptible changes in his personality and behaviors
  - When he was 11 years old, he sustained two black eyes and a suspected head trauma
    - Per available records, he exhibited symptoms of psychosis including visual hallucinations, delusions, hyperactivity, insomnia, and disorientation
  - He received psychiatric treatment from when he was 5 years to 17 years of age
    - He was first psychiatrically hospitalized when he was 8 years old
    - Per record review, he attempted suicide by overdose when he was 12 years old
    - He was diagnosed with conduct disorder, Attention-Deficit/Hyperactivity Disorder (ADHD), psychosis, and bipolar disorder, and demonstrated impulsive, hyperactive, inattentive, hypersexual, and unprovoked aggressive behaviors per record review
    - He was treated with valproic acid, clonidine, and olanzapine, and identified valproic acid and clonidine as therapeutically beneficial or helpful
    - Following acute inpatient stabilization, the patient decompensated multiple times in the community, which resulted in his placement in long-term residential care

PATIENT FILE

- He underwent neuropsychologic evaluation and testing when he was 12 years and 16 years old
  - Neuropsychologic testing revealed a constellation of findings or results consistent with cerebral dysfunction, dyspraxia, dysgraphia, dyslexia, and his intelligence was deemed average
    - The patient had deficits in reality testing and in the ability to think clearly and process and handle emotions
      - Deficits in reality testing were akin to or paralleled the findings of those suffering with psychotic symptoms
    - The patient's characterological traits were suggestive of severe psychopathology
  - He was described as exhibiting persistent affective and behavioral dysregulation
- He completed 11 years of formal education and trade school
- The patient has an extensive history of violence with multiple arrests, charges, and in-custody violent acts
- The patient was not previously hospitalized in forensic psychiatric facilities
- He was not prescribed trials of various scheduled medications while hospitalized in forensic facilities
- Substance use history: the patient reported that his drug of choice is cannabis, but relayed daily crystal methamphetamine use for approximately 10 years and at the time of the instant offense leading to his hospitalization

Social and personal history

- His parents divorced when he was young, and, because of impaired mother–child bonding, the patient's father was the primary caregiver and custodian for an unknown length of time
- The patient was raised in a group home setting because of his behavioral difficulties
- Multiple encounters with law enforcement noted with first documented arrest and incurred charge when he was 12 years of age
- He worked as a crane operator
- He intermittently received Social Security benefits for his medical diagnoses
- He was never married and has three children

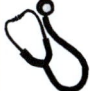

Medical history

- Traumatic brain injury
- Hypertension

PATIENT FILE

Family history
- There is no known familial history to report

Medication history
- He reported treatment with various medication trials, including antipsychotics, mood stabilizer, and alpha-agonist medication, as a child. However, he denied receiving treatment with psychiatric medications as an adult

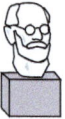

Psychotherapy history
- There is no known psychotherapy history to report

Mechanism of action moment
- Haloperidol
  - Blocks D_2 receptors
    - Reduces positive symptoms and aggressive behaviors
    - In the nigrostriatal pathway, D_2 blockade improves tics and associated symptoms of Tourette's
- Hydroxyzine
  - Blocks histamine (H1) receptors

Attending physician's mental notes
- The patient has a history of experiencing psychotic symptoms including persecutory delusions
- His history of head trauma and psychiatric symptoms contributed to his placement in residential settings, inability to engage in prosocial behaviors, and multiple contacts with law enforcement
- The patient's history is notable for deficits in multiple cognitive domains including that of complex attention, social cognition, language, and executive functioning
- The patient currently denies experiencing overvalued versus persecutory beliefs and thoughts of jealousy
- The patient has the right to refuse medications and does not provide informed consent for prescribed psychiatric medications
- As-needed medications including haloperidol and hydroxyzine were prescribed to the patient

Further investigation
- The month following his hospitalization, the patient was verbally redirected by staff when he over-personalized unit rules and identified said rules as unjust or unfair

PATIENT FILE

- Three months after he was admitted, the patient was evaluated by psychology
  - The patient scored high on scales measuring psychopathy. He exhibited superficiality, glibness, deceitfulness, interpersonal manipulation, increased sense of self-worth, and he externalized blame. He demonstrated deficits in his affective range and ability to empathize
  - In lifestyle domains, his behaviors coincided with narcissistic and antisocial traits in that he took advantage of others financially, was impulsive and irresponsible, set unrealistic expectations, participated in risky behaviors, and had difficulty modulating his anger
- Five months after the patient was admitted, he was placed in restraints for fighting with a peer and breaking his peer's jaw. During the encounter and ensuing evaluation, the patient did not demonstrate psychotic symptoms. He presented as glib, controlling, and superficial
- The patient did not demonstrate symptoms of psychosis, voice thoughts related to themes of jealousy or persecution, and psychiatrically decompensate or destabilize during his hospitalization
- He engaged in multiple verbally or physically violent acts that were associated with a defined outcome
- The patient refused to provide informed consent for medications and was not court-ordered to involuntarily take medications

Attending physician's mental notes

- The patient has a history of experiencing psychotic symptoms including persecutory delusions; however, he has not demonstrated mood, affective, or psychotic symptoms during his hospitalization
- During his hospitalization, he had difficulty engaging in prosocial behaviors, made verbally disparaging comments to other patients and staff, and behaved violently
- The patient has the right to refuse medications and has only taken hydroxyzine as needed for sleep on occasion
- As-needed medications including haloperidol and hydroxyzine will continue to be offered
- The patient will be monitored and assessed for precursors of violence, violence risk, and victimization of his peers and staff
- Verbally and physically aggressive and violent behaviors likely stem from character pathology, his history of traumatic brain injury, and resultant frontotemporal neurocognitive disorder

PATIENT FILE

Case outcome
- The patient's case is followed monthly
- Through his hospitalization, the patient engaged in multiple verbally and physically violent behaviors that resulted in his placement in seclusion and/or restraints once, but he refused to provide informed consent for treatment with psychiatric medications and did not demonstrate psychotic or affective symptoms

Case debrief
- The patient was administratively transferred from one forensic state hospital to a forensic hospital within the same state system
- The patient was not prescribed scheduled psychiatric medications upon admission to our facility
- Our patient was diagnosed with stimulant – methamphetamine-type use disorder, mild frontotemporal neurocognitive disorder, and unspecified personality disorder with antisocial and narcissistic traits
- The patient did not demonstrate psychotic and affective symptoms during his hospitalization, and he refused to provide informed consent for treatment with medications to reduce his behaviors
- He participated in multiple purposeful acts of violence which were attributed to his characterological and personality structure as well as his history of mild frontotemporal neurocognitive disorder

Take-home points
- Aggression is defined as any act with the potential to harm self or others, whereas violence is a subcategory of aggression that results in harm to others
- Comparative percentages attributed to impulsive, predatory, and psychotic violence in forensic settings are: impulsive (54%) > predatory (29%) > psychotic (17%)
  - Although impulsive violence is represented in greater proportions in forensic settings when compared to other subtypes of violence, psychopathy associated with predatory violence is present in 1% of the population, and 15–25% of the carceral population, and is associated with a national cost of $460 billion annually
  - Meloy's forensic criteria for distinguishing predatory violence include:
    - There is minimal to no autonomic arousal
      - Individuals who engage in predatory violence are less responsive to noxious stimuli and may have a lowered heart rate in response to stressful stimuli

PATIENT FILE

- There is lack of conscious emotion and the act occurs in the absence of a perceived threat
  - It is not necessarily a response to threatening or noxious stimuli
- Because the act is not a response to a threatening or noxious stimulus, it is not time-limited or displaced onto an intervening target
- It is a planned or purposeful act with an intended or anticipated outcome
  - Cognitive (versus emotional) act and intentional attack (not a defensive or protective behavior)
- The act may be preceded by private preparation and accompanied with intense focus and attention
- Different individuals engaging in predatory violence have differing goals
  - Examples of goals include: gratification (fantasy, omnipotence, sexual sadism) or provision of relief in the context of an ego-dystonic compulsion
- Classifying the subtype of violence aids with treatment management
  - Predatory violence
    - Represents the most severe and least treatable of the subtypes of aggressive acts
    - Identifying and managing predatory violence includes evaluation of the offender or patient with risk assessments, and for physical, medical, and psychiatric conditions as well as medication side effects, and assessing the contribution of environmental, scheduling, staff, and institutional factors
      - Violence risk assessments
        - Structured professional judgment
          - Historical Clinical Risk Management 20 (HCR-20)
          - Short-Term Assessment of Risk and Treatability (START)
          - Violence Risk Screening-10 (V-RISK-10)
        - Actuarial risk assessments
          - Violence Risk Appraisal Guide (VRAG)
          - Classification of Violence Risk (COVR)
        - Psychopathy assessments
          - Psychopathy Checklist Revised (PCL-R)
      - Patient factors
        - Labs / vital signs:
          - Electrolytes: sodium, calcium, glucose
          - Infection: white blood cell count (WBC), infectious disease serologies

PATIENT FILE

- Endocrine: thyroid stimulating hormone (TSH)
- Ammonia
- Erythrocyte sedimentation rate (ESR)
- Vital signs: O_2 saturation, blood pressure, temperature, heart rate
  - Medical conditions: pain, substance withdrawal or intoxication, seizure disorder, delirium, insomnia
  - Medication side effects:
    - Antipsychotics: sedation, extrapyramidal symptoms (EPS), orthostasis
    - Neuroleptics: ataxia, sedation, cognitive effects
    - B blockers: hypotension, bradycardia, bronchospasm
    - Lithium: tremor, polyuria, cognitive effects
  - Psychiatric symptomatology
- Environmental factors
  - Physical space:
    - Example: patients in close proximity while waiting in line
  - Unit population
    - Examples: unsafe population mix, younger patient population
- Scheduling
  - Unstructured, unplanned events, groups, and activities
  - Increased frequency of patient:staff interactions
  - Contact during patient movement
- Staff factors
  - Examples: high staff turnover, staff burnout
- Institutional factors
  - Inability to house patients in settings reflective of behavior
    - Example: inability to transfer a patient with multiple violent behaviors to a unit with increased programming and security
  - Inability to identify patient risk factors because of inaccessible patient information
  - Acceptance of high-risk practices and lack of or ineffective crisis management planning
    - Medications target anxiety and tension, mood swings, and anger and impulsivity
      - Mood stabilizers can assist with anger, mood swings, and impulsivity

> **PATIENT FILE**

- SSRIs and antidepressants are utilized to reduce anxiety and tension
- Clozapine treatment is associated with a reduction in aggression and violence
- It is important and vital to address and treat comorbid psychiatric symptoms and disorders
- Psychological and social interventions
    - Risk need responsivity determines the patient's level of risk treatment needs, and optimal modalities of treatment delivery
        - Risk: identifies patient risk factors, and behaviors that can precipitate violence
        - Need: identifies needs or desired outcomes of patients engaging in violence
        - Responsivity: involves modification of individual treatment plans based on the patient strength, motivation, and learning style
- Review medications, violence risk assessments, psychosocial interventions, and treatment plans in cases of persistent violence

Performance in practice: confessions of a psychopharmacologist

What could have been done better?

- In this case, the patient did not exhibit psychotic or psychiatric symptomatology although his psychiatric history was notable for various mental health diagnoses, psychiatric hospitalization, and treatment with psychotropic medication. The patient reported perceived therapeutic benefit with clonidine and valproic acid. Given the patient's report of positive treatment response, a therapeutic modality could include trial of these medications
- While in the forensic hospital setting, the patient engaged in multiple acts of predatory violence and did not consent to treatment with antipsychotic medication. Familiarity with local hospital policy and state and federal law governing involuntary treatment can aid the practitioner in determining if a patient may qualify for involuntary treatment with psychotropic medications

What are clinical considerations when treating predatory violence?

- Predatory violence can be distinguished from impulsive and psychotic violence in that predatory violence *is* a cognitive, planned act and *is not* time-limited, displaced on an object or person, and in response to a threatening or painful stimulus

PATIENT FILE

- Nonpharmacological interventions include performance of violence risk assessments and risk need responsivity planning as well as optimizing the patient's environment, staffing, schedule, and security requirements
- Be familiar with statutory requirements and respective recommendations for prescribing psychiatric medications involuntarily and emergently
- Clozapine antagonizes D_2 receptors, which reduces positive symptoms of psychosis and provides mood stabilization; and serotonin 2A receptors, which enhances dopamine release in brain regions to minimize motor side effects and improve cognitive and affective symptoms. Clozapine also interacts with $5\text{-}HT_{2C}$ and $5\text{-}HT_{1A}$ receptors which may promote increased efficacy in treatment of cognitive and affective symptoms
- Clozapine may be associated with reduction in aggressive and violent behaviors irrespective of etiology (i.e., psychotic, impulsive, and predatory)

Tips and pearls
- The various subtypes of violent behaviors are linked to different neurochemical and neuroanatomical deviations
  - Violent behaviors are linked to the dorsolateral prefrontal cortex and orbitofrontal circuit
    - The dorsolateral prefrontal cortex modulates executive functioning including the ability to plan, sequentially plan, problem-solve, and adapt behaviors to associated cognitive processes
    - The orbitofrontal circuit connects frontal processing cortical centers to emotional limbic centers and directs responses to social cues and interpersonal responsiveness
  - Neurodevelopmentally, early damage to the ventromedial prefrontal cortex impedes moral development
  - Predatory violence is associated with:
    - Normal to increased prefrontal activity and intrafrontal connectivity
    - Hypometabolism in the limbic system including the amygdala, hippocampal formation and parahippocampal gyrus, ventral striatum, and anterior and posterior cingulate gyrus
      - Hypometabolism in the limbic system manifests as shallow affect and lack of affective empathy
      - Hypermetabolism in the limbic system presents as aggressive impulsivity

PATIENT FILE

- Increased collosal white matter volume and length and hemispheric connectivity which contributes to deficiencies in affect
- Alterations in steroid hormone interactions with the insula, anterior cingulate cortex, and amygdala which decreases the perception of stress and increases callousness
  - Potential treatment options associated with neuroanatomical and neurochemical deviations include:
    - Targeting hypoarousal in the limbic region
    - Cognitive reappraisal and reframing
    - Mindfulness
      - Short term (8 weeks): associated with increased attention, emotional modulation, perspective of self and others, and body awareness
        - Abbreviated mindfulness practices can promote changes in neuroplasticity of the anterior cingulate cortex, insula, temporoparietal junction, and frontolimbic circuitry
      - Long term: associated with increased volume of the insula, amygdala, and right temporoparietal junction, fostering increased empathy

Two-minute tutorial

- Classifying the type and nature of aggressive patient behaviors enables the practitioner to identify potential treatment options
- Identifying and managing predatory violence includes performance of violence risk assessments and evaluating the offender or patient for physical, medical, and psychiatric conditions as well as medication side effects, and assessing the contribution of environmental, scheduling, staff, and institutional factors
  - Medications target anxiety and tension, mood swings, and anger and impulsivity
    - Mood stabilizers can assist with anger, mood swings, and impulsivity
    - SSRIs and antidepressants are utilized to reduce anxiety and tension
    - Clozapine treatment is associated with a reduction in aggression and violence
  - It is important and vital to address and treat comorbid psychiatric symptoms and disorders

- Ascertaining the reasons underlying predatory violence, utilizing risk assessments and risk need responsivity strategies, avoiding countertransference, reevaluating treatment progress, maintaining appropriate security, and providing staff and patients with training on de-escalation and prevention strategies can assist with establishing and maintaining safe and therapeutic interactions and milieus

Post-test question

What type of violence in forensic hospital settings is the most severe, least treatable, and associated with increased costs?

A. Interpersonal
B. Psychotic
C. Impulsive
D. Predatory
E. None of the above
F. Intimate partner

Answer: D

References

1. Chialant, D., Edersheim, J., & Price, B. H. (2016). The dialectic between empathy and violence: an opportunity for intervention? *Journal of Neuropsychiatry and Clinical Neuroscience*, 28(4), 273–285. https://doi.org/10.1176/appi.neuropsych.15080207.
2. Declercq, F. & Audenaert, K. (2011). Predatory violence aiming at relief in a case of mass murder: Meloy's criteria for applied forensic practice. *Behavioral Sciences & the Law*, July 11, 29(4), 578–591. https://doi.org/10.1002/bsl.994.
3. Meyer, J. M., Cummings, M. A., Proctor, G., & Stahl, S. M. (2016). Psychopharmacology of persistent violence and aggression. *Psychiatric Clinics of North America*, 39(4), 541–556. https://doi.org/10.1016/j.psc.2016.07.012.
4. Stahl, S. M. (2014). *Stahl's Essential Psychopharmacology: Prescriber's Guide*, 5th ed. New York: Cambridge University Press.
5. Stahl, S. M., Morrissette, D. A., Cummings, M., et al. (2014). California State Hospital Violence Assessment and Treatment (Cal-VAT) guidelines. *CNS Spectrums*, October, 19(5), 449–465. https://doi.org/10.1017/S1092852914000376.

SECTION II
Self-Injurious Behaviors (SIB) or Non-suicidal self-injury (NSSI)

PATIENT FILE

4

Self-injurious behavior (SIB) and violence: Inward and outward

The Psychopharmocological Dilemma: Clozapine-resistant schizoaffective disorder bipolar type

Jennifer O'Day

Pretest self-assessment question

What is the next step in treating a primary psychotic illness with aggression when high-dose/high-level clozapine treatment only provides a partial response?

A. Add a mood stabilizer
B. Start individual psychotherapy
C. Combine with ECT
D. Discontinue the clozapine because it's not working

Answer: C

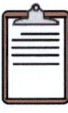

Patient evaluation on intake

Ms. C is a 32-year-old single, conserved, Caucasian female admitted to a state hospital for continued care due to ongoing SIB, aggression toward others, impulsivity, somatic delusions, tangential and illogical thought process, as well as other maladaptive behaviors.

Psychiatric history

- Ms. C was first hospitalized in 1995 when she was an adolescent after running away from her foster home. She told staff she was "seeing things and hearing voices" that were telling her to harm others
- She was started on psychotropic medications and discharged back to her foster home, but was ultimately hospitalized 6 months later, again for verbalizations of a paranoid nature and extreme agitation
- Ms. C has stated in the past that, if she does not like a particular placement, she knows she can become angry, break windows, and falsely claim to "hear voices" telling her to hurt others so that she will be moved to another facility. Ms. C was placed in multiple community-based psychiatric facilities for children since her adolescent years. She has repeatedly engaged in fire-setting, property destruction, aggressive and self-injurious behaviors, and made several suicide attempts

PATIENT FILE

- She has been admitted to state hospitals repeatedly since 2000 as an early adult. Available records on admission to state hospital confirmed that she has an extensive history of aggression and SIB. Historically, these behaviors have included cutting her wrists, head banging, punching and slapping herself and tying items around her neck
- She has been hospitalized at various state hospitals at least four times for periods of 2 months to 2 years at a time

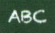
Social and personal history

Ms. C was born and raised in a mid-sized city. She and her five siblings were placed in foster care in 1988, when she was a young child. She was in foster care or youth placement settings until she was a legal adult, at which point she briefly regained contact with an older brother and her father.

Ms. C reported dropping out of high school in tenth grade but was actually placed in juvenile hall after assaulting two teachers' aides, one of whom was pregnant at the time. She said she was in special education classes because she had "ADHD and I couldn't pay attention in school."

Her only work experience is holding a job serving coffee at a community-based psychiatric facility.

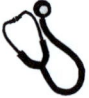
Medical history
- Dyslipidemia
- Hypothyroidism
- Hypertension
- Gastroesophageal reflux disease (GERD)
- Obesity

Family history
Ms. C's biological mother abused illicit substances.

Medication history
She has a history of poor response to olanzapine and risperidone, and only a partial response to clozapine.

Current history
Ms. C's primary working diagnoses include schizoaffective disorder – bipolar type, borderline personality disorder (BPD), and post-traumatic stress disorder (PTSD) due to early childhood trauma.

Over the past year, her psychotropic medications included clozapine (serum levels in the 1000s ng/mL), divalproex (serum levels in the 80s mcg/dL), and lithium (serum levels ranged from 0.7–1.1 mmol/L)

PATIENT FILE

Despite adequate mood stabilization and antipsychotic medication treatment, she continued to have resistant symptoms including repeated aggression toward herself, staff, and peers, and fixed delusions such as "I was born today"; "I don't want heart surgery"; or identifying staff as family members. The aggression was deemed to be psychotic and impulsive in nature. Specific post-traumatic stress-related symptoms were not elucidated. It is likely there is some degree of underlying cognitive impairment; however, there is no formal neuropsychological testing documented.

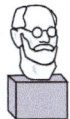

Psychotherapy history
- There was no documented history of psychotherapy treatment

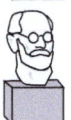

Psychotherapy moment
Dialectical behavioral therapy is a well-known and studied treatment for self-injurious behavior.

Cognitive behavioral therapy for psychosis could also be considered in this case.

Mechanism of action moment
ECT involves inducing a generalized tonic–clonic seizure by applying electricity to the brain via electrodes placed on the scalp. ECT is conducted with general anesthesia and muscular paralysis to protect the body from the motor convulsion.

The exact mechanism of action is not clear. Seizures change many aspects of brain chemistry, neural activity, and connectivity, which produce an exceptionally broad therapeutic spectrum of action – for example in depression, psychosis, catatonia, repetitive injurious behaviors, status epilepticus, etc.

Attending physician's mental notes
Due to ongoing aggression to self and others despite maximizing serum levels of clozapine and mood stabilizers, ECT augmentation treatment was started. After initiation of ECT, Ms. C began to show improvement in her aggressive acts to herself, peers, and staff.

After several months, ECT was stopped due to legal delay. Symptoms worsened quickly without ECT treatment and she began requiring PRNs and five-point restraints due to psychotic and impulsive aggression.

ECT was restarted several weeks later, after court approval, at the frequency of three times a week. Once ECT resumed, Ms. C's behavior

PATIENT FILE

improved. She was less impulsive, agitated, and aggressive. She continued to have fixed delusions.

As of approximately one year later, Ms. C had received a total of 52 ECT treatments.

Case outcome; use of outcome measures

ECT augmentation of clozapine showed a definitive improvement in Ms. C's aggressive behaviors to herself and others, based on a substantial decline in PRN use and Incident Reports (IRs) for aggressive behavior prior to, compared to after, the initiation of ECT treatment. However, aggression resumed quickly when ECT treatment was not maintained. Her fixed delusions showed minimal improvement while receiving ECT.

Case debrief

Upon resuming ECT, there were no further aggressive behaviors. However, she continued to be intrusive, hypersexual, and delusional with bouts of yelling and screaming, along with impulsivity at times.

Over the course of several months after reinitiating ECT, Ms. C remained intrusive, getting in the personal space of others when communicating, but was easier to verbally redirect when that occurred. She was still receiving maintenance ECT once a week. She still had no aggressive behavior since restarting ECT. Nevertheless, she remained highly delusional, believing she had died, her mother died "yesterday," and believing she's a "dog."

Over the course of several more months, she decompensated after being assigned a new conservator who delayed signing off on her ECT consent. As a result, Ms. C had a drastic increase in bouts of aggression toward others, requiring PRNs and five-point restraints and seclusion. The treating psychiatrist quickly started the process to resume ECT.

Since then, she was found to have the capacity to consent for ECT and subsequently refused it.

Over the past several months, she began to display aggression toward herself and others, including the need for increased supervision, with a one-on-one (1:1) staff for 24 hours for dangerousness to self (DTS) / safety. In another incident, she attempted to charge at her 1:1 staff and an intramuscular (IM) PRN and five-point restraints were required. In the past 30 days, she required 6 PRNs for agitation, and 5 PRNs for insomnia.

PATIENT FILE

Take-home points

ECT can be helpful alone or as an adjunctive treatment to clozapine or a non-clozapine antipsychotic for treatment-resistant psychosis and aggression toward self and others.

The combination of ECT and antipsychotic drugs is associated with better outcomes than ECT alone or antipsychotic drugs alone during the acute phase of treatment. This finding holds true during the continuation phase of ECT as well. There is also anecdotal evidence that ECT may exert additive or synergistic effects with antipsychotic agents.

From 1% to 3% of state hospital patients may be candidates for ECT treatment.

Performance in practice: confessions of a psychopharmacologist

Night-time doses of lithium may need to be held or decreased prior to ECT treatment in order to decrease the trough serum level during the ECT course, as this decreases the risk of post-ECT delirium.

Night-time doses of divalproex may need to be held or lowered prior to ECT treatment to decrease the trough serum level during the ECT course in order to decrease seizure threshold and improve chances of adequate seizures.

Benzodiazepine doses may need to be decreased or tapered off during ECT treatment to decrease seizure threshold and improve chances of adequate seizures.

Tips and pearls

Often, patients with severe treatment-resistant mental illness and aggression who respond to ECT treatment will require ongoing maintenance ECT to maintain their treatment response after their initial acute ECT course.

In patients with psychiatric disorders there is no apparent long-term adverse cognitive consequence even after several hundred treatments administered as frequently as weekly or bi-weekly over several consecutive years.

Reasons for choosing continuation or maintenance ECT:

- Lack of adequate response to medication
- Good response to ECT in the past
- Aggression
- Self-injury
- Refusal to eat or drink
- Physical problems limiting the ability to change the psychopharmacological regimen
- Attempt to prevent severe exacerbations evident in the past

PATIENT FILE

Two-minute tutorial

The exact mechanism of action of ECT is not clear. Seizures change many aspects of brain chemistry, neural activity, and connectivity, which produce an exceptionally broad therapeutic spectrum of action.

In cases where underlying mood and psychotic illnesses are aggressively treated with mood stabilizers and antipsychotics, including clozapine, with residual treatment-resistant aggression toward self or others, ECT should be considered as an augmentation strategy.

Night-time doses of lithium may need to be held or decreased prior to ECT treatment in order to decrease the trough serum level during the ECT course, as this decreases the risk of post-ECT delirium.

Night-time doses of divalproex may need to be held or lowered prior to ECT treatment to decrease the trough serum level during the ECT course to decrease seizure threshold and improve chances of adequate seizures.

Benzodiazepine doses may need to be decreased or tapered off during ECT treatment to decrease seizure threshold and improve chances of adequate seizures.

Often, patients with severe treatment-resistant psychotic illness and aggression who respond to ECT treatment will require ongoing maintenance ECT to maintain their treatment response after their initial acute ECT course.

References

1. Andrade, C. & Kurinji, S. (2002). Continuation and maintenance ECT: a review of recent research. *Journal of ECT*, 18(3), 149–158.
2. Chanpattana, W. and Andrade, C. (2006). ECT for treatment-resistant schizophrenia: a response from the Far East to the UK – NICE report. *Journal of ECT*, 22, 4–12.
3. Deng, Z. D., Robins, P. L., Regenold, W., Rohde, P., Dannhauer, M., & Lisanby, S. H. (2024). How electroconvulsive therapy works in the treatment of depression: is it the seizure, the electricity, or both? *Neuropsychopharmacology: Official Publication of the American College of Neuropsychopharmacology*, 49(1), 150–162. https://doi.org/10.1038/s41386-023-01677-2.
4. Iancu, I., Pick, N., Seener-Lorsh, O., & Dannon, P. (2015). Patients with schizophrenia or schizoaffective disorder who receive multiple electroconvulsive therapy sessions: characteristics, indications, and results. *Neuropsychiatric Disease and Treatment*, 11, 853–862.

PATIENT FILE

5. Lally, J., Tully, J., Robertson, D., Stubbs, B., Gaughran, F., & MacCabe, J. H. (2016). Augmentation of clozapine with electroconvulsive therapy in treatment resistant schizophrenia: a systematic review and meta-analysis. *Schizophrenia Research*, 171(1–3), 215–224.
6. McCall, W. V., Weiner, R. D., Shelp, F. E., & Austin, S. (1992). ECT in a state hospital setting. *Convulsive Therapy*, 8(1), 12–18.
7. Petrides, G., Malur, C., Braga, R. J., et al. (2015). Electroconvulsive therapy augmentation in clozapine-resistant schizophrenia: a prospective, randomized study. *American Journal of Psychiatry*, 172(1), 52–58.
8. Sadock, B. J., Sadock, V. A., Ruiz, P., & Kaplan, H. I. (2017). *Kaplan and Sadock's Comprehensive Textbook of Psychiatry* (10th ed.). Kingston upon Thames: Wolters Kluwer.
9. Witzel, J., Held, E., & Bogerts, B. (2009). Electroconvulsive therapy in forensic psychiatry –ethical problems in daily practice. *Journal of ECT*, 25(2), 129–132.
10. Zheng, W., Cao, X. L., Ungvari, G. S., et al. (2016). Electroconvulsive therapy added to non-clozapine antipsychotic medication for treatment resistant schizophrenia: meta-analysis of randomized controlled trials. *PloS One*, 11(6), e0156510.

PATIENT FILE

5

Non-suicidal self-injury (NSSI): Death by a thousand cuts

The Psychopharmacological Dilemma: What are the treatment options for non-suicidal self-injurious behaviors?

Maanasi Chandarana

Pretest self-assessment question

Which of the following statements about non-suicidal self-injurious behaviors are true?

A. Medical and psychiatric literature reflects self-injurious behaviors are medically managed by combination therapies including antipsychotic, mood stabilizer, and antidepressant medications
B. Behavioral therapies may reduce non-suicidal self-injurious behaviors
C. The prevalence of non-suicidal self-injurious behavior is highest in the general, community population
D. The most common type of non-suicidal self-injurious behaviors in correctional settings is inserting foreign objects
E. Individuals who engage in non-suicidal self-injurious behaviors are less likely to harm others and more likely to die by suicide

Answer: B

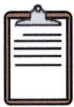

Patient evaluation on intake

The patient is a 43-year-old male with previous diagnoses of Schizoaffective Disorder, borderline personality disorder (BPD), antisocial personality traits, and Stimulant – Methamphetamine-type Use Disorder. Due to his persistent violent behaviors, the patient was conserved and committed to a state forensic hospital. While hospitalized, the patient engaged in a serious violent act which prompted the patient's administrative transfer from one forensic hospital to another forensic state hospital. The patient was subsequently admitted to the specialized unit of the receiving forensic hospital that provides increased programming, structure, and security measures and is reserved for the most unstable and violent patients. Despite maintenance in a more highly structured and secure environment, the patient engages in multiple externalized violent acts as well as self-injurious behaviors, including ingesting and swallowing foreign, nonfood objects.

PATIENT FILE

Psychiatric history
- Mental health history with onset in childhood
  - Per record review, the onset of the patient's psychotic symptoms began when he was 11 years old
  - He reported command auditory hallucinations (CAH) and visual hallucinations. Per record review, he demonstrated persecutory delusions, symptoms of mania and depression, and aggression
  - He was described as prone to affective dysregulation, behavioral destabilization, and multiple acts of violence
  - He was psychiatrically involuntarily hospitalized multiple times in the community; however, necessitated a more restrictive care environment due to his aggression toward hospital and care staff
- He said he repeated the second grade but denied placement in special education classes
- He reported that he graduated high school
- Behaviorally, the patient exhibited impulsive and aggressive acts
  - The patient has a history of self-injurious, physical, and verbally threatening behavior and interpersonal conflict
    - The patient has a history of head banging and head butting
    - It was thought that some of his behaviors were attempts to obtain identifiable goals or outcomes
- The patient has an extensive history of violence with multiple arrests, charges, and in-custody offenses
- The patient has been hospitalized in forensic psychiatric facilities multiple times
- He was prescribed multiple trials of medications, including antipsychotics and mood-stabilizer medications
- Substance use history
  - The patient reported that his drug of choice is methamphetamine, age of first use as 20 years old, and characterized use as daily for three years
  - He relayed using cannabis occasionally when he was 16–20 years of age
  - He said that he drank approximately two 40-ounce beers daily from the age of 17 to 39 or 40 years
  - He reported last substance use of alcohol about 3–4 years prior to current hospitalization
  - He denied lysergic acid diethylamide (LSD), mushroom, opiate, MDMA, prescription pill, and intravenous drug use

PATIENT FILE

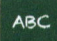
Social and personal history
- Multiple encounters with law enforcement noted, with first documented arrest and incurred charge when he was 22 years of age
- He reported working as a forklift driver, in a warehouse, and in the fast-food industry
- He was never married; he reported having an adult child

Medical history
- Hypothyroidism
- Gastroesophageal reflux disease
- History of pneumonia and asymptomatic positive tuberculin purified protein derivative (PPD) test
- History of malignant catatonia with aspiration
- The patient reported a history of seizure disorder, with the last seizure-like activity experienced 4–5 years prior to this current hospitalization

Family history
- The patient reported a maternal familial history of substance use and medical history of asthma

Medication history
- The patient was prescribed multiple trials of medications including antipsychotics and mood-stabilizer medication

Current history
- The patient presented to the evaluation as calm, polite, and cooperative
- He was dressed in hospital attire, and his grooming and hygiene were deemed fair
- His speech rate, rhythm, and volume were normal
- The patient did not demonstrate psychomotor agitation, retardation, and abnormal involuntary movements
- He reported good mood, and he exhibited a broad affective range. He denied suicidal thoughts. He denied experiencing homicidal ideations
- He denied experiencing auditory and visual hallucinations and symptoms of thought insertion or extraction. Overt delusional content was not reported or observed
- His thought process was linear and goal-directed
- The patient was alert, and oriented to person, time, and place. His recent and remote memory and attention were deemed fair. His fund of knowledge was thought to be adequate
- He demonstrated deficits in his cognition, insight, and judgment

PATIENT FILE

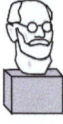

Psychotherapy history
- There is no known psychotherapy history to report

Mechanism of action moment
- Clozapine
    - Antagonizes D_2 receptors and serotonin 2A receptors
        - Blocking D_2 receptors reduces positive symptoms of psychosis and provides mood stabilization
        - Blocking serotonin 2A receptors enhances dopamine release in brain regions to minimize motor side effects and improve cognitive and affective symptoms
    - Interacts with $5-HT_{2C}$ and $5-HT_{1A}$ which may promote increased efficacy in treatment of cognitive and affective symptoms
- Divalproex
    - Stabilizes neuronal membrane by optimizing K+ efflux and Na+ influx
        - Decreases the glutamate:GABA ratio
            - Decreases glutamate by stimulating glutamine synthetase
            - Increases GABA by increasing GABA levels, GABA release, $GABA_B$ receptor density, and neuronal responsiveness to GABA; and decreases GABA catabolism and turnover
    - Dampens excitatory systems by decreasing aspartate release, CSF somatostatin, and NMDA mediated circuits
    - Increases dopamine turnover
- Fluphenazine decanoate
    - Antagonizes D_2 receptors and decreases positive symptoms of psychosis
- Lithium carbonate
    - Mechanism of action is complex and not well understood
    - Thought to recruit second messenger signaling pathway including that of cAMP and cGMP
    - Involved in genetic transcription and post-translational modification
        - Competes with other cations involved in signal transduction
    - Decreases the glutamine : gamma aminobutyric acid (GABA) ratio
        - Prevents loss of phosphorylated cAMP Response Element Binding Protein
            - Inhibits glutamate activation of protein kinases
                - Provides neuroprotective effects

PATIENT FILE

Attending physician's mental notes
- The patient has a history of experiencing psychotic symptoms, including auditory and visual hallucinations as well as persecutory delusions and aggression
  - During this evaluation, the patient reported that he did not experience CAH
  - His previous mental health provider documented that the patient identified that his violent acts prevented his release from the hospital (i.e., the patient's motivation for engaging in specific behaviors was to attain specific goals or outcomes)
- The patient reported a history of depressive episodes and episodic mania
- The patient exhibits a pervasive pattern of instability in his self-image, interpersonal relationships, affect, and impulse control which impairs his social, occupational, and educational functioning
- Medications prescribed by the referring facility appear to be targeting his symptoms
  - Clozapine 50 mg p.o. daily and 375 mg p.o. qHS
  - Divalproex 1500 mg p.o. daily and 2000 mg p.o. qHS
  - Fluphenazine decanoate 50 mg intramuscularly (IM) every 2 weeks

Further investigation
- The patient engaged in multiple acts of violence requiring placement in restraints and seclusion, as well as multiple instances of administration of emergency or PRN medications
  - The patient continues to engage in acts of violence, often directed at care staff following the discontinuation of seclusion or restraints, despite multiple therapeutic interventions and strategies
  - A divalproex level resulted as 118.7 ug/mL
- Clozapine and fluphenazine decanoate were both increased in dosage to optimize treatment effect
  - Following the changes in his medications, the patient engaged in persistent self-injurious behaviors including head banging, ingesting nonfood objects, and hitting inanimate objects, and violent acts directed toward his peers and hospital staff
    - His behavior prompted his treatment with emergency medications and placement in seclusion or restraints
- About 2 months after administrative transfer, the patient was diagnosed with aspiration pneumonia and divalproex and fluphenazine decanoate were decreased and discontinued
- Lithium was added to the patient's medication regimen to treat his persistent self-injurious behaviors

PATIENT FILE

- With continued observation and treatment, it was thought that the etiology of the patient's symptoms, including aggressive and violent acts, was not related to psychotic symptoms, but rather associated with his characterological and personality traits
  - Approximately 6 months after admission, psychiatric medications – clozapine and lithium – were decreased to observe the patient's behaviors and for diagnostic clarification
  - By the ninth month of hospitalization, treatment with lithium and clozapine therapy was stopped
  - Six weeks after medications were discontinued, the patient inquired if he could have certain privileges if he engaged in violent behaviors. He proceeded to verbally and physically threaten and assault staff. Clozapine was restarted to treat the patient's persistent aggressive symptoms

Case outcome

- The patient's case is followed monthly
- Through his hospitalization, the patient engaged in multiple aggressive behaviors that resulted in his placement in seclusion and/or restraints, benefited from treatment with as-needed (PRN) medications, prompted increase in his prescribed medications to therapeutic dosing, and warranted his continued treatment on the specialized unit reserved for the most unstable and violent patients
- The patient's diagnoses were amended to intermittent explosive disorder and antisocial and borderline personality disorder
- The patient exhibited persistent impulsive aggressive behaviors, including verbal aggression / verbal threats, physical aggression, repetitive self-harm behaviors, eating nonfood items, and punching and kicking inanimate objects
- During his previous and current hospitalization, the patient questioned whether and reported that participating in acts of violence resulted in specific, defined, and desired outcomes

Case debrief

- Our patient was diagnosed with intermittent explosive disorder, antisocial and borderline personality disorder, and Stimulant – Methamphetamine-type Use Disorder
- Due to his persistent violent behaviors, the patient was transferred from one forensic hospital to the unit reserved for the most unstable and violent patients of another forensic state hospital

PATIENT FILE

- Despite increased dosing of prescribed medications – including clozapine, divalproex, fluphenazine decanoate, and lithium – and a drug holiday for diagnostic clarification and to determine whether the patient's behaviors could be clinically explained by characterological or personality traits, and reintroduction and titration of clozapine, the patient exhibited impulsive aggressive behaviors which posited him as a danger to himself and others, and benefited from multiple psychopharmacological and nonpharmacologic therapeutic interventions

Take-home points

- The International Society for the Study of Self-Injury defines self-injurious behaviors as intentional self-directed tissue injury
- The prevalence of self-injury in the United States ranges from 2200 to 3700 per 100,000
  - There is a greater incidence of self-injury in forensic and correctional settings than in the general population
    - Self-injury in the mentally ill carceral population is about 68%, versus 4% in the general population
    - 30–48% of those incarcerated report a history of self-injurious behaviors
    - Environmental conditions in the correctional setting may contribute to greater incidence of self-harm events
      - Solitary confinement, disciplinary interventions, and victimization are examples of environmental stressors experienced by offenders
- Self-injurious behaviors in correctional settings include:
  - Scratching (95.7%)
  - Cutting with an item/object (94.3%)
  - Head banging (84.8%)
  - Scratching with an item/object (82.2%)
  - Reopening a wound (81.3%)
  - Inserting an object (70.9%)
- Factors influencing non-suicidal self-injury
  - Demographic
    - The prevalence of self-harm acts is not gender specific
  - Psychiatric symptoms and illnesses
    - Self-harm behaviors are associated with impulsivity, PTSD, and depressive and psychotic symptoms
  - Substance use
    - Male inmates with substance use disorder have an increased likelihood of self-injuring compared to those without substance use disorder (30% versus 21%)

PATIENT FILE

- Individual characteristics
  - Non-suicidal self-injury is associated with BPD, antisocial personality disorder, and psychopathy
    - Higher prevalence of self-injurious behaviors in females diagnosed with BPD (approximately 73%) versus females not diagnosed with this disorder (in whom the rate of NSSI is estimated to be between 6 and 17%)
  - Personal emotions and behaviors
    - Self-injurious behaviors are associated with negative emotional states and feeling less in control, anger, shame, and frustration
    - Self-injury is associated with avoidant, aggressive, and impulsive behaviors
  - Coping style
    - Avoidant coping styles, fewer coping strategies, and less problem-solving skill correlates with an increased risk of NSSI, and this has been demonstrated in prisoners
- Childhood adverse events
  - Increased incidence of self-directed injury by individuals with a history of physical and sexual abuse, especially if associated with the survivor's feeling or experience of shame
- Interpersonal relationships
  - An interpersonal conflict preceded 42% of performed self-harm acts
- Motivation
  - To regulate emotions
    - It is postulated that self-harm behaviors are attempts to reduce negative emotional states and restore emotional balance
      - 31.6% of male offenders identified emotional relief, and 21.1% of male offenders cited release of anger, as the reason for self-harming
      - 31% of non-suicidal self-injury is preceded by angry, guilty, and hopeless mood states in male offenders
      - 72% of female inmates demonstrate anger and aggression prior to harming themselves
  - To decrease arousal
    - Emotions prior to self-injurious behaviors are described as intense, negative, and intolerable, and patients report increased affective arousal
    - After the self-harm act, emotions are characterized as calm to euphoric and patients report a subjective sense of decreased physical tension and arousal

- To punish oneself
- To cope with the external environment
  - Self-directed injury may represent a means of controlling the surrounding environment
- For a socially reinforced goal or outcome
  - Self-injurious behaviors may represent an attempt to modify the surrounding environment, attract attention, and achieve a specific outcome or goal
    - 20–40% of polled male and female offenders who self-harmed identified manipulation as the purpose of their behaviors
      - Examples include exerting interpersonal influence or change in physical location
- Assessing non-suicidal self-injury
  - Currently there is no standardized measure to determine a patient's risk for non-suicidal self-injury
  - Violence risk assessments may be helpful when performing a comprehensive clinical formulation of self-harm
    - Increased total score, historical subscale score (H10), risk management score (R5), and summary judgment (SJ) for violence of the Historic Clinical Risk Management 20 (HCR-20) potentially distinguish those who engage in self-injurious behaviors from those who do not
  - Characterizing the nature of the self-harm act, identifying potential secondary gain, and evaluating the offender's environment can assist when developing a behavior plan
    - The medical and motivational seriousness of the performed self-harm act can illuminate contributory or provocative thought and behavioral patterns
      - Medical seriousness refers to the individual's understanding of the potential physical outcomes of the behavior
      - Motivational seriousness refers to the veracity of the individual's desire for a specific outcome
        - For example, how motivated the individual who harmed themselves was to end their life, to receive help, or to change their circumstances and environment
- Treatment
  - Currently, there is no singular efficacious treatment option or strategy to reduce self-injury
  - Pharmacologically, medical literature and evidence do not support the use of SSRIs, mood stabilizers, and antipsychotic treatment

PATIENT FILE

- Psychologically, manual-assisted cognitive behavioral therapy (CBT) and dialectical behavioral therapy (DBT) may mitigate factors that influence non-suicidal self-injury
  - CBT fosters problem-solving skills, emotional regulation, and cognitive restructuring
  - DBT can improve interpersonal effectiveness, emotional regulation, and distress tolerance
    - DBT is associated with reduction in suicidal ideation (SI) and self-injurious behaviors in patients diagnosed with BPD

Performance in practice: confessions of a psychopharmacologist

What are clinical considerations when treating non-suicidal self-injurious behaviors?

- Non-suicidal self-injurious behaviors (NSSI) may be distinguished from other types of violence in that non-suicidal self-injurious acts are preceded by interpersonal conflict in approximately half of the incidents (42% of events); an individual may experience negative emotional states associated with the act; and individual motivators include regulation of emotions and arousal, punishment, coping strategy, and secondary gain
- There isn't a singular psychopharmacological approach to treat these behaviors
- Performing violence and suicidal risk assessments can assist with risk stratification and identify clinical factors that can further guide potential therapeutic interventions
- Behavioral therapies can improve individual emotional and cognitive regulation, coping skills and distress tolerance, and interpersonal interactions

Tips and pearls

- Current limitations for assessing and treating individuals who engage in self-harm or injurious behaviors are opportunities for future investigation and research, including:
  - Distinguishing and assessing suicidal from non-suicidal self-injury
  - Developing empirical and validated instruments or assessment tools to diagnose self-harm behaviors
  - Identifying etiologic risk factors and mechanisms that contribute to an individual's risk of performing self-injurious behaviors
  - Determining the effectiveness of interventions and staff training on the incidence of self-harm events

PATIENT FILE

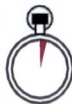

Two-minute tutorial
- 30% of offenders self-harm while in custodial settings
  - The incidence of non-suicidal self-injury is higher in forensic and correctional settings than in the general population
  - Reports of self-injury or threat to oneself represent the fourth and fifth reasons, respectively, for observation enhancement
- Individuals who engage in self-injurious behaviors are more likely to demonstrate physical violence toward others
  - Self-harm is a strong predictor of repetitive and severe violent acts, including when controlled for confounding factors of impulsivity, antisocial personality disorder, and BPD
- Multiple factors influence self-directed injury
- Non-suicidal self-injury is associated with psychological, physical safety, financial, and occupational costs
  - Psychologically, self-harm behaviors are associated with negative emotions and can be associated with depressed mood
    - 50% of individuals who complete suicide in both the carceral and general population have a history of self-injurious behaviors
  - Individuals who self-harm are transferred to more secure levels of care, including acute or specialized mental health facilities. This in turn increases risks associated with transfers and more invasive procedures, as well as financial considerations related to transportation, escort, and care costs
    - 23% of mentally ill offenders who engaged in self-injurious behaviors were admitted to mental health hospitals, and 48–67% of admitted mentally ill offenders reported a history of self-injury
    - Staff providing care for patients who harm themselves can experience professional burnout, absences from work, and decreased emotional well-being
- Currently, there is no standardized assessment and treatment for non-suicidal self-injurious behaviors
  - However, development of a behavioral plan, participation in individualized therapy, and cognitive and dialectical behavioral therapy may assist with individual emotional resilience, cognitive restructuring, distress tolerance, and affective regulation

PATIENT FILE

Post-test question

Which of the following outcomes is NOT associated with non-suicidal self-injurious behaviors?

A. Increased institutional cost
B. Increased risk for a patient death by suicide
C. Patient engagement in externalized acts of violence
D. Decreased supervision by staff
E. Staff burnout, work absence, and emotional distress

Answer: D

References

1. de Vogel, V. & Verstegen, N. (2021). Self-injurious behavior in forensic mental health care: a study into the prevalance and characteristics of incidents of self-injury. *Journal of Forensic Practice*, 23(2), 106–116. https://doi.org/10.1108/JFP-12-2020.
2. Dixon-Gordon, K., Harrison, N., & Roesch, R. (2012). Non-suicidal self-injury within offender populations: a systematic review. *International Journal of Forensic Mental Health*, 11(1), 33–50. https://doi.org/10.1080/14999013.2012.667513.
3. Jeglic, E. L., Vanderhoff, H. A., & Donovick, P. J. (2005). The function of self-harm behavior in a forensic population. *International Journal of Offender Therapy and Comparative Criminology*, April, 49(2), 131–142. https://doi.org/10.1177/0306624X04271130.
4. Lohner, J. & Konrad, N. (2006). Deliberate self-harm and suicide attempt in custody: distinguishing features in male inmates' self-injurious behavior. *International Journal of Law and Psychiatry*, Sept.-Oct., 29(5), 370–385. https://doi.org/10.1016/j.ijlp.2006.03.004.
5. O'Shea, L. E., Picchioni, M. M., Mason, F. L., Sugarman, P. A., & Dickens, G. L. (2014). Predictive validity of the HCR-20 for inpatient self-harm. *Comprehensive Psychiatry*, Nov., 55(8), 1937–1949. https://doi.org/10.1016/j.comppsych.2014.07.
6. Richmond-Rakerd, L. S., Caspi, A., Arseneault, L., et al. (2019). Adolescents who self-harm and commit violent crime: testing early-life predictors of dual harm in a longitudinal cohort study. *American Journal of Psychiatry*, 176(3), 186–195. https://doi.org/10.1176/appi.ajp.2018.18060740. Epub 2019 Jan 4. PMID: 30606048; PMCID: PMC6397074.

PATIENT FILE

7. Sahlin, H., Kuja-Halkola, R., Bjureberg, J., et al. (2017). Association between deliberate self-harm and violent criminality. *JAMA Psychiatry*, 74(6), 615–621. https://doi.org/10.1001/jamapsychiatry.2017.0338.
8. Shafti, M., Taylor, P. J., Forrester, A., & Pratt, D. (2021). The co-occurrence of self-harm and aggression: a cognitive–emotional model of dual-harm. *Frontiers in Psychology*, 12(24 February). https://doi.org/10.3389/fpsyg.2021.586135.
9. Stahl, S. M. (2014). *Stahl's Essential Psychopharmacology: Prescriber's Guide*, 5th ed. New York: Cambridge University Press.

6
Prolonged fasting: Starved for care

The Psychopharmocological Dilemma: Treating prolonged fasting and determining decisional capacity to continue fasting

Amanie Salem and Carolina A. Klein

Pretest self-assessment question
What evidence-based treatment is first line for addressing prolonged fasting secondary to a delusional belief?
A. Antipsychotics
B. Cognitive behavioral therapy (CBT)
C. Electroconvulsive therapy (ECT)
D. None of the above

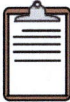

Patient evaluation on intake
- A 47-year-old male charged with the first-degree murder of his wife
  - He was transferred to the state hospital after being found not competent to stand trial
- The patient began a full fluid and food fast and had to be transferred from jail to the medical center twice due to malnutrition, orthostatic hypotension, and dehydration
  - He fasts to "be resurrected in a clean soul"
  - He lost 50 pounds in 3 months
- He exhibits positive symptoms of psychosis
  - He sees holographic images of angels
  - He is not concerned about dying because he has "everlasting life"
- He briefly started eating again following a "request from the Archangel Gabriel," then reinitiated fasting following the Archangel Gabriel's reappearance and command
  - He had been communicating with this archangel since 1979 and notified the Vatican of the communication, noting the Pope had seen the archangel as well
- He denies symptoms of depression

Psychiatric history
- The patient denied any psychiatric history prior to the initiation of his fasting
  - He stated he was evaluated by a psychiatrist once before the initiation of his fasting in the context of a workplace evaluation

PATIENT FILE

- ○ He specified no diagnosis was made and no treatment was recommended at the time
- However, records indicate two previous hospitalizations, both prompted by prolonged fasting
  - ○ Length of stay is unclear
- He reported never experiencing significant symptoms of depression, anxiety, or psychosis
- Collateral information was provided
  - ○ He develops a variety of personas that assist him in social relationships with political figures who believe his false narrative on background, credentials, and notoriety

Social and personal history
- He was born in Germany and is the youngest of three siblings
- He was raised by his mother and uncle in Germany and the United States; his father died weeks after he was born
- He joined the military shortly after graduating from high school
- He obtained a Bachelor's degree in international relations and was one credit short of completing a master's degree
- The patient started drinking alcohol in his late teen years and has been drinking little over the previous 3 years
  - ○ Records indicate that the patient drinks alcohol frequently and family describes a history of problematic drinking
- He has never used marijuana, heroin, cocaine, methamphetamine, or any other illicit substances
- His legal history includes several domestic violence charges filed against him by his wife

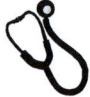

Medical history
- There are no known allergies
- There is no known surgical history
- He has experienced several head injuries
  - ○ He fell off a changing table as an infant – no treatment received
  - ○ He fell off a horse as a child
  - ○ He hit his head during a car accident and was hospitalized for 1 week

Family history
- There is no family history of psychiatric illness, substance use, or suicide in the family

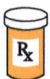

Medication history
- The patient has been on antipsychotics including haloperidol and quetiapine

PATIENT FILE

- The dosages and adherence are unclear
- He has also been administered benztropine and clonazepam in the past
- There is no record of any treatment for depression or anxiety

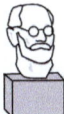

Psychotherapy history
- Intermittent therapy during previous hospitalizations; unclear level of engagement

Mechanism of action moment
- Antipsychotics block dopamine and other chemicals in the brain
- Haloperidol is a conventional (first-generation) antipsychotic
  - Blocks dopamine-2 receptors
  - Reduces positive symptoms of psychosis such as hallucinations
- Quetiapine is an atypical (second-generation) antipsychotic
  - Blocks dopamine-2 receptors and serotonin 2A receptors
  - Interactions at other neurotransmitter receptors may contribute to efficacy in treatment of depression and other affective symptoms

Attending physician's mental notes: initial evaluation
- The patient exhibits symptoms of psychosis but does not seem to meet full diagnostic criteria for schizophrenia
  - He is verbalizing clear delusions, and delusional disorder is a differential diagnosis
  - His history of head trauma may be contributing to his presentation, and unspecified neurocognitive disorder is a differential diagnosis
  - Additional differential diagnoses include a personality disorder, factitious disorder, and malingering
- His history of alcohol use may also be contributing to his current presentation
- He may benefit from an antipsychotic to treat his symptoms of psychosis

Further investigation
What are the options for treatment?
- This patient meets criteria for alcohol use disorder (AUD)
  - He will require B12, thiamine, and folate to address any nutritional deficiencies from alcohol use
  - He needs to be on Clinical Institute Withdrawal Assessment (CIWA) protocol to prevent adverse effects of withdrawal
- He may benefit from an antipsychotic to treat his symptom of delusion
  - Although he has received haloperidol and quetiapine in the past, it is unclear if he has had adequate trials of any antipsychotic

PATIENT FILE

- One option includes an adequate dose and duration of either of the medications he has already been trialed on
- He currently demonstrates the capacity to consent to treatment

Case outcome: 2-week follow-up

- Quetiapine has been initiated and gradually increased over 2 weeks
- The patient is currently refusing to eat solid food or drink any liquid
- He is currently refusing vital sign checks and fingerstick glucose monitoring
- There are no notable changes in his symptoms of psychosis since admission
  - However, he has started to exhibit physical symptoms including weakness, falls, and hypotension

Attending physician's mental notes

- The patient's quetiapine will need to be discontinued due to his current physical symptoms
- The patient requires close monitoring of physical and mental symptoms
  - His physical symptoms are consistent with prolonged starvation
- He will need transfer to a medical center for management of symptomatic hypoglycemia, hypotension, and neurological symptoms associated with prolonged starvation
- He will receive a forensic evaluation to determine decisional capacity for nourishment and will require an evaluation for capacity to stand trial once he is medically stable

Case outcome: 2-month follow-up

- The patient was transferred back to psychiatry 1 week ago
- He is intermittently accepting solid food and fluid
- There have been no adverse events observed from renourishment or refeeding
- He is able to manage his hygiene independently
- The patient remains on a high-risk list for falls because of his weakened state
  - However, he has appeared stronger over the last week due to intermittent eating
- A forensic evaluation was conducted upon transfer back to psychiatry
  - It was determined that the patient lacked capacity to refuse treatment
- Olanzapine was initiated to address symptoms of psychosis and increased to 10 mg at night since his transfer
  - Oral olanzapine is offered first, with an option for injection should he refuse to take the oral dose of medication

Case outcome: 4-month follow-up

- The patient has been compliant with his medication
- He is compliant with nourishment, but his delusional thinking persists
- Another forensic evaluation was conducted to determine his capacity to refuse nourishment
  - He demonstrated an understanding of the risks discussed with him, including multiorgan dysfunction, long-term neurological damage, and death
  - He was unable to appreciate these risks as it pertained to his situation
- An additional forensic evaluation found him competent to stand trial
  - Psychological testing was administered (the Test of Memory Malingering [TOMM], the Rey 15-Item Test, and the b Test)
    - Testing indicated that he was not feigning cognitive symptoms
  - Both the Georgia Court Competency Test and the Competency Assessment Instrument – Revised were administered to assist in determining competency to stand trial

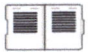

Case debrief

- This patient's history of psychiatric illness is complicated by unclear diagnosis on presentation and contradictory information between the patient's self-report, collateral information, and available records
- After being found incompetent to stand trial, he was transferred to a psychiatric hospital
- However, his persistent delusion resulted in prolonged fasting and self-starvation that required discontinuation of psychiatric medication and acute transfer for medical intervention
- After medical stabilization and transfer back to psychiatry, it was determined the patient lacked capacity to refuse nourishment or psychiatric medication
  - He was started on olanzapine with no adverse side effects noted
- Though he continued to verbalize delusions around fasting, his symptoms improved, and he no longer refused food and drink
- He was also deemed competent to stand trial

Take-home points

- Prolonged fasting can be a life-threatening consequence of a firmly held delusional belief and requires close medical and psychiatric monitoring

PATIENT FILE

Performance in practice: confessions of a psychopharmacologist

Could this patient be delusional without a primary psychotic disorder?

- Delusions can be present in a range of psychiatric illnesses and disorders even without a primary psychotic disorder
- The patient's differential diagnoses throughout hospitalization included delusional disorder, schizophrenia, factitious disorder, malingering, and a neurocognitive disorder

Could we have tried monotherapy with another agent?

- Delusions can be treated with antipsychotic medication
- Although literature is limited, there seems to be no clear benefit or increased efficacy between antipsychotics administered to treat delusions
- Symptom response to treatment and monitoring of side effects may assist in choosing an appropriate antipsychotic medication

Tips and pearls

- Prolonged fasting and self-starvation stemming from a delusional belief can be challenging to treat
- It is important to rule out any organic etiology and treat any medical issues that have arisen secondary to the prolonged fasting
- Treatment of delusions includes antipsychotic medication

Two-minute tutorial

Self-starvation and psychosis

- There have been few case studies on starvation secondary to psychosis reported in the literature, and evidence-based intervention and treatment are limited
- Additional study is warranted to develop specific guidelines

Delusions and their treatment

- A delusion is defined as a belief that is often not amenable to change even when presented with conflicting evidence
- Delusions are one of the defining symptoms of psychosis
- Delusions have a variety of themes including persecutory, grandiose, somatic, and religious
- Delusions are deemed bizarre if they are clearly implausible and do not derive from ordinary life experiences
- Clinicians should distinguish between a delusion and a strongly held idea

PATIENT FILE

- ○ This should be determined in part by the degree of conviction held in light of clear or reasonable contradictory evidence
- ○ Consider cultural, religious, and historical experiences
- Some research suggests plasticity in delusional beliefs
  - ○ Delusions can fade or disappear with resolution of an acute psychotic episode
  - ○ Longitudinal studies suggest variability in delusions over time
- First-line treatment of delusions generally includes antipsychotic medication
- Cognitive behavioral therapy has also been shown to improve delusions as an adjunct to medication in some evidence-based studies

Post-test question

What evidence-based treatment is first line for addressing prolonged fasting secondary to a delusional belief?

A. Antipsychotics
B. Cognitive behavioral therapy
C. Electroconvulsive therapy
D. None of the above

Answer: A

References

1. American Psychiatric Association. (2022). *Diagnostic and Statistical Manual of Mental Disorders* (5th ed., text rev.). Washington, DC: American Psychiatric Association. https://doi.org/10.1176/appi.books.9780890425787.
2. Appelbaum, P. S., Robbins, P. C., & Vesselinov, R. (2004). Persistence and stability of delusions over time. *Comprehensive Psychiatry*, 45(5), 317–324.
3. Lincoln, T. M. & Peters, E. (2019). A systematic review and discussion of symptom-specific cognitive behavioural approaches to delusions and hallucinations. *Schizophrenia Research*, 203, 66–79.
4. Manschreck, T. C. & Khan, N. L. (2006). Recent advances in the treatment of delusional disorder. *Canadian Journal of Psychiatry*, 51(2), 114–119. https://doi.org/10.1177/070674370605100207.
5. Pacilio, R. M., Coverdale, J. H., Siddiqui, S., David, E. H., & Gordon, M. R. (2020). Food refusal secondary to psychosis: a case series and literature review. *Journal of Nervous and Mental Disease*, September, 208(9), 654–657. | https://doi.org/10.1097/NMD.0000000000001174. PMID: 32868687.

PATIENT FILE

6. Rodgers, E., Marwaha, S., & Humpston, C. (2022). Co-occurring psychotic and eating disorders in England: findings from the 2014 Adult Psychiatric Morbidity Survey. *Journal of Eating Disorders*, 10, 150. https://doi.org/10.1186/s40337-022-00664-0.
7. Stahl, S. M. (2005). *Essential Psychopharmacology: The Prescriber's Guide*. New York: Cambridge University Press.

PATIENT FILE

7

Severe suicidality: To die at any cost

The Psychopharmocological Dilemma: Treating persistent self-injurious behavior and chronic suicidality

Amanie Salem and Carolina A. Klein

Pretest self-assessment question

Meta-analyses of symptom-focused medication management suggest that impulsive and behavioral dysregulation in borderline personality disorder (BPD) is best treated by which of the following classes of psychotropics?

A. Antidepressants
B. Antipsychotics
C. Mood stabilizers
D. Alpha-antagonists

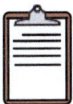

Patient evaluation on intake

- A 52-year-old female with severe treatment-refractory BPD and intellectual disability
  - She is under Lanterman–Petris–Short (LPS) conservatorship and does not have the capacity to leave against medical advice or request a "Do not resuscitate" code status

Psychiatric history

- The patient has a long-standing history of mental illness and has been hospitalized for self-injurious behavior several times
- She has engaged in self-injurious behavior since the age of 11 years old
- She was first hospitalized in adolescence after cutting her wrist in a self-reported suicide attempt
  - She has since had dozens of emergency department visits and inpatient medical and psychiatric hospitalizations for SI and self-injurious behavior
  - She has various instances and modalities of self-harm during hospitalizations
    - During a 2-month hospitalization, she harmed herself 15 times
    - The events included self-inflicted shoulder dislocation, digging into a surgical wound, re-opening a wound on her left arm while in mittens, stabbing herself with a plastic spoon, digging into her forearm with her nails, and scratching into her knee

PATIENT FILE

- She has been discharged to various outpatient modalities, including partial hospitalization, intensive outpatient treatment, and outpatient clinics after each hospitalization
  - Adherence to and engagement with both therapy and medication management have varied over the years

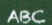
Social and personal history
- The patient was adopted at age 4
- She was raised by her adoptive mother and father, and lived with them and one adopted sibling
- She experienced sexual abuse by a close family member from the ages of 6–11 years old
- Her highest level of education is high school
  - She was in special education classes starting from elementary school
  - She had an individualized education plan (IEP) from first grade to twelfth grade
- She is divorced and has no children
- She states she has never smoked cigarettes, drunk alcohol, or used illicit substances
- She was placed under LPS conservatorship in her early 20s

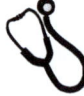
Medical history
- The patient has a history of recurrent urinary retention and urinary tract infections
- The patient is obese and has sleep apnea
- The patient has diabetes mellitus type 2
- She has required surgical intervention for self-inflicted wounds
  - Most recently, she required surgical intervention for a left lower quadrant abdominal wound after stabbing herself and inserting a foreign object into the wound
  - The patient also has a history of recurrent, self-inflicted shoulder dislocation
- She has no known history of drug allergies

Family history
- The patient's biological mother had a history of alcohol use disorder (AUD) and major depressive disorder
- The patient's biological father's history is unknown

PATIENT FILE

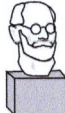

Psychotherapy history

- Intermittent therapy during previous hospitalizations with varying levels of engagement
- Has been discharged to a partial hospitalization program that integrated intense dialectical behavioral therapy techniques – however, the patient did not meaningfully participate in individual or group therapy portions

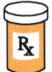

Medication history

- The patient has been trialed on various medications with unclear benefit
    - In childhood, she was on an unknown dose of escitalopram for symptoms of anxiety and behavioral dysregulation, with partial efficacy
    - After her initial hospitalization in adolescence, she was on fluoxetine, guanfacine, and carbamazepine, all of unknown doses and efficacy
- She has received antipsychotic augmentation to medication during previous hospitalizations but frequently self-discontinues these when outpatient due to self-reported side effects
- She has also received benzodiazepines while inpatient on an as-needed (PRN) basis, with some benefit
- She has never exhibited evidence of extrapyramidal symptoms (EPS) or long-term movement disorders, excessive daytime sedation, or metabolic syndrome during hospitalizations

Current history

- The patient presents with a self-inflicted left lower quadrant abdominal wall wound which appears to be a re-opening of the wound from her most recent hospitalization
- She verbalizes persistent thoughts of wanting to harm herself
    - She reports voices in her head that tell her to hurt herself
    - She states these voices sound like her own voice
- She exhibits symptoms of BPD, including affective instability and impulsivity
    - In the emergency department she required four patient restraints after attempting to assault a staff member who was checking her wound
    - She also asked for "heavy-duty" PRN medication and attempted to "tear [her] breasts off" when she felt like no one was listening

PATIENT FILE

- She says that none of her medication has worked for 6 years and that she wants to go to jail so she can "cut there and kill [her]self"
- Her current medication regimen includes fluoxetine 80 mg once daily, risperidone 9 mg at night, and prazosin 2 mg at night

Mechanism of action moment

- Fluoxetine is a selective serotonin reuptake inhibitor (SSRI) often used to treat depression and anxiety, as well as obsessive compulsive disorder, premenstrual dysphoric disorder, panic disorder, and bipolar depression and treatment-resistant depression (in combination with olanzapine)
  - Boosts the neurotransmitter serotonin and blocks serotonin reuptake
  - Desensitizes serotonin receptors, especially serotonin 1A
  - Has antagonist properties at $5\text{-}HT_{2C}$ receptors which may increase norepinephrine and dopamine neurotransmission

Attending physician's mental notes

- This patient has a chronic history of persistent symptoms consistent with BPD
- Her history is such that she has been in hospitals for the majority of her adult life, yet her symptoms are still poorly managed due to a limited response to treatment
- Although she has been on various medications in the past, it is unclear if these have been true medication trials, and efficacy of each medication is unclear
  - She is currently on an antidepressant, antipsychotic, and alpha-antagonist with limited benefit
  - Although a long-acting injectable would be helpful for a patient with medication non-adherence, the benefit of administering a long-acting injectable for a medication that lacks adequate response is limited
- Therapy is first-line treatment for patients with BPD, and medication management is used for symptomatic treatment
- In patients with frequent emergency department visits and hospitalizations, as well as persistent symptoms and unclear medication benefit, a consistent behavioral plan is important
- The patient also has a history of intellectual disability that is likely exacerbating her behavioral symptoms and contributing to limited medication efficacy

PATIENT FILE

Further investigation

What is a reasonable immediate plan for this patient? What are the long-term goals?

- This patient requires an assessment of acute versus chronic risk of suicidality, and a safety plan for her acute risk
- This patient is on the maximum dose of an SSRI, as well as an antipsychotic and an alpha-antagonist, and remains symptomatic
- A mood stabilizer is indicated for impulsivity and behavioral dysregulation
- Other options include an antipsychotic for cognitive perceptual symptoms or an antipsychotic and/or antidepressant for affective dysregulation
- A consistent behavioral plan needs to be in place for any in-hospital behavioral dysregulation

Is there anything else you would like to know about the patient? What about the voices she says she hears?

- She describes these voices as something she has heard since childhood
- She says the voices sound like her own voice and tell her to hurt herself
- She states she has never heard voices that sound like anyone else

Case outcome: 2-week follow-up

- Consent for work-up and treatment was obtained by the patient's LPS conservator
- The patient has been assessed by the surgical team that has provided wound care for the abdominal injury
- Risperidone has been gradually tapered and discontinued
- Fluoxetine has been gradually tapered and is now at 40 mg once daily
- A safety plan has been implemented and the treatment team is aware of consistency in enforcement
- There have been no notable changes in symptoms since admission

Case outcome: 2-month follow-up

- The patient has had one significant incident of self-harm during which she self-dislocated her shoulder
  - The dislocation was complicated by hemorrhagic shock and she required immediate surgical intervention
  - She was transferred to the surgical intensive care unit (SICU) for 1 week, then transferred back to the psychiatry unit

PATIENT FILE

- Lithium has been started to address impulsive and behavioral dysregulation, as well as affective instability
- Fluoxetine has been further tapered and discontinued
- Prazosin has been increased to 5 mg at night to address sleep quality and contribute to behavior regulation

Attending physician's mental notes

- Lithium both can assist in regulating mood and has some evidence suggesting anti-suicidal properties
- Before initiating treatment with lithium, kidney function tests, thyroid function tests, and an electrocardiogram (EKG) were checked
- Lithium has a narrow therapeutic window, so initial monitoring will be completed every 1–2 weeks until the desired serum concentration is achieved
- Side effects of lithium include weight gain, polyuria, polydipsia, diarrhea, renal impairment, and ataxia
  - Lithium toxicity can be life threatening
  - If any side effects occur, collect a serum concentration to determine the patient's level
- As the patient has been on several SSRIs in the past with limited efficacy, will start a serotonin–norepinephrine reuptake inhibitor (SNRI) to address underlying mood symptoms

Case outcome: 6-month follow-up

- The patient continues to verbalize SI
- She has had intermittent instances of self-harm but these seem to be relatively minor compared to her admitting event
- She received several PRN medications over the last few months; however, this seems to make her behavioral dysregulation worse
- Although the lithium seems to be helpful, she has verbalized increased thirst and started refusing the medication
- Chlorpromazine was initiated and gradually increased to 100 mg twice daily
- Duloxetine 20 mg once daily was started and gradually increased to 60 mg once daily

Question

How would you address the non-adherence to lithium due to a side effect that does appear to be bothering the patient?

- Discontinue the lithium and start another mood stabilizer
- Decrease the dose of lithium

PATIENT FILE

Case outcome: 8-month follow-up
- The patient continues to verbalize SI
- She continues to engage in instances of self-harm but these seem to be relatively minor compared to her admitting event
- She continues to have some behavioral dysregulation
- The lithium was discontinued and divalproex was initiated
- Chlorpromazine has been gradually increased to 300 mg twice daily
- Duloxetine remains at 60 mg once daily and prazosin remains at 5 mg nightly

Case outcome: 1-year follow-up
- The patient continues to verbalize SI
- She continues to engage in instances of self-harm, including scratching her forearm and hitting her head
- Divalproex appeared to be helping her mood but there was concern for peripheral edema and divalproex was subsequently discontinued
- Her current medication regimen remains chlorpromazine 300 mg twice daily, duloxetine 60 mg once daily, and prazosin 5 mg nightly
- She will likely require long-term placement after hospitalization

Case debrief
- This patient has a long history of psychiatric illness, specifically affective instability and self-injurious behavior, complicated by intellectual disability
- Due to her limited cognitive functioning and early psychiatric symptoms, she was placed under LPS conservatorship in her early 20s
- She had been trialed on several medications including various antidepressants, anticonvulsants, and antipsychotics
- Although she remained at elevated chronic risk for suicide, her symptoms were improved with a combination of an SNRI, an antipsychotic, and an alpha-antagonist

Take-home points
- Patients with BPD represent a large population of individuals seen in the emergency department with SI
- Clinicians must use their judgment to determine acute versus chronic risk of suicide when assessing these patients and avoid reinforcing any suicidal behavior through hospitalization or as-needed medication management
- A consistent behavior plan can provide positive reinforcement for the patient

PATIENT FILE

Performance in practice: confessions of a psychopharmacologist

What is the role of medication in patients with chronic suicidality?
- Medication should be used in combination with psychotherapeutic interventions
- Medication management is important for symptomatic treatment in patients with chronic suicidality
- While there is some evidence that lithium and antipsychotics may address self-harm, additional studies are needed to substantiate the limited quality of evidence and small number of trials

Can medication exacerbate the problem of chronic suicidality?
- While there is no evidence that medication itself exacerbates suicidality, in patients with symptoms consistent with BPD and chronic suicidality, frequent medication changes and PRN medication can exacerbate and reinforce affective and behavioral dysregulation
- Providers should use their clinical judgment and follow a consistent behavior plan when changing medications or administering PRN medication

Tips and pearls
- Suicidal behavior in patients with BPD is often chronic and recurrent in nature
- Patients with BPD express higher suicidal intent but often with lower lethality. Individuals with BPD will attempt suicide an average of 3.3 times in their lifetime

Two-minute tutorial

Borderline personality disorder
- BPD is an illness marked by instability in affect, self-image, and interpersonal relationships. Patients also exhibit marked impulsivity
- These patients frequently engage in suicidal behavior
- Onset occurs in adolescence or early adulthood
- Treatment of BPD
  - Treatment should start with dialectical behavioral therapy (DBT), particularly for self-destructive patients
    - DBT includes individual and group components that focus on increasing coping skills, building resistance to affective instability, and providing practical suggestions on how to manage symptoms

PATIENT FILE

- Some patients with BPD experience severe symptoms even with therapy. In these patients, adjunctive medications can be used for symptomatic treatment. However, studies on pharmacological interventions for BPD remain limited
  - Anticonvulsants have been shown to improve anger, aggression, and affective lability
  - Antipsychotics can address perceptual disturbances, including paranoid ideation and unstable self-image and identity
  - Mood stabilizers have shown efficacy for impulsivity and behavioral instability
  - Antidepressants may address co-occurring symptoms of depression and anxiety
- Chronic suicidality in BPD
  - Suicidality can take the form of threats, gestures, attempts, and non-suicidal self-injury
  - Patients with BPD have a high rate of suicide completion
  - Suicide threats and attempts peak early in the course of the illness. However, this is not always when suicide completion occurs
  - Clinicians should differentiate between chronic and acute suicide risk
    - The suicidality of patients with BPD can vary over time
    - Chronic suicidality is often seen in patients who are treatment seeking
    - Acute suicidality may occur during episodes of co-occurring psychiatric illness or particularly high periods of stress

Post-test question

Meta-analyses of symptom-focused medication management suggest that impulsive and behavioral dysregulation in borderline personality disorder (BPD) is best treated by which of the following classes of psychotropics?

A. Antidepressants
B. Antipsychotics
C. Mood stabilizers
D. Alpha-antagonists

Answer: C

References

1. American Psychiatric Association. (2022). *Diagnostic and Statistical Manual of Mental Disorders* (5th ed., text rev.). Washington, DC: APA. https://doi.org/10.1176/appi.books.9780890425787.

PATIENT FILE

2. Bozzatello, P., Rocca, P., De Rosa, M. L., & Bellino, S. (2019). Current and emerging medications for borderline personality disorder: is pharmacotherapy alone enough? *Expert Opinion on Pharmacotherapy*, 21(1), 47–61. https://doi.org/10.1080/14656566.2019.1686482.
3. Choi-Kain, L. W., Finch, E. F., Masland, S.R., et al. (2017). What works in the treatment of borderline personality disorder. *Current Behavioral Neuroscience Reports*, 4, 21–30. https://doi.org/10.1007/s40473-017-0103-z.
4. Gunderson, J. G. & Choi-Kain, L. W. (2018). Medication management for patients with borderline personality disorder. *American Journal of Psychiatry*, 175(8), 709–711. https://doi.org/10.1176/appi.ajp.2018.18050576.
5. Stahl, S. M. (2005). *Essential Psychopharmacology: The Prescriber's Guide*. New York: Cambridge University Press.
6. Watt-McMahon, K., Mildred, H., King, R., Craigie, G., Hyder, S., & Hall, K. (2023). Understanding chronic suicidality in borderline personality disorder through comparison with depressive disorder: a systematic review. *Clinical Psychologist*, 27(2), 232–258. https://doi.org/10.1080/13284207.2023.2190879.
7. Witt, K. G., Hetrick, S. E., Rajaram, G., et al. (2021). Pharmacological interventions for self-harm in adults. *Cochrane Database of Systematic Reviews*, 1. Art. No.: CD013669. https://doi.org/10.1002/14651858.CD013669.pub2.

SECTION III
Critical Associated Syndromes of Severe Mental Illness (SMI)

SECTION III

Critical Assessment and Special Issues of the North Atlantic Blooms (SIBM)

PATIENT FILE

8

Who's who? Misidentification syndromes in severe mental illness (SMI)

The Psychopharmocological Dilemma: Treating high-risk psychosis – misidentification syndrome and treatment-resistant schizophrenia

Carolina A. Klein and Amanie Salem

Pretest self-assessment question

A patient on clozapine has an absolute neutrophil count (ANC) of 1200. What do the prescribing guidelines recommend as the next step?

A. Continue clozapine at its current dose and continue the current blood draw schedule
B. Continue clozapine at its current dose and increase monitoring to three times weekly
C. Decrease the dose of clozapine by 50%, initiate lithium, and continue the current blood draw schedule
D. Discontinue clozapine, initiate lithium, and increase monitoring to three times weekly

Patient evaluation on intake

- A 26-year-old male who was adjudicated not guilty by reason of insanity (NGRI) for the charge of aggravated malicious wounding. He was transferred to a state hospital after being found NGRI
  - His charge involved stabbing his mother because he "thought she was someone else" and "can't be trusted"
- The patient exhibits positive symptoms of psychosis
  - He has auditory hallucinations, visual hallucinations, and olfactory hallucinations
  - He has delusions that he is infected with an undiagnosed disease and has a foreign object in his abdomen
  - He has grandiose delusions with hyperreligiosity
- He has thought and behavior disorganization
- He exhibits symptoms of misidentification syndromes including Capgras syndrome and Fregoli syndrome involving multiple family members, such as his mother, brother, and sister
  - Voices told the patient his mother was "Jezebel"
  - It is reported he stated his mother "can't be trusted," because he thought she was "someone else"
  - It is reported he threatened to kill his sister saying she was taken over by someone else that looked like his sister

85

- He was aggressive in his behavior on transfer to the hospital and reports indicate a history of threats and aggression directly correlated with distress from his symptomatology
- His current regimen includes a combination of olanzapine 90 mg total daily dose and lurasidone 160 mg with food
- Continue his current medication regimen with plan to cross-taper to clozapine

Psychiatric history

- The patient has a long-standing history of mental illness dating back to childhood
  - He reports symptoms of psychosis throughout his entire life, stating he was born with them
  - His records indicate that he exhibited rocking back and forth and pounding his head against the wall in childhood
- He was first diagnosed with psychiatric illness at the age of 15 when he was admitted to a psychiatric hospital with a presentation of suicidal ideation (SI) and feelings of depression
- Since then he has experienced persistent positive symptoms of psychosis that have not been well controlled
- He was discharged from the Army due to reported symptoms of psychosis
  - At the time, he reported "people could hear [his] thoughts" and were hacking into his social media page, and that he felt someone "touching [him] and holding [him] on the bed"
- He has been hospitalized a total of four times previously and has been hospitalized for the majority of his adult life, with no more than about 1 year of continuous community placement (3 years prior)
  - His first hospitalization was at the age of 15 years, with unclear medication trial doses and durations
  - His second hospitalization was at the age of 18 years; trialed on olanzapine 30 mg total daily dose, only partially effective
  - His third hospitalization was at the age of 21 years; trialed on haloperidol without response, and risperidone with partial response – doses and duration unclear
  - His fourth hospitalization was at the age of 23 years; trialed on risperidone
- He has never received consistent outpatient treatment and has generally been nonadherent to medication
- He has never received a long-acting injectable, despite the limited responses to antipsychotic trials and medication nonadherence
- He has received diagnoses of schizophrenia and schizoaffective disorder

PATIENT FILE

Social and personal history
- The patient was raised by his mother and lived with three brothers, four sisters, and one stepbrother when growing up
- Experienced verbal and physical abuse by his mother and stepfather from ages 11–15 years
- He dropped out of school in tenth grade and eventually earned a GED
- His only employment was for 5 months at a fast-food restaurant
- He is single and has never been married or in any romantic relationships
- His maternal grandmother is his authorized representative
- His legal history includes an assault charge in 2007 and an assault charge in 2011
- He started using marijuana and alcohol on a daily basis at the age of 14 until he joined the Army at the age of 18
- It is reported he tried cocaine and methamphetamine twice each

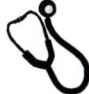
Medical history
- He has a history of hypothyroidism
- There is no history of head injury or loss of consciousness
- There is no history of surgeries
- He has no known drug allergies

Family history
- Father has a history of schizophrenia
- Mother has a history of Attention-Deficit/Hyperactivity Disorder (ADHD)

Medication history
- The patient has been on numerous psychotropic medications, including antipsychotics, mood stabilizers, antiepileptics, benzodiazepines, and antidepressants
- He has received two adequate trials of clozapine (maximum dose up to 900 mg total daily dose) with a positive response
  - Both trials were discontinued due to severe adverse reactions (including a seizure episode, neutropenia, and dilated cardiomyopathy)
- He has received antipsychotic augmentation in the forms of N-acetyl cysteine, famotidine, naltrexone, fish oil, and vitamin D
- He has never exhibited evidence of extrapyramidal symptoms (EPS) or long-term movement disorders, excessive daytime sedation, or metabolic syndrome

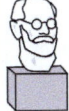
Psychotherapy history
- Intermittent therapy during previous hospitalizations, unclear level of engagement

PATIENT FILE

Mechanism of action moment
- Clozapine is a second-generation antipsychotic
  - Blocks dopamine-2 receptors
  - Blocks serotonin 2A receptors
  - Interacts at various other receptors that might contribute to its efficacy

Attending physician's mental notes: initial visit
- This patient has tried a variety of antipsychotics for his significant history of hallucinations and delusions
- He is on a high dose of olanzapine and is still experiencing symptoms of psychosis as well as behavioral aggression
- His history is such that he has been in hospitals for the majority of his adult life, yet his symptoms are still poorly managed due to a limited response to treatment
- Although a long-acting injectable would be helpful for a patient with medication nonadherence, the benefit of administering a long-acting injectable for a medication that lacks adequate response is limited
- The patient requires complete blood counts (CBCs) to monitor his absolute neutrophil count (ANC) while on clozapine
- Clozapine initiation guidelines recommend continuing existing medication regimen for 1 week while clozapine is titrated, prior to tapering existing medication

Further investigation
Is this a reasonable plan? Are there other options for treatment? What are the concerns with clozapine for this patient specifically?
- This patient is on a high dose of olanzapine with lurasidone and remains symptomatic
- His history suggests he has had at least two adequate trials of antipsychotic medications with minimal or partial relief of his delusions and hallucinations
  - This suggests he has treatment-resistant schizophrenia
- Clozapine is indicated for treatment-resistant schizophrenia
- Other options include an adequate dose and duration trial of an antipsychotic that the patient has partially responded to (on an unknown dose) or has not been trialed on; increasing the lurasidone; or adding another medication as adjunct to his current regimen
- This patient currently lacks capacity to consent to treatment and has a history of nonadherence to his treatment and overall management

PATIENT FILE

Case outcome: 1-week follow-up

- Consent for medication changes and lab work was obtained by the patient's grandmother who is now his authorized representative
- Clozapine has been initiated and gradually increased for 1 week, and is now at 100 mg daily
  - His ANC is 4800
- The patient is receiving olanzapine 90 mg total daily dose and lurasidone 160 mg with food
- There are no notable changes in his symptoms since admission

Attending physician's mental notes

- Now that he has had 1 week of clozapine, will gradually decrease olanzapine and lurasidone
- Side effects of clozapine include constipation, sialorrhea, hypotension, tachycardia, decreased seizure threshold, myocarditis, and neutropenia
- He will require close monitoring of response to the clozapine as well as any emergence of side effects

Question

How frequently should the patient receive blood draws to monitor ANC in the first month?

- Daily
- Weekly
- Every 2 weeks
- Monthly

Case outcome: 1-month follow-up

- The patient has been seen daily
- Nursing staff have reported seeing the patient frequently responding to internal stimuli
- The patient reports derogatory and persecutory auditory hallucinations
  - He states the voices tell him "you are dead," "you are gonna get killed," "you are the devil"
- His olanzapine and lurasidone have been tapered and discontinued
- He is receiving 400 mg total daily dose of clozapine
- He has received weekly blood draws to monitor ANC as per clozapine prescription guidelines
  - ANC has remained between 3000 and 4000 on CBC
- He has been started on a laxative due to constipation from clozapine

PATIENT FILE

Case outcome: 2-month follow-up
- The patient has been seen daily
- The patient continues responding to internal stimuli
- He reports, "these annoying voices still bother me," and states they are trying to kill him and he "felt a chainsaw" go through his back
- He voices delusions regarding "end times" and "demons that owe [him] money"
- He is receiving 600 mg total daily dose of clozapine
- He has received weekly blood draws to monitor ANC as per clozapine prescription guidelines
  - His most recent ANC was 1200

Question
What would you do next?
- Start lithium to address decrease in ANC
- Change ANC monitoring to three times weekly until ANC gets back to 1500

Case outcome: 4-month follow-up
- The patient has been seen daily
- The patient was started on lithium to address the decrease in ANC. His ANC returned to above 1500, so weekly blood draws were initiated again as per guidelines
  - His most recent ANC was 3200
- His clozapine has been increased to 650 mg total daily dose
- He reports his auditory hallucinations "are less there"
- He continues to respond to internal stimuli but less frequently than before

Case outcome: 6 months
- The patient has been seen daily
- He appears less aggressive than previously and there have been no behavioral disturbances on the unit in 2 weeks
- His ANC is within normal limits and he is now able to transition blood draws from weekly to every 2 weeks
- Last week, he had a seizure

Attending physician's mental notes
- Both lithium and clozapine decrease seizure threshold
- His symptoms seem to be improving on clozapine more than on any previous medication trial
- The lithium did assist in normalizing his ANC

PATIENT FILE

- A meeting with the treatment team may be beneficial in weighing the risks and benefits of continuing clozapine as part of the patient's management
- Although more commonly used for affective disorders, ECT can be a useful augmentation strategy for managing psychosis

Further investigation

What additional information would you like to know? How about the patient's seizure history?

- The patient had no known seizure history prior to this episode

What next steps should be taken?

- As clozapine is known to decrease seizure threshold in a dose-dependent manner, a decrease in the clozapine may prevent medication-induced seizures in the future
- The patient would also be able to continue clozapine while being treated with ECT

Case outcome: 8 months

- The patient received 12 sessions of ECT over 4 weeks
- He is now in the maintenance phase of treatment and is scheduled for ECT once per week
- He continues to describe auditory hallucinations but notes they are much less frequent than at the time of admission
- He continues to voice delusions regarding his family members being "someone else" – however, he has recently voiced uncertainty in these beliefs
- The patient remains on clozapine 450 mg total daily dose and lithium 600 mg
  - As per guidelines, he gets blood drawn every 2 weeks to check his ANC
  - Most recent ANC was 3200
- He has not had another seizure episode

Case debrief

- This patient had a long history of psychiatric illness, specifically psychosis, and treatment with a variety of antipsychotic medications, with limited benefit
- After being found NGRI for stabbing his mother, whom he thought was "someone else," he was transferred to a state hospital
- Due to having at least two adequate trials of other medication with limited efficacy at best, he was deemed to have treatment-resistant schizophrenia

PATIENT FILE

- He was started on clozapine and, although his symptoms improved, his treatment course was complicated by adverse side effects including neutropenia and seizure
- Due to the benefits he experienced from clozapine, the dose was decreased and the side effect of lowering seizure threshold was optimized by administration of ECT
- Although he continued to exhibit symptoms of psychosis including hallucinations and delusions, his symptoms were improved with the combination of clozapine and ECT when compared to symptoms on admission

Take-home points

- Misidentification syndromes are seen in individuals who are diagnosed with a psychotic illness, an affective illness, or a general medical illness

Performance in practice: confessions of a psychopharmacologist

What could have been done better here?

- Should another antipsychotic with an option for a long-acting injectable have been trialed while the patient was in the hospital?
  - The patient had an extensive history of psychosis and was trialed on various antipsychotics. He had never been trialed on a long-acting injectable. A long-acting injectable might have addressed his medication nonadherence – however, his history suggested limited benefit from previously trialed antipsychotics that are offered in a long-acting form

Should the patient have been put on an antiepileptic and kept on a higher dose of clozapine to address persistent symptoms of psychosis?

- The risks of a seizure need to be weighed against the benefit of treating the patient's symptoms. In some cases, adding an antiepileptic may be beneficial in protecting the patient from future seizure activity while allowing continued treatment with clozapine. This patient's treatment team utilized the decrease in seizure threshold to their advantage by initiating ECT as an adjunct to his medication

What is the mechanism of action of clozapine thought to contribute to its benefit?

- Clozapine blocks the dopamine-2 receptors, reducing positive symptoms of psychosis and stabilizing affective symptoms

PATIENT FILE

- It blocks serotonin 2A receptors, causing enhancement of dopamine release in certain brain regions and reducing motor side effects, and possibly improving cognitive and affective symptoms
- The mechanism of efficacy for psychotic patients who do not respond to conventional antipsychotics is unknown

Tips and pearls

- Misidentification syndromes are rare psychopathological phenomena that may occur within the context of schizophrenia or affective or organic illnesses. They include Capgras syndrome, Fregoli syndrome, intermetamorphosis syndrome, syndrome of subjective doubles, mirrored self, delusional companions, and clonal pluralization of the self
  - All have a common theme of the "double," or one person being an exact likeness of another
- Treatment-resistant schizophrenia is characterized by persistence of symptoms despite adequate treatment trials of antipsychotics
- Clozapine remains the gold standard for people with treatment-resistant schizophrenia or persistent symptoms of schizophrenia
  - In patients with refractory schizophrenia, 50–60% of patients will respond to clozapine
  - The response rate to other atypical antipsychotics in a patient with refractory schizophrenia ranges from 0% to 9%
- Additional research is needed to guide treatment for treatment-resistant individuals partially responsive or nonresponsive to clozapine

Two-minute tutorial

Treatment-resistant schizophrenia

- Treatment-resistant schizophrenia is defined as an inadequate response to two antipsychotics, each taken with adequate dose and duration
- Between 75% and 87% of patients with first-episode psychosis (FEP) responded to the first treatment with an antipsychotic medication by 4 weeks to 1 year
- Treatment-resistant schizophrenia occurs in approximately 30% of patients with schizophrenia
- Due to clozapine's widely known side-effect profile, it is often avoided by many practitioners, even in cases of treatment-resistant schizophrenia. Alternative treatment strategies include increasing antipsychotic trial duration, using higher doses of a non-clozapine antipsychotic, or augmenting with a non-clozapine antipsychotic or mood stabilizer

PATIENT FILE

- Studies demonstrate limited clinical benefit to using non-clozapine pharmacological strategies to address inadequate treatment response to antipsychotics

Treatment with clozapine
- Clozapine has been shown in studies to be more effective than other antipsychotics in the treatment of treatment-resistant schizophrenia, and it lowers hospital readmission rates and all-cause mortality. This has been borne out both in randomized control trials and in cohort studies of antipsychotic use in the general population
- Clozapine requires a slow titration and close monitoring to avoid complications associated with potentially serious side effects, including orthostatic hypotension, tachycardia, benign hyperthermia, risk of myocarditis, pneumonia, and seizures
- The recommendation is to trial clozapine for at least 12 weeks to evaluate a response
- Providers must monitor a patient's ANC while they are prescribed clozapine
  - Patients must obtain a lab work, specifically CBC with differential
  - The first 6 months require weekly collection
  - The second 6 months require collection every other week
  - Thereafter, a CBC is obtained once monthly
  - The patient and provider must both enroll in the clozapine REMS program, an online database where all of the patient's ANC data must be entered. Pharmacies dispensing clozapine must also be enrolled in the program, and will not be able to dispense clozapine if ANC data is not up to date in the system and appropriate
- If the patient develops neutropenia
  - ANC 1000–1500: continue treatment, monitor the patient's CBC three times weekly; when ANC is above 1500, resume CBC schedule prior to neutropenia
  - ANC < 1000: discontinue clozapine, monitor the patient's CBC daily until CBC is above 1000; when above 1000, restart clozapine and monitor CBC three times weekly; when above 1500, monitor once weekly for a month, then resume CBC schedule prior to neutropenia
  - ANC < 500: discontinue clozapine and do not rechallenge unless prescriber determines the benefits significantly outweigh the risks
    - If a prescriber chooses to restart clozapine, do not restart until the ANC is above 1000. Monitor the patient's CBC daily until CBC is above 1000; when above 1000, can restart clozapine and monitor CBC three times weekly; when above 1500, reinitiate the standard ANC monitoring protocol

PATIENT FILE

- Myocarditis and cardiomyopathy secondary to clozapine do not appear to be dose dependent, nor do they appear related to titration schedule
- Gastrointestinal hypomotility is another side effect that needs to be closely monitored, as clozapine can cause paralytic ileus or gastroparesis, which can progress to aspiration or toxic megacolon. It is important to monitor concomitant medications, such as anticholinergics or opiates. Often, patients who are already at risk for constipation are put on prophylactic laxatives along with clozapine to reduce this risk
- Clozapine is also associated with an increased risk of pneumonia and lowers seizure threshold in a dose-dependent manner. If high doses of clozapine are required, often a prophylactic antiepileptic will be started to lower this risk
- Even more than other second-generation antipsychotics (SGAs), clozapine carries a risk of contributing to metabolic syndrome

Post-test question

A patient on clozapine has an ANC of 1200. What do the prescribing guidelines recommend as the next step?

A. Continue clozapine at its current dose and continue the current blood draw schedule
B. Continue clozapine at its current dose and increase monitoring to three times weekly
C. Decrease the dose of clozapine by 50%, initiate lithium, and continue the current blood draw schedule
D. Discontinue clozapine, initiate lithium, and increase monitoring to three times weekly

Answer: B

References

1. Agid, O., Arenovich, T., Sajeev, G., et al. (2011). An algorithm-based approach to first-episode schizophrenia: response rates over 3 prospective antipsychotic trials with a retrospective data analysis. *Journal of Clinical Psychiatry*, 72(11), 1439–1444.
2. Ali, S., Mathur, N., Malhotra, A., & Braga, R. (2019). Electroconvulsive therapy and schizophrenia: a systematic review. *Molecular Neuropsychiatry*, 5(2), 75–83. https://doi.org/10.1159/000497376.

PATIENT FILE

3. Aydin, M., Ilhan, B. C., Calisir, S., Yildirim, S., & Eren, I. (2016). Continuing clozapine treatment with lithium in schizophrenic patients with neutropenia or leukopenia: brief review of literature with case reports. *Therapeutic Advances in Psychopharmacology*, Feb., 6(1), 33–8. https://doi.org/10.1177/2045125315624063. PMID: 26913176; PMCID: PMC4749743.
4. Correll, C. U., Agid, O., Crespo-Facorro, B., et al. (2022). A guideline and checklist for initiating and managing clozapine treatment in patients with treatment-resistant schizophrenia. *CNS Drugs*, July, 36(7), 659–679. https://doi.org/10.1007/s40263-022-00932-2. Epub 2022 Jun 27. Erratum in: CNS Drugs. 2022 Aug. 17; PMID: 35759211; PMCID: PMC9243911.
5. Kane, J. M., Agid, O., Baldwin, M. L., et al. (201). Clinical guidance on the identification and management of treatment-resistant schizophrenia. *Journal of Clinical Psychiatry*, 80(2), 18com12123.
6. Klein, C., & Hirachan, S. (2014). The mask of identities: who's who? Delusional misidentification syndrome. *Journal of the American Academy of Psychiatry and the Law*, 42, 369–378.
7. Stahl, S. M. (2005). *Essential Psychopharmacology: The Prescriber's Guide*. New York: Cambridge University Press.

PATIENT FILE

9

Primary polydipsia: Unquenchable thirsts

The Psychopharmacological Dilemma: Identifying biological treatments for primary polydipsia

Shrey Patel and Seth Judd

Pretest self-assessment question

Which of the following is associated with increased risk for primary polydipsia?

A. Alcohol use disorder (AUD)
B. Lithium
C. Fluoxetine
D. Lead poisoning
E. All of the above

Patient evaluation on intake

- 49-year-old male with a long history of schizophrenia, moderate AUD, and antisocial personality disorder (ASPD), who was transferred from a community outpatient program to a forensic state hospital after reporting increasing paranoia and persecutory delusions of feeling that the outpatient program director was "out to get him"
- Patient has a long history of primary polydipsia (formerly known as *psychogenic* polydipsia)
  - Patient reports drinking excessive water when feeling anxious or bored
  - Polydipsia episodes coincide with reemergence of psychotic symptoms and aggression
  - Patient denies dry mouth as a factor
  - Patient is an unreliable narrator regarding his history of water intoxication, acknowledging that symptoms of polydipsia were a problem in the past, but he is unsure of when he last experienced polydipsia behaviors or when the symptoms began
- Patient requested to be at the state hospital and reports "feeling better" now that he is here
- The patient states that he had been adherent with medications at the community outpatient program but is a poor historian and has a documented history of nonadherence
- Patient minimizes his substance use and the consequences related to his substance use

97

PATIENT FILE

- Specific gravity on intake was found to be very dilute (low specific gravity), indicating that polydipsia behaviors were present at time of admission
    - On the unit the patient was observed to be drinking excessively, leading to sodium (Na+) levels of 118. Patient was placed on 1:1 observation
- Mental status examination (MSE)
    - General: in hospital attire, fairly kempt, cooperative
    - Motor: no abnormal movements
    - Speech: normal latency, volume, amount, difficulty with pronunciation
    - Mood/affect: "good"/congruent, full range
    - Thought process: linear
    - Thought content: he denies suicidal and homicidal thoughts; paranoid delusions
    - Insight/judgment: fair/fair
- Plan: patient was placed in a unit with a polydipsia wing. Patient's water intake and weight were monitored daily and electrolytes monitored weekly. No medication changes were made. He was continued on olanzapine 15 mg twice daily (BID) and buspirone at 15 mg three times daily (TID)

Psychiatric history

- He has a history of psychiatric treatment since his early teens and has been treated in both inpatient and outpatient settings. His first hospitalization was in his late teens
    - Historically, his symptoms have included auditory hallucinations, paranoia, delusions of thought insertion, pressured speech, and negative symptoms, including lack of initiative and flat affect
    - He has failed multiple trials of psychotropic medications, including antipsychotic and mood-stabilizing agents
- He has been hospitalized in different levels of mental health facilities and has received mental health treatment during periods of incarceration. He has more than 10 admissions to forensic hospitals
- He has a history of violence and aggression secondary to his mental illness

Social and personal history

- His parents divorced when he was a toddler, and his mother remarried
- He is the second of five siblings
- He dropped out of high school in the twelfth grade, but later received a GED. He reportedly attended some college. No history of learning disability

- He worked for a few months as a truck driver
- He has no known history of trauma or abuse
- He has extensive nonviolent and violent criminal history, including robbery, burglary, possession of substances, and parole violations
- He has a history of substance use, including alcohol, cannabis, cocaine, heroin, methamphetamine, and inhaling metallic paint in his late teens

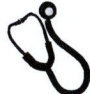

Medical history

- He developed transient hyperthyroidism suspected to be correlated to lithium use, now resolved after discontinuation of lithium
- Records suggest he may have sustained brain damage from inhalant abuse with lead-based/metallic paints
  - As evaluated by Wide Range Achievement Test 4 (WRAT4), the patient was "below average to average" in the 25th percentile for reading and comprehension skills
- He has a history of hepatitis C (in remission, post-treatment)
- He has a history of hyponatremia/polydipsia dating back to at least his early 30s, when he had his first polydipsia-related seizure
  - He was also transferred to another local hospital in his mid-40s for hyponatremic coma due to polydipsia
- Patient is prediabetic with A1c of 6.3%, stable without medication
- He has history of hypertension, stable without medication

Family history

- He has no family history of mental illnesses. Patient's family is not involved with care but has been contacted by the treatment team in the past to confirm medical history

Medication history

- Antipsychotics: clozapine 275 mg twice a day, fluphenazine 2.5 mg daily, haloperidol 10 mg twice a day, olanzapine 30 mg twice a day, quetiapine fumarate 300 mg three times a day, risperidone 3 mg twice a day, loxapine 50 mg twice a day
- Antidepressants: fluoxetine 60 mg, paroxetine 60 mg, trazodone 200 mg
- Anticonvulsant / mood stabilizer: divalproex 1000 mg, lithium 900 mg, and valproic acid 250 mg three times a day
- Patient was also prescribed benztropine 2 mg twice for extrapyramidal symptoms (EPS), clonazepam 2 mg twice a day for anxiety/agitation, lorazepam 2 mg for agitation
- Adverse reactions: lithium – transient hyperthyroidism

PATIENT FILE

Current Medications
- Fluoxetine 40 mg every morning
- Hydroxyzine 50 mg every 8 hours as needed for anxiety
- Olanzapine 30 mg twice a day

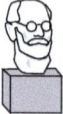
Psychotherapy history
- Patient resides in a designated polydipsia unit, and, given the therapy focus on restricting his excessive water intake, groups were limited to the following: community re-entry, coping skills, library, movies, therapeutic community, and symptom management / water-intake group talk
- Patient has poor attendance with group therapy (25–50%) as he feels he already knows the information

Mechanism of action moment

What are the potential benefits of lithium? What is lithium's mechanism of action?

- Lithium is a mood-stabilizing medication that may also reduce suicide and suicidal behavior
- There are multiple proposed mechanisms for lithium's mood-stabilizing effects
    - Reduced dopamine and glutamate neurotransmission, as well as modulation of the adenylyl-cyclase, phosphoinositide, and protein kinase C pathways leading to dampened excitatory response
    - Increased inhibitory gamma aminobutyric acid (GABA) neurotransmission
    - Reduces oxidative stress that occurs with multiple episodes of mania and depression, through increased protective proteins such as brain-derived neurotrophic factor (BDNF) and B-cell lymphoma-2 (BCL-2), as well as reduced apoptotic processes through inhibition of glycogen synthase kinase 3 and decreased autophagy

Attending physician's mental notes: initial assessment
- Our patient developed symptoms of schizophrenia in his mid-teens and was noted to have his first polydipsia-related hospitalization in his early 30s. Just prior to his admission to our forensic hospital, he had been medically hospitalized for hyponatremic coma secondary to polydipsia. He was on lithium during this time period, which may have also exacerbated his polydipsia. His other risk factors for polydipsia include his psychotic disorder and AUD

PATIENT FILE

- Although it can be observed with other psychiatric conditions, primary polydipsia is most commonly observed in schizophrenia, with estimates of up to 20% in this population
- At the time of his admission, the patient continued to present with psychotic symptoms, including delusions
- Given his primary risk factor for polydipsia is schizophrenia, we recommend changes to current antipsychotic regimen. By reducing the presence of psychotic symptoms, this could reduce the frequency and intensity of his polydipsia behaviors

Further Investigation

Is there anything else you would like to know about this patient? Does the patient have any other risk factors for polydipsia?

- While we do not have medical information from this patient's early life, including blood lead levels or exposure to lead-based paints, we do know that the patient had a history of paint inhalation in his teens during a time period in which lead paints may have been available, as they were phased out in 1978. Although the exact mechanism is unknown, human and animal studies have shown that there is a link between heavy metal toxicity and polydipsia/polyuria, as well as neuropsychiatric effects, especially in children. Lead toxicity is associated with nephritis and accumulation in the proximal renal tubules, although in rats there was no effect on arginine vasopressin release observed as would be seen in central diabetes insipidus. Additionally, lead exposure in infancy was linked to increased polydipsia in rats that were later administered lithium. Perhaps exposure may have predisposed our patient toward lithium-induced polydipsia
- In patients with AUD and comorbid schizophrenia, roughly one in four will develop primary polydipsia, compared to roughly one in two of institutionalized patients with the same conditions. There may also be a genetic component as these patients are also more likely to have a first-degree relative with AUD

Case outcome; use of outcome measures (8 years post-admission)

- Patient has been calm and cooperative with staff except when he is struggling with water-seeking behaviors, when he becomes disgruntled and argumentative
- Patient states that he feels he "is never getting out of the hospital" and that is why he goes against the rules and drinks an excessive amount of water

PATIENT FILE

- His polydipsia has been associated with worsening psychotic symptoms
- Over the years, patient has intermittently passed the polydipsia rehabilitation program and been placed in a general treatment unit only to fail and be returned to the polydipsia unit
    - Notably, the patient was seen to circumvent a 1:1 sitter and drank from the toilet
    - Na+ level was 137
- In the general treatment unit, patient has poor therapeutic group attendance
- Patient received another trial of lithium but quickly redeveloped hyperthyroidism
    - After discontinuation, thyroid panels have been normal, and no abnormalities have been seen on ultrasound
- Patient's medication regimen:
    - Olanzapine 30 mg twice a day
    - Fluoxetine 60 mg daily

Attending physician's mental notes: interim progress report

- The patient's polydipsia behaviors continue to impair his ability to progress in treatment
- Discontinuing the lithium was appropriate given the patient developed hyperthyroidism and the potential for this medication increasing the risk for polydipsia behaviors
- The patient is also on fluoxetine, a selective serotonin reuptake inhibitor (SSRI)
    - SSRIs carry risk for development of Syndrome of Inappropriate Antidiuretic Hormone secretion (SIADH), which may present with hyponatremia or worsening of existing electrolyte abnormalities
    - SIADH is also seen with other antidepressants such as serotonin/norepinephrine reuptake inhibitors (SNRIs), tricyclics, monoamine oxidase inhibitors (MAOIs), and mirtazapine, but the greatest risk has been shown with SSRIs
    - Symptoms of SIADH can mimic primary polydipsia and include excessive thirst, polydipsia, and increase in urinary frequency
- At this point, fluoxetine may pose more of a risk than benefit
    - The indication for the SSRI is also unclear as the patient's record did not indicate a history of a major depressive disorder, obsessive–compulsive disorder (OCD), or an anxiety disorder
- Treatment goals should focus on improving group attendance

PATIENT FILE

- Patient also displays a pattern of rule breaking. We recommend exploring the factors leading to rule breaking in greater detail as they could be related to poor impulse control secondary to his psychotic illness, or could be due to his antisocial personality traits. Determining the factors leading to rule breaking can assist the team in designing a treatment plan to address these factors

Further Investigation

What changes to the treatment plan would you recommend?

- Based on records of this patient's polydipsia, his symptoms are highly correlated to the severity of his underlying psychosis
  - His psychotic symptoms have not sufficiently improved with antipsychotic medications
  - The initiation of clozapine would be the likely next best step to treat his psychosis, given that he has failed trials of multiple antipsychotics

When might it be appropriate to use SSRIs in patients who have polydipsia?

- Although there is risk for SSRI-associated SIADH, fluoxetine has shown benefit in the management of polydipsia secondary to OCD or anxiety-related disorders

Case outcome: interim follow-up progress report (9 years post-admission)

- The patient decompensated due to "disliking his roommate" and had an episode of polydipsia
  - Patient was found to be drinking out of faucet despite having a 1:1 sitter
  - Patient was found to have an Na+ level of 119 and was transferred to an outside local hospital for monitoring. He returned to the forensic hospital once levels stabilized. He was placed in a polydipsia unit
- He was started on clozapine but subsequently requested to be taken off this medication as he opposed the frequent blood draws
- Group attendance was highly variable. In the first quarter of the year, he had 100% attendance, but afterward his group attendance rate significantly dropped
- Current medication regimen:
  - Clozapine 275 mg twice a day
  - Olanzapine 30 mg twice a day
  - Fluoxetine 40 mg daily
  - Hydroxyzine 50 mg every 8 hours as needed for anxiety

PATIENT FILE

Attending physician's mental notes: second interim progress report

- Patient has been on clozapine for about 5 months with only marginal improvement. Given the patient's history of nonadherence with medication, it is important that routine clozapine levels are monitored
  - In males, the expected level would be about 1.08 x the daily oral dose, and in females, the level should be about 1.32 x the daily oral dose
  - If serum levels are sub-therapeutic, consider switching from tablet form to disintegrating tablet or oral suspension (liquid) form
- This patient expressed wanting to stop clozapine due to frequent blood draws, a common complaint among patients prescribed this medication. Psychoeducation about the efficacy of clozapine and lab draw schedule can help alleviate those concerns. This patient has been on clozapine for 5 months. It is important the patient understands that, after 6 months, blood draws will be reduced to every other week (if absolute neutrophil count [ANC] levels are appropriate)
- Patient is currently on two antipsychotic medications, clozapine and olanzapine. Because these two medications are structurally and pharmacologically similar, there may be benefit in switching olanzapine to a typical antipsychotic such as haloperidol
- In addition, the use of a long-acting injectable antipsychotic could help increase medication adherence
- This patient reported fatigue as an additional reason for stopping clozapine. He is currently on a twice-a-day dosing schedule. Switching to once-a-day (bedtime) dosing only could help reduce daytime fatigue and sedation

Further investigation

What else would you like to know? Clozapine was recently added but could this medication contribute to or worsen polydipsia? What other factors can contribute to a patient's nonadherence with clozapine?

- Second-generation antipsychotics (SGAs), such as clozapine, have shown efficacy in the management of patients with primary polydipsia
- One concern with clozapine (along with some other antipsychotics) in patients with polydipsia is its strong anticholinergic properties
  - Antipsychotics have been associated with dose-dependent anticholinergic effects such as dry mouth
  - The development of dry mouth could lead to increased water intake
  - There have been some reports of clozapine-induced polydipsia, although most reports show clozapine can ameliorate symptoms associated with polydipsia

PATIENT FILE

- It is important to assess for other clozapine side effects that may be contributing toward nonadherence. Sialorrhea and constipation are two common side effects leading to nonadherence
    - Sialorrhea is not dose dependent. Treatment options include off-label use of medications such as diphenhydramine, glycopyrrolate, and atropine drops, among others. Botulinum toxin has also shown to be an effective treatment
    - Clozapine-induced constipation is a dose-related effect and can lead to serious or life-threatening consequences such as paralytic ileus and/or toxic megacolon. This side effect can be managed as follows
        - Emollient laxatives such as docusate should be started in conjunction with clozapine
        - If emollients fail, start an osmotic laxative such as polyethylene glycol, lactulose, magnesium hydroxide, or magnesium citrate
        - If osmotics fail, start stimulant laxatives such as bisacodyl or senna
        - If all else fails, consider an enema, manual disimpaction, or surgical disimpaction if indicated
        - Bulk-forming agents such as psyllium and methylcellulose are not used due to risk of inspissation, exacerbating constipation

Case outcome: interim follow-up progress report (10 years post-admission)

- After the last interim evaluation, the patient successfully completed the polydipsia rehabilitation program again and was placed in the general treatment unit until he contracted coronavirus (COVID-19).
- Due to asymptomatic COVID-19 positivity, the patient was placed in an isolation unit. Upon release, he did not appear more psychotic but was found to be drinking from the faucet
    - Patient was placed back in the polydipsia unit, where he has had minimal symptoms for approximately 1 year
- Patient thyroid panel continued to be normal
- Patient group participation has increased to 65%
- Current medications
    - Olanzapine 30 mg twice a day
    - Fluoxetine 40 mg daily
    - Hydroxyzine 50 mg every 8 hours as needed for anxiety
    - PRNs for constipation (senna, docusate, lactulose, etc.)

PATIENT FILE

Attending physician's mental notes: final interim progress report

- Patient has shown a pattern that he has been unable to maintain stability off the polydipsia wing
- While olanzapine appears to have markedly reduced his psychotic symptoms, his polydipsia behaviors remained unchanged
- Clozapine failed to reduce his polydipsia behaviors and other treatment options should be considered
- Treatment options for primary polydipsia include pharmacological, supportive, behavioral, and interventional
  - Pharmacologic management
    - There is no Federal Drug Administration-approved medication for polydipsia
    - Although antipsychotics and mood stabilizers are the most studied, no preference for any particular pharmacotherapy has been demonstrated
    - Some smaller studies have shown naltrexone resulted in a significant reduction in diurnal weight change and polydipsia behaviors
  - Supportive treatment
    - Frequent weight checks, a balanced diet, and minimizing medications that can cause dry mouth
  - Behavioral therapy
    - Biofeedback, education, and group therapy have been used but results have been mixed
    - Relaxation, response prevention, and cognitive behavioral therapy have shown some success in small case studies
  - Interventional treatments
    - Electroconvulsive therapy (ECT) may be another possible treatment option given its ability to reduce psychotic symptoms, although additional research is needed

Case debrief

- Patient has a long, well-documented history of schizophrenia and primary polydipsia. In addition, he has a history of using and abusing multiple substances such as alcohol, cannabis, cocaine, heroin, and methamphetamine. He also inhaled paint as a teenager.
- He has a history of hyponatremia/polydipsia for over a decade and a half, and has had several episodes of severe hyponatremia resulting in seizure and even coma
- His polydipsia behaviors appear to stem from psychotic illness and not develop secondary to psychotropic medications

PATIENT FILE

- He has failed multiple trials of psychotropic medications, including clozapine, fluphenazine, haloperidol, olanzapine, quetiapine, risperidone, loxapine, fluoxetine, paroxetine, trazodone, buspirone, divalproex, lithium, and valproic acid
- On the other hand, his adherence with medication and individual/group therapy has been consistently inconsistent
- He has been able to demonstrate the ability to graduate from a polydipsia unit but has been unable to maintain stability off the polydipsia unit for more than a year

Take-home points

- Primary polydipsia is a disorder characterized by excessive water intake
- Primary polydipsia is not uncommon in inpatient psychiatric facilities
- Primary polydipsia is most commonly seen in schizophrenia and can occur in up to 20% of this population
  - Polydipsia can also lead to decompensation and worsening of psychotic symptoms
- AUD is also a risk factor for primary polydipsia
- Other risk factors include medications such as lithium and SSRIs
- Management of primary polydipsia requires a multimodal approach:
  - Psychotropic medications to address the underlying psychiatric condition
  - For medications with high anticholinergic burden, patients should be monitored closely for excessive dry mouth as this could lead to excessive water intake
  - Supportive treatment such as frequent weight checks and monitoring Na+ levels
  - Behavioral therapy such as individual and group therapy, biofeedback, and psychoeducation
  - Interventional treatments such as ECT

Performance in practice: confessions of a psychopharmacologist

What could have been done better?

- In this case, the patient had failed multiple trials of antipsychotic medications, including clozapine, at therapeutic doses. In such cases of treatment-resistant schizophrenia, ECT would be the next appropriate step.
  - ECT can ameliorate psychotic symptoms and can potentially reduce polydipsia behaviors
- Other non-pharmacological approaches should also be considered

PATIENT FILE

- Patient reported feeling anxious, bored, and hopeless (e.g., expressing that he was never going to leave the hospital) as risk factors for polydipsia behaviors
    - Treatment plan should consider these risk factors and develop strategies to target anxiety, boredom, and feelings of helplessness
- The patient also has a diagnosis of ASPD, which may be contributing toward his impulsivity and rule-breaking behaviors
    - The patient may benefit from participating in dialectical behavioral therapy (DBT) groups offered at the hospital to help manage such behaviors

What are some concerns about the use of fluoxetine in this patient and in a forensic hospital in general?

- As mentioned previously, SSRIs increase the risk for hyponatremia and polydipsia behaviors
- Our patient has been on fluoxetine since the date of his admission. Although it is unlikely to be a contributor to his polydipsia, as his polydipsia has been stable at times while on this medication, it is important that, as psychiatrists, we periodically review a patient's medication regimen to assess appropriateness for each medication. This is particularly important in a forensic hospital, where patients are likely to have longer admissions and be under the care of multiple psychiatrists during their admission
    - From the medical records there was not a clear indication for prescribing fluoxetine. He did not carry diagnoses suggestive of the need for it, such as schizoaffective disorder – depressive type, anxiety disorder, trauma-related disorder, or OCD, etc.
- Fluoxetine inhibits several liver enzymes, such as Cytochrome P450 – 2D6 and 3A4, which can lead to drug-to-drug interactions. Given fluoxetine's extensive inhibition of liver enzymes, it should be used with caution in this population to avoid drug-to-drug interactions
- Patients in forensic settings are typically complex and require polypharmacy to target a myriad of disorders or a disorder resistant to treatment

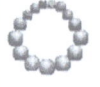

Tips and pearls

What are risk factors for polydipsia?

- Risk factors for polydipsia include psychiatric and medical conditions, and medications
    - The most common psychiatric condition associated with polydipsia is schizophrenia, and polydipsia can occur in up to 20% of this population

PATIENT FILE

- The most common medical conditions associated with polydipsia are diabetes insipidus and SIADH
- Medications can also increase the risk for polydipsia/polyuria
  - Psychotropic medications include lithium, SSRIs, and other antidepressants
  - Other medications include cidofovir, foscarnet, amphotericin B, demeclocycline, ifosfamide, and ofloxacin, among others

What are the treatment options for primary polydipsia?

- Treating primary polydipsia requires a multi-model approach involving psychotropic medications which target the underlying psychiatric condition
- A structured treatment plan which includes individualized therapy, daily weight monitoring, and weekly Na+ levels
- Off-label use of medications to target impulsive behaviors associated with polydipsia
  - Antidepressants or naltrexone
- ECT is recommended if patient develops treatment-resistant symptoms

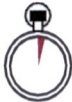

Two-minute tutorial

Primary polydipsia

- Primary polydipsia is characterized by an excessive intake of fluid, with symptoms typically manifesting after an acute ingestion of 3 liters
- A diagnosis of primary polydipsia can only be made after other causes of excessive water intake have been ruled out, such as diabetes insipidus and SIADH
  - Work-up includes a history and physical examination, as well as laboratory tests including: low serum electrolytes, low serum and urine osmolality, and low urine specific gravity (consistently below 1.020)
  - The gold standard for diagnosis is the water deprivation test
    - Those with primary polydipsia will have a very concentrated urine (> 600 mOsm/L) and an elevated Antidiuretic Hormone (ADH)
- There are three stages in primary polydipsia:
  1. Polydipsia and polyuria
  2. Hyponatremia
  3. Water intoxication
- Untreated primary polydipsia can lead to several complications
  - Hyponatremia has been associated with increased morbidity and mortality

PATIENT FILE

- Initial neurological complications of water intoxication include: ataxia, tremors, nausea, vomiting, and disorientation, as well as deficits in concentration and memory. If left untreated, complications include: seizure, coma, and death
- Psychiatric complications such as exacerbation of pre-existing psychiatric symptoms, including psychotic symptoms. Patients with untreated polydipsia may also exhibit mood lability and anger
- Given the multiple and potentially life-threatening complications arising from primary polydipsia, early recognition and treatment are essential

What other conditions can present with polydipsia?

- Polydipsia/polyuria may present in other conditions leading to osmotic diuresis:
  - Hyperglycemic conditions: the hyperosmolar state of elevated blood glucose levels in diabetes mellitus, as well as water loss due to glycosuria-related polyuria, leads to the activation of the ventromedial nuclei of the hypothalamus which controls hunger/satiety and thirst
  - Renal defects: genetic glycosuria or Fanconi syndrome
  - Excessive sodium intake or intravenous saline
  - Urea diuresis: resolving acute kidney injury, urea therapy for SIADH, high-protein intake, or glucocorticoid therapy
- Polydipsia/polyuria may also present in conditions leading to free water loss
  - Central diabetes insipidus: patients with this condition do not produce sufficient quantities of vasopressin, leading to polyuria. Testing for this condition is by administration of desmopressin which will decrease urine output. Follow-up brain MRI is indicated if this test is positive, as the most common causes are tumors of/near the sella turcica. The progression of tumors, infiltrative disease, structural abnormalities, or the sequelae of trauma and neurosurgery may produce a wide spectrum of severity called partial central diabetes insipidus
  - Nephrogenic diabetes insipidus: patients with this condition may have inadequate response to vasopressin in the principal cells. Testing for this condition by administration of desmopressin will not improve urine output. However, there are multiple etiologies:
    - Genetic conditions including sickle cell disease, Sjögren's syndrome, polycystic kidney disease, or V2-vasopressin (antidiuretic hormone) receptor abnormalities
    - Medications such as lithium, cidofovir, foscarnet, amphotericin B, demeclocycline, ifosfamide, and ofloxacin, among others

PATIENT FILE

- Electrolyte disturbances such as hypercalcemia or hypokalemia
- Damage to the nephron via heavy metal toxicity, ureteral obstruction, or transiently in post-obstructive diuresis

What is the proposed pathophysiology of lithium-induced polydipsia and its other potential side effects?

- Potential adverse effects of lithium include the following:
  - Polyuria/polydipsia, nausea, diarrhea, tremor, weight gain, cognitive impairment (particularly in language and memory), sexual dysfunction, worsening psoriasis/acne
- Lithium-induced polydipsia
  - In rat models, lithium-induced polydipsia appeared to be dependent on intact nigrostriatal dopaminergic fibers, but not on other monoaminergic systems in the brain. Lithium also increased plasma renin, angiotensin I and II reactivity. In other studies, renin appeared to have a strong correlation as well
  - In humans, nephrogenic diabetes insipidus appears to be the underlying cause of polydipsia/polyuria in lithium use via disruption of antidiuretic hormone effect: specifically, interference in the ability of the V2-vasopressin receptors in the principal cells of the collecting tubules to generate cyclic adenosine monophosphate in response to stimulation
- Chronic effects associated with high-dose lithium use include renal dysfunction, hypothyroidism, and, more uncommonly, hyperthyroidism and hyperparathyroidism
  - Lithium-associated hypothyroidism is multifactorial, including inhibition of hormone release from the thyroid gland, decreased iodine trapping with the gland, and inhibition of hormone synthesis
  - Hyperthyroidism, such as in our patient, is thought to be due to the direct toxic effect of lithium on the thyroid due to disturbance of iodine kinetics. Patients have also been found to have an increased titer of antithyroid peroxidase antibodies

Post-test question

Which of the following is associated with increased risk for primary polydipsia?

A. Alcohol use disorder (AUD)
B. Lithium
C. Fluoxetine
D. Lead poisoning
E. All of the above

Answer: E

PATIENT FILE

References

1. Ahmadi, L. & Goldman, M. B. (2020). Primary polydipsia: update. Best practice & research. *Clinical Endocrinology & Metabolism*, 34(5), 101469. https://doi.org/10.1016/j.beem.2020.101469.
2. Ahmed, A. G., Heigh, L. M., & Ramachandran, K. V. (2001). Polydipsia, psychosis, and familial psychopathology. *Canadian Journal of Psychiatry*, 46, 522–527.
3. Ali, S. N. & Bazzano, L. A. (2018). Hyponatremia in association with second-generation antipsychotics: a systematic review of case reports. *Ochsner Journal*, 18(3), 230–235.
4. Andrew, R. D. (1991). Seizure and acute osmotic change: clinical and neurophysiological aspects. *Journal of the Neurological Sciences*, 101(1), 7–18.
5. Behl, T., Kotwani, A., Kaur, I., & Goel, H. (2015). Mechanisms of prolonged lithium therapy-induced nephrogenic diabetes insipidus. *European Journal of Pharmacology*, 755, 27–33. https://doi.org/10.1016/j.ejphar.2015.02.040.
6. Bhatia, M. S., Goyal, A., Saha, R., & Doval, N. (2017). Psychogenic polydipsia – management challenges. *Shanghai Archives of Psychiatry*, 29(3), 180–183.
7. Brookes, G. & Ahmed, A. G. (2006). Pharmacological treatments for psychosis-related polydipsia. *Cochrane Database of Systematic Reviews*, 4, CD003544.
8. Chen, S. Y., Ravindran, G., Zhang, Q., Kisely, S., & Siskind, D. (2019). Treatment strategies for clozapine-induced sialorrhea: a systematic review and meta-analysis. *CNS Drugs*, March, 33(3), 225–238. https://doi.org/10.1007/s40263-019-00612-8.
9. Chisolm, J. (1971). Lead poisoning. *Scientific American*, 224(2), 15–23. JSTOR, www.jstor.org/stable/24927721. Accessed 26 Feb. 2023.
10. Czarnywojtek, A., Zgorzalewicz-Stachowiak, M., Czarnocka, B., et al. (2020). Effect of lithium carbonate on the function of the thyroid gland: mechanism of action and clinical implications. *Journal of Physiology and Pharmacology*, April, 71(2). https://doi.org/10.26402/jpp.2020.2.03.
11. Deas-Nesmith, D. & Brewerton, T. D. (1992). A case of fluoxetine-responsive psychogenic polydipsia: a variant of obsessive–compulsive disorder? *Journal of Nervous and Mental Disease*, May, 180(5), 338–339.
12. DeHaven, D. L., Krigman, M. R., Gaynor, J. J., & Mailman, R. B. (1984). The effects of lead administration during development on lithium-induced polydipsia and dopaminergic function. *Brain*

Research 297(2), 297–304. https://doi.org/10.1016/0006-8993(84)90570-5.
13. de Leon. J. (2003). Polydipsia – a study in a long-term psychiatric unit. *European Archives of Psychiatry and Clinical Neuroscience*, 253, 37–39.
14. de Leon, J., Verghese, C., Tracy, J. I., Josiassen, R. C., & Simpson, G. M. (1994). Polydipsia and water intoxication in psychiatric patients: a review of the epidemiological literature. *Biological Psychiatry*, March 15, 35(6), 408–419. https://doi.org/10.1016/0006-3223(94)90008-6.
15. Dundas, B., Harris, M., & Narasimhan, M. (2007). Psychogenic polydipsia review: etiology, differential, and treatment. *Current Psychiatry Reports*, 9, 236–241.
16. Evenson, R. C., Jos, C. J., & Mallya, A. R. (1987). Prevalence of polydipsia among public psychiatric patients. *Psychological Reports*, 60, 803–807.
17. Fenske, W., Refardt, J., Chifu, I., et al.(2018). A copeptin-based approach in the diagnosis of diabetes insipidus. *New England Journal of Medicine*, 379(5), 428–439. https://doi.org/10.1056/nejmoa1803760.
18. Flanagan, R. J., Lally, J., Gee, S., Lyon, R., & Every-Palmer, S. (2020). Clozapine in the treatment of refractory schizophrenia: a practical guide for healthcare professionals. *British Medical Bulletin*, Oct. 14, 135(1), 73–89. https://doi.org/10.1093/bmb/ldaa024.
19. Gill, M. & McCauley, M. (2015). Psychogenic polydipsia: the result, or cause of, deteriorating psychotic symptoms? A case report of the consequences of water intoxication. *Case Reports in Psychiatry*, 2015, 846459. https://doi.org/10.1155/2015/846459.
20. Gitlin, M. (2016). Lithium side effects and toxicity: prevalence and management strategies. *International Journal of Bipolar Disorders*, 4(1). https://doi.org/10.1186/s40345-016-0068-y.
21. Goldman, M. (2009). The mechanism of life-threatening water imbalance in schizophrenia and its relationship to the underlying psychiatric illness. *Brain Research Reviews*, 61(2), 210–220.
22. Gutman, Y., Benzakein, F., & Livneh, P. (1971). Polydipsia induced by isoprenaline and by lithium: relation to kidneys and renin. *European Journal of Pharmacology*, 16(3), 380–384. https://doi.org/10.1016/0014-2999(71)90042-2.
23. Hernandez, L. & Briese, E. (1972). Analysis of diabetic hyperphagia and polydipsia. *Physiology & Behavior*, 9(5), 741–746. https://doi.org/10.1016/0031-9384(72)90044-3.

PATIENT FILE

24. Hogg, S. & Dalvi, A. (2004). Acceleration of onset of action in schedule-induced polydipsia: combinations of SSRI and 5-HT1A and 5-HT1B receptor antagonists. *Pharmacology Biochemistry and Behavior*, 77(1), 69–75. https://doi.org/10.1016/j.pbb.2003.09.020.
25. Illowsky, B. P. & Kirch, D. G. (1998). Polydipsia and hyponatremia in psychiatric patients. *American Journal of Psychiatry*, 145, 675–683.
26. Kim, G.-H. (2022). Pathophysiology of drug-induced hyponatremia. *Journal of Clinical Medicine*, 11, 5810. https://doi.org/10.3390/jcm11195810.
27. Kirino, S., Sakuma, M., Misawa, F., et al. (2020). Relationship between polydipsia and antipsychotics: a systematic review of clinical studies and case reports. *Progress in Neuro-psychopharmacology and Biological Psychiatry*, Jan. 10, 96, 109756. https://doi.org/10.1016/j.pnpbp.2019.109756.
28. Kruse, D., Pantelis, C., Rudd, R., et al. (2001). Treatment of psychogenic polydipsia: comparison of risperidone and olanzapine, and the effects of an adjunctive angiotensin-II receptor blocking drug (irbesartan). *Australian and New Zealand Journal of Psychiatry*, Feb., 35(1), 656–8. https://doi.org/10.1046/j.1440-1614.2001.00847.x.
29. Lieberman, J. A. (2004). Managing anticholinergic side effects. *Primary Care Companion to the Journal of Clinical Psychiatry*, 6(Suppl. 2), 20–23.
30. Lightfoot, T. L. & Yeager, J. M. (2008). Pet bird toxicity and related environmental concerns. *Veterinary Clinics of North America: Exotical Animal Practice*, May, 11(2), 229–259, vi. https://doi.org/10.1016/j.cvex.2008.01.006. PMID: 18406386.
31. Mailman, R. B., Krigman, M. R., Mueller, R. A., Mushak, P., & Breese, G. R. (1978). Lead exposure during infancy permanently increases lithium-induced polydipsia. *Science*, Aug. 18, 201(4356), 637–639. https://doi.org/10.1126/science.675249.
32. Mailman, R. B. (1983). Lithium-induced polydipsia: dependence on nigrostriatal dopamine pathway and relationship to changes in the renin-angiotensin system. *Psychopharmacology*, 80, 143–149. https://doi.org/10.1007/BF00427958.
33. Malhi, G. S., Tanious, M., Das, P., Coulston, C. M., & Berk, M. (2013). Potential mechanisms of action of lithium in bipolar disorder: current understanding. *CNS Drugs*, Feb., 27(2), 135–153. https://doi.org/10.1007/s40263-013-0039-0.
34. Mercier-Guidez, E. & Loas, G. (2000). Polydipsia and water intoxication in 353 psychiatric inpatients: an epidemiological and psychopathological study. *European Psychiatry*, 15(5), 306–311.

35. Moncrieff, A. A., Koumides, O. P., Clayton, B. E., Patrick, A. D., Renwick, A. G. C., & Roberts, G. E. (1964). Lead poisoning in children. *Archives of Disease in Childhood*, Feb., 39(203), 1–13. https://doi.org/10.1136/adc.39.203.1.
36. Moreno, M. & Flores, P. (2012). Schedule-induced polydipsia as a model of compulsive behavior: neuropharmacological and neuroendocrine bases. *Psychopharmacology (Berlin)*, Jan., 219(2), 647–659. https://doi.org/10.1007/s00213-011-2570-3.
37. Nagashima, T., Inoue, M., Kitamura, S., et al. (2012). Brain structural changes and neuropsychological impairments in male polydipsic schizophrenia. *BMC Psychiatry*, Nov. 26, 12, 210. https://doi.org/10.1186/1471-244X-12-210.
38. Nigro, N., Grossmann, M., Chiang, C., & Inder, W. J. (2018). Polyuria–polydipsia syndrome: a diagnostic challenge. *Internal Medicine Journal*, March, 48(3), 244–253. https://doi.org/10.1111/imj.13627.
39. Ogilvie, A. D. & Croy, M. F. (1992). Clozapine and hyponatraemia. *Lancet*, Sept. 12, 340(8820), 672. https://doi.org/10.1016/0140-6736(92)92206-u.
40. Ozbilen, M., Adams, C. E., & Marley, J. (2012). Anticholinergic effects of oral antipsychotic drugs of typicals versus atypicals over medium- and long-term: systematic review and meta-analysis. *Current Medicinal Chemistry*, 19(30), 5214–5218. https://doi.org/10.2174/092986712803530476.
41. Plasencia-García, B. O., Rodríguez-Menéndez, G., Rico-Rangel, M. I., Rubio-García, A., Torelló-Iserte, J., & Crespo-Facorro, B. (2021). Drug–drug interactions between COVID-19 treatments and antipsychotic drugs: integrated evidence from 4 databases and a systematic review. *Psychopharmacology (Berlin)*, Feb., 238(2), 329–340. https://doi.org/10.1007/s00213-020-05716-4.
42. Poirier, S., Legris, G., Tremblay, P., et al. (2010). Schizophrenia patients with polydipsia and water intoxication are characterized by greater severity of psychotic illness and a more frequent history of alcohol abuse. *Schizophrenia Research*, May, 118(1–3), 285–291. https://doi.org/10.1016/j.schres.2009.12.036.
43. Riblet, N. B., Shiner, B., Young-Xu, Y., & Watts, B. V. (2022). Lithium in the prevention of suicide in adults: systematic review and meta-analysis of clinical trials. *BJPsych Open*, Nov. 17, 8(6), e199. https://doi.org/10.1192/bjo.2022.605.
44. Rizvi, S., Gold, J., & Khan, A. M. (2019). Role of naltrexone in improving compulsive drinking in psychogenic polydipsia. *Cureus*, 11(3), e5320.

45. Sailer, C., Winzeler, B., & Christ-Crain, M. (2017). Primary polydipsia in the medical and psychiatric patient: characteristics, complications and therapy. *Swiss Medical Weekly*, 147, 14514.
46. Sawant, N. S., Kate, N. S., Rupani, K. I., et al. (2015). Amelioration of psychogenic polydipsia in schizophrenia with risperidone & ECT. *Indian Journal of Research*, 4(4).
47. Shutty, M. S., Jr., Hundley, P. L., Leadbetter, R. A., Vieweg, V., & Hill, D. (1992). Development and validation of a behavioral observation measure for the syndrome of psychosis, intermittent hyponatremia, and polydipsia. *Journal of Behavior Therapy and Experimental Psychiatry*. Sept., 23(3), 213–219. https://doi.org/10.1016/0005-7916(92)90038-k.
48. Taube, M. (2021). Hyponatremia caused by water intoxication: successful treatment of psychiatric disturbances with olanzapine and fluoxetine. *Oxford Medical Case Reports*, Jan. 23, 2021(1), omaa127. https://doi.org/10.1093/omcr/omaa127.
49. Torres, I. J., Keedy, S., Marlow-O'Connor, M., Beenken, B., & Goldman, M. B. (2009). Neuropsychological impairment in patients with schizophrenia and evidence of hyponatremia and polydipsia. *Neuropsychology*, May, 23(3), 307–314. https://doi.org/10.1037/a0014481.
50. Verghese, C., de Leon, J., & Josiassen, R. C. (1996). Problems and progress in the diagnosis and treatment of polydipsia and hyponatremia. *Schizophrenia Bulletin*, 22, 455–464.
51. Winzeler, B., Jeanloz, N., Nigro, N., et al. (2016). Long-term outcome of profound hyponatremia: a prospective 12 months follow-up study. *European Journal of Endocrinology*, Dec., 175(6), 499–507. https://doi.org/10.1530/EJE-16-0500.
52. Yoshida, K. & Takeuchi, H. (2021). Dose-dependent effects of antipsychotics on efficacy and adverse effects in schizophrenia. *Behavioral Brain Research*, March 26, 402, 113098. https://doi.org/10.1016/j.bbr.2020.113098.
53. Zafonte, R. D., Watanabe, T. K., Mann, N. R., & Ko, D. H. (1997). Psychogenic polydipsia after traumatic brain injury: a case report. *American Journal of Physical Medicine & Rehabilitation*, May–June, 76(3), 246–248. https://doi.org/10.1097/00002060-199705000-00018.

10
Catatonia: Turning into stone

The Question: How do we treat catatonia in a man with an otherwise limited psychiatric history?
The Psychopharmacological Dilemma: How aggressively do we treat catatonia in a patient without a clear etiology?

Amanie Salem and Carolina A. Klein

Pretest self-assessment question
What is the first-line treatment for catatonia?
A. Antipsychotics
B. Benzodiazepines
C. ECT
D. Supportive medical treatment

Patient evaluation on intake
- 38-year-old single male with a history of HIV, reactive inflammatory polyarthritis, who presents with new-onset psychosis and catatonia resulting in two psychiatric hospitalizations in the past 12 months. His psychiatric history is otherwise limited. He was admitted to internal medicine services for treatment of malignant catatonia. His elevated blood pressure, heart rate, and temperature improved with lorazepam and discontinuation of benztropine. He was transferred to inpatient psychiatry for continued management of underlying catatonia.

Psychiatric history
- He was psychiatrically hospitalized 12 months ago and 5 months ago for catatonia
  - A consult note from a previous hospitalization reads: "severe depressive episode vs. acute psychosis beginning October 2020 following a workplace accident and brief psychotic episode in March 2021 (while on steroids as well)"
  - He was treated with antipsychotics which he self-discontinued
- He is nonadherent with outpatient medication and has never seen an outpatient psychotherapist

PATIENT FILE

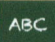
Social and personal history
- He lives at home with his mother
- His highest level of education is a Bachelor's degree
- He enjoys building websites and working on the computer
- There is no reported history of alcohol or other substance use

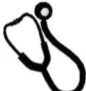
Medical history
- He has HIV and is compliant with antiretroviral therapy
- He has reactive inflammatory polyarthritis and is compliant with treatment
- There is no history of head injury, loss of consciousness, seizures, thyroid problems, or cardiac problems

Family history
- It is reported he has a younger brother with autism spectrum disorder

Medication history
- Paliperidone injectable for psychosis, most recently administered 5 months ago

Current history
- The patient exhibits notable catatonic symptoms including immobility and mutism
- His temperature is 98.7, heart rate is 76, and blood pressure is 123/79
- It is reported he is eating minimally but requires significant encouragement and assistance with meals
- He is able to nod and shake his head but does not respond verbally
  - These movements seem slowed
- Continue lorazepam 2 mg three times daily
- Continue 1:1 observation for safety monitoring
- ECT referral placed

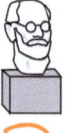
Psychotherapy history
- He has never had any previous outpatient therapy

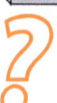
Question
Does this choice of medication make sense?
- Yes
- No

PATIENT FILE

Mechanism of action moment
- Lorazepam binds to benzodiazepine receptors at the gamma aminobutyric acid (GABA)-A ligand-gated chloride channel complex
  - It enhances the inhibitory effect of GABA and boosts chloride conductance through GABA-regulated channels

Attending physician's mental note: initial evaluation
- This patient exhibits symptoms without a previous significant psychiatric history
- He is older than the average age for most individuals with first-episode psychosis (FEP), although his high level of premorbid functioning may have been protective
- The differential etiology for malignant catatonia is broad and his medical issues may also be contributing
- He does not appear to have a history of developmental disorder, in which 15–20% of individuals develop unexplained catatonia
- Treatment for catatonia may require higher doses of benzodiazepines than what he is currently prescribed
- Bush–Francis Catatonia Rating Scale (BFCRS) scores may help keep track of his symptoms changing
- He would benefit from ECT given his significant negative symptoms

Case outcome: first interim follow-up visit the next day
- Lorazepam was increased to 3 mg three times daily for treatment of catatonia
- Nursing notes indicate that the patient improves with benzodiazepine administration but improvement is not maintained, remains catatonic, and requires continued nursing assistance and 1:1 observation
- He was tachycardic overnight and required IV bolus treatment
- He still has limited fluid and food intake
- His BFCRS score is 9 with limited examination
- ECT referral is pending

Question
What would be your next step?
- Maintain lorazepam dose and wait for ECT referral to go through
- Increase lorazepam

PATIENT FILE

Attending physician's mental note: initial evaluation
- The etiology of his catatonia remains unclear but it may be a combination of his medical conditions and an affective disorder; it is unclear if there is an underlying psychotic disorder
- He responds positively to lorazepam but the effects of it are insufficiently maintained
- It may be helpful to dose the lorazepam more frequently since there is partial response that is insufficiently maintained
- Catatonia often requires much higher doses of benzodiazepines for a longer period of time
- Close monitoring of his vital signs is important

Case outcome: at 1 week
- Lorazepam has been changed to 2 mg four times daily
- Clinical presentation continues to be consistent with malignant catatonia
- He exhibits mutism, rigidity, staring, catalepsy, waxy flexibility, withdrawal, autonomic alterations
- His BFCRS score has risen to over 18

Attending physician's mental note: 1 week after admission
- The etiology of his catatonia remains unclear
  - Collateral information may be helpful in understanding chronology of symptoms and any underlying psychosis
- The response to benzodiazepines has not been sufficient
- It may be helpful to dose the lorazepam even more frequently since there is partial response that is insufficiently maintained
- There have been several case reports of valproic acid having prophylactic and ameliorating effects on symptoms of catatonia
- Single case reports also cite lithium, carbamazepine, topiramate, and levetiracetam as beneficial for acute catatonic symptoms; however, levetiracetam has also been noted to provoke symptoms
- There needs to be a follow-up as ECT is urgently needed

Question
Which of the following would be your next step?
- Increase the dose of lorazepam
- Increase the frequency of lorazepam
- Increase lorazepam dose and frequency
- Add a second agent to treat the catatonia

PATIENT FILE

Case outcome: at 4 weeks
- Consent for valproic acid was declined; lorazepam has been increased to 3 mg every 4 hours
- The patient remains withdrawn at times but is also more interactive and has been seen slowly walking and speaking in one-to-two-word sentences
- His blood pressure is low

Further investigation
What additional information would you especially like to know in order to make a decision about the next step in his treatment? How long do the periods of increased interactivity last? What behaviors is he exhibiting during this time? Is the patient exhibiting symptoms of low blood pressure?

- The patient is seen walking in the halls and making eye contact with staff and other patients
- One staff member reported he saw the patient trying to play ping-pong
- He has been able to increase the size of bites of food he takes and has worked with speech therapy on this
- His systolic blood pressure ranges from 100 to 115 and diastolic blood pressure ranges from 65 to 70; he has not endorsed any dizziness or lightheadedness and has not fallen

Attending physician's mental notes
- There has been significant progress over the past few days – however, he needs to continue to be aggressively treated so that his symptoms do not worsen
- He remains at risk if his medication is lowered too quickly
- Even though his blood pressure has been low, he has not had any falls and the treatment for catatonia outweighs the risk of falls at the current time
- Encouraging hydration will help maintain his blood pressure
- He will remain on 1:1 for safety to help minimize the risk of any falls

Case outcome: at 6 weeks
- He has been approved for ECT treatment
- Lorazepam has been slowly lowered from 18 mg daily to 15 mg daily without incident in preparation for ECT treatment
- Spoke with infectious disease specialist who ruled out antiretroviral therapy as cause
- Continue slowly tapering lorazepam over the next few weeks

PATIENT FILE

Case outcome: at 8 weeks
- The patient has had no behavioral issues and continues responding to lorazepam
- Lorazepam was tapered to 12 mg daily with resurgence of catatonic symptoms; 15 mg appears to be a sort of threshold
  - Symptoms worsen when lorazepam is dosed at less than 15 mg daily
- ECT pending

Case outcome: at 10 weeks
- Lorazepam has been held at 15 mg daily with improvement
- The patient reports feeling better on current dose of lorazepam
- His communication, movement, and independent activity have improved
  - His rate of speech is unremarkable
  - He is tending to activities of daily living independently
  - There is no psychomotor agitation or retardation noted
- ECT pending

Further investigation
Given the improvement on lorazepam, would you still want or need to pursue ECT? What other information would you want to know to make an informed decision? How would you decrease the lorazepam?

- The patient is not having any noted side effects from lorazepam and although he still exhibits low blood pressure, this is not causing any symptoms
- In order to provide ECT treatment, he would need to be transferred to an outside hospital inpatient unit
- The patient is still agreeable to ECT treatment
- The plan would be to taper the lorazepam by 2–3 mg per week and closely monitor for recurrent symptoms of catatonia

Attending physician's mental notes
- Increasing suspicion that catatonia is a result of a general medical condition, autoimmune versus infectious versus iatrogenic (medication-induced)
- Many causes have already been ruled out
- He has improved significantly over the last few weeks and, given the overall improvement, can attempt to decrease the dose of lorazepam
- Decreasing the lorazepam will have to be done slowly to avoid decompensation and withdrawal symptoms as seen earlier during the hospitalization

PATIENT FILE

Case outcome: at 12 weeks

- Lorazepam has been tapered to 12 mg daily, with no resurgence of catatonic symptoms
- Nursing staff report meaningful socialization and activities – still not at baseline
- The patient is aware of plan to aim for transfer for ECT
- Spoke with family who is aware of the plan but expressed interest in the patient being discharged home

Case outcome: at 16 weeks

- Continues to not have any catatonic symptoms
- Lorazepam has been tapered to 6 mg daily, with no worsening of catatonic symptoms
- Family continues to express interest in the patient being discharged to home
- Blood pressure is within normal limits

Attending physician's mental notes

- The patient continues to show improvement with no medication side effects
- He presents as fully stable now, and collateral information suggests he is improved compared to his worst catatonic moments outside the hospital
    - At his baseline, he is a high-achieving entrepreneur and holds multiple managerial-level positions
    - Illness and prolonged hospitalization have impacted his functionality as he has presented with catatonia intermittently for almost a year
- Although he presents well now, it is important to have follow-up in place due to his decompensation outside the hospital
- The etiology of his catatonia remains unchanged – possibly from autoimmune diseases, associated with HIV and its treatment – and is likely to recur if lorazepam taper is completed
- Therefore, ECT continues to be medically necessary

Question

Does this patient still require ECT?

- Yes
- No

PATIENT FILE

Case outcome: at 18 weeks
- The patient remains stable without notable symptoms of catatonia
- Lorazepam has been tapered to 4 mg daily, no reemergence of symptoms and no signs of benzodiazepine withdrawal
- Treatment team met in regard to updated plan; given marked improvement in his symptoms, plan to defer ECT and continue with medication management
- Plan for discharge with lorazepam
- ECT referral is still pending but is not necessary at this time

Case debrief
- With no significant psychiatric history, this patient developed catatonia of unclear etiology and experienced symptoms for about 1 year, for which he required three total hospitalizations. His symptoms never fully resolved in between hospitalizations
- During this most recent hospitalization, the patient developed malignant catatonia, was medically stabilized, then transferred to psychiatry for management of his symptoms
- The patient was treated with benzodiazepines with partial success, and an ECT referral was placed
- Benzodiazepines were titrated to a high dose while the patient waited for ECT
- The patient's symptoms improved with high dose of benzodiazepines over the course of about 4 months and he no longer required ECT
- He was discharged home with outpatient follow-up and ECT was deferred

Take-home points
- Catatonia is a motor syndrome
- Symptoms of catatonia include catalepsy, waxy flexibility, stupor, agitation, mutism, negativism, posturing, mannerisms, stereotypies, grimacing, echolalia, and echopraxia
- Malignant catatonia can be life threatening and is characterized by a fever and autonomic disturbances
- The treatment of catatonia often involves the use of benzodiazepines, such as lorazepam, that can be used in combination therapy with antipsychotics
- Patients with long-standing catatonia may not respond as rapidly or robustly to benzodiazepines

PATIENT FILE

- ECT is a highly effective treatment for catatonia, and may be the definitive treatment
  - Even patients who do not respond to benzodiazepines may respond to ECT

Performance in practice: confessions of a psychopharmacologist

What could have been done better here?

- Was enough information gathered regarding the patient's history to help establish an etiology?
- Should the patient have been started on an additional medication?
- Should the benzodiazepines have been titrated more quickly or titrated to a higher dose?

Is there anything else that could have contributed to the patient's symptoms?

- There was a suspicion for underlying psychosis in this patient, but should there have been a more thorough exploration of additional mental illnesses (for example, affective disorders) or other medical conditions that might have contributed to the symptoms?
- The patient is a high-functioning entrepreneur, and first-break psychosis is more common in an individual's early 20s. The DSM-5-TR no longer diagnoses catatonia as a subtype of schizophrenia, and there is a possibility that the patient may have experienced an affective disorder that contributed to his catatonia

Is there a chance the patient may develop symptoms of catatonia in the future?

- It is possible this patient may develop symptoms of catatonia again in the future. He still requires tapering of the remaining lorazepam on an outpatient basis. His symptoms will have to be monitored closely for resurgence

What is the neurological mechanism underlying catatonia?

- The exact mechanism is not well understood
- Reduced GABA activity, specifically GABA-A receptor activity, is thought to be a driver of the dysfunction seen in catatonia
- Excitatory glutamatergic N-methyl-D-aspartate receptor (NMDA-R) appears to be associated as well. Glutamate hyperactivity is thought to be the cause of catatonia symptoms in this case
- There is some evidence that dopamine dysfunction contributes to catatonic symptoms

PATIENT FILE

Tips and pearls
How do you diagnose catatonia?
- When catatonia is suspected, a lorazepam challenge can be performed
  - This is done by giving a dose of lorazepam, either through IM or IV, and watching for a response. A response indicates the need for high suspicion of catatonia

What are the risk factors for catatonia?
- Catatonia is associated with mental illness and general medical conditions
- Roughly 20% of individuals with catatonia have an underlying medical cause
- About 35% of patients with schizophrenia will show symptoms of catatonia at some point in their life
- Patients with bipolar disorder, autism, schizophrenia, or major depressive disorder all have a higher incidence of catatonia than the general population
- General medical conditions – such as strokes, neoplasms, infections, autoimmune disorders, neurodegenerative diseases, and metabolic derangements – and certain drugs have all been associated with catatonia
- Infectious and autoimmune etiologies account for roughly 29% of cases associated with general medical causes
- Meningitis and encephalitis as well as bacterial, viral, or fungal infections may result in catatonia
- Autoimmune processes, particularly N-methyl-D-aspartate receptor (NMDA-R) encephalitis and systemic lupus erythematosus (SLE) also have a strong association with catatonia

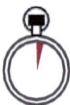

Two-minute tutorial
Catatonia
- Catatonia is a severe motor syndrome with an estimated prevalence among psychiatric inpatients of about 10%
- Catatonia was originally diagnosed as a subtype of schizophrenia; however, it may be diagnosed as: a specifier for depressive, bipolar, and psychotic disorders; as a separate diagnosis in the context of another medical condition; or as another specified diagnosis
  - Catatonia should be considered in any patient with a deterioration in psychomotor functioning and responsiveness
- Catatonia is also seen in children and adolescents. As many as 15–20% of children with developmental disorder may develop catatonia of unknown etiology

PATIENT FILE

Only 3 of 12 symptoms (catalepsy, waxy flexibility, stupor, agitation, mutism, negativism, posturing, mannerisms, stereotypies, grimacing, echolalia, and echopraxia) need to be present in order to diagnose catatonia

Treatments for catatonia

- The first part of effective treatment for catatonia is its quick and correct diagnosis
  - General medical conditions may mask symptoms of catatonia
- Rating scales, such as the BFCRS, can be used to detect and quantify catatonia and may help guide treatment
  - The BFCRS is a 23-item scale, with ratings for each item made solely based on observed behavior
  - Each item is ranked on a Likert scale
  - Immobility/stupor: is the patient extremely hypoactive, immobile, minimally engaged?
  - Mutism: is the patient verbally responsive or minimally responsive?
  - Staring: does the patient have a fixed gaze, little or no visual scanning of the environment, decreased blinking?
  - Posturing/catalepsy: does the patient spontaneously maintain posture, including mundane (sitting or standing) for long periods of time without reacting?
  - Grimacing: does the patient maintain odd facial expressions?
  - Echopraxia/echolalia: does the patient mimic the examiner's movement (echopraxia) or speech (echolalia)?
  - Stereotypy: does the patient engage in repetitive, non-goal-directed motor activity (e.g., finger-play; repeatedly touching, patting or rubbing self)?
    - The abnormality is not inherent in the act itself but the frequency
  - Mannerisms: does the patient exhibit odd, purposeful movements (hopping or walking tiptoe, saluting passers-by, or exaggerated caricatures of mundane movements)?
    - The abnormality is inherent in the act itself
  - Stereotyped and meaningless repetition of words and phrases (verbigeration): does the patient engage in repetition of phrases or sentences (like a scratched record)?
  - Rigidity: does the patient maintain a rigid position despite efforts to be moved (exclude if cog-wheeling or tremor present)?
  - Negativism: does the patient exhibit apparently motiveless resistance to instructions or attempts to move/examine them?

PATIENT FILE

- Do they exhibit contrary behavior, in which the behavior is the exact opposite of instruction?
  - Waxy flexibility: during repositioning of patient, does the patient offer initial resistance before allowing themselves to be repositioned, similar to that of a bending candle (also defined as slow resistance to movement as the patient allows the examiner to place their extremities in unusual positions – the limb may remain in the position in which they are placed, or not)
  - Withdrawal: does the patient refuse to eat, drink, and/or make eye contact?
  - Excitement: does the patient exhibit extreme hyperactivity, constant motor unrest which is apparently non-purposeful? (Not to be attributed to akathisia or goal-directed agitation)
  - Impulsivity: does the patient suddenly engage in inappropriate behavior (e.g., runs down hallway, starts screaming, or takes off clothes) without provocation? (Afterwards, they can give no, or only a facile, explanation)
  - Automatic obedience: does the patient exhibit exaggerated cooperation with examiner's request or spontaneous continuation of movement requested?
  - Passive obedience (*mitgehen*): does the patient raise their arm in response to light pressure of finger despite instructions to the contrary
  - Muscle resistance (*gegenhalten*): does the patient have involuntary resistance to passive movement of a limb to a new position? (Resistance increases with the speed of the movement)
  - Motorically stuck (ambitendency): does the patient appear stuck in indecisive, hesitant motor movements?
  - Grasp reflex: does striking the patient's open palm with two extended fingers of the examiner's hand result in automatic closure of patient's hand?
  - Perseveration: does the patient repeatedly return to same topic or persist with the same movements?
  - Combativeness: does the patient exhibit belligerence or aggression, usually in an undirected manner, without explanation?
  - Autonomic abnormality: does the patient have abnormality of body temperature (fever), blood pressure, pulse, respiratory rate, inappropriate sweating, flushing?
- The first-line treatment of catatonia is generally high-dose benzodiazepines

PATIENT FILE

- A treatment response is usually seen within 3–7 days
- There is no agreement on how long to administer benzodiazepines. Tapering can cause the catatonia symptoms to return, which necessitates the continuation of benzodiazepines for an unknown length of time
- ECT is an established treatment for catatonia that has been shown to be highly effective

Post-test question

What is the first-line treatment for catatonia?

A. Antipsychotics
B. Benzodiazepines
C. ECT
D. Supportive medical treatment

Answer: B

References

1. Bush, G., Fink, M., Petrides, G., Dowling, F., & Francis, A. (1996). Catatonia. I. Rating scale and standardized examination. *Acta Psychiatrica Scandinavica*, 93(2), 129–136.
2. Edinoff, A. N., Kaufman, S. E., Hollier, J. W., et al. (2021). Catatonia: clinical overview of the diagnosis, treatment, and clinical challenges. *Neurology International*, 13(4), 570–586. https://doi.org/10.3390/neurolint13040057.
3. Pelzer, A., van der Heijden, F., & den Boer, E. (2018). Systematic review of catatonia treatment. *Neuropsychiatric Disease and Treatment*, 14, 317–326. https://doi.org/10.2147/NDT.S147897.
4. Rajagopal, S. (2007). Catatonia. *Advances in Psychiatric Treatment* 13(1), 51–59. https://doi.org/10.1192/apt.bp.106.002360.
5. Sienaert, P., Dhossche, D. M., Vancampfort, D., De Hert, M., & Gazdag, G. (2014). A clinical review of the treatment of catatonia. *Frontiers in Psychiatry*, Dec. 9, 5, 181. https://doi.org/10.3389/fpsyt.2014.00181. PMID: 25538636; PMCID: PMC4260674.

PATIENT FILE

11

Negative syndrome: Nothing and nobody

The Psychopharmocological Dilemma: Once the positive symptoms of schizophrenia have been stabilized, what can clinicians do to alleviate persistent negative symptoms?

Michael McGee and Rocco Marotta

Pretest self-assessment question

What treatment poses the best likelihood of ameliorating the negative symptoms of schizophrenia?

A. Cognitive behavioral therapy (CBT), cognitive remediation, and social skills training
B. Antidepressants
C. A change of antipsychotic
D. Oxytocin
E. A combination of the above

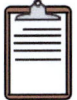

Patient evaluation on intake

- A 21-year-old single upper-middle-class Caucasian male who was a student at an elite college, with self-reported history of bipolar disorder, obsessive–compulsive disorder (OCD), and alcohol dependence in remission, who presents for stabilization of his worsening mood instability, escalating paranoia, and suicidal ideation (SI). Patient reports, "My meds are just not working. I am bipolar. I have anxiety issues, paranoia and get overwhelmed"

Psychiatric history

- At age 20, patient has "very intense mood swings" that happen over the course of a day. He felt the newspaper was talking to him and isolated in his room. Started ziprasidone and then switched to aripiprazole. Had SI, and acted on it once, going to the top floor of a building at school. Patient reports racing thoughts and thought issues triggered by interpersonal relationships, where he may become paranoid. Denies A/V hallucinations, referential ideation, or thought broadcasting. Started using alcohol at 17 and by 20 began binging frequently, vomiting and blacking out. Has used cannabis for 3 years
- Patient completed a residential program for mood lability, alcohol, and cannabis dependence. He was diagnosed with bipolar II disorder as well as OCD during this stay, with informal testing

PATIENT FILE

- Patient readmitted to the hospital after an increase in anxiety and paranoia led him to mistrust everyone so that he was unable to leave the house. He isolated and was convinced that headlights behind him while in the car were always the police; a phone ringing was to tell him he was in trouble. The increased anxiety led to anhedonia where he was no longer able to read. He could not concentrate, had racing thoughts, restlessness, and an increase in energy. He had a constant sense of doom. Sleep disturbance. Periods of mania followed by depression with SI. Diagnosed with schizoaffective disorder, bipolar type. Once stabilized on clozapine, had persistent avolition, asociality, and anhedonia, and was unable to function

Social and personal history

He attended excellent schools. Always described as highly intelligent with excellent verbal skills. Began using drugs and alcohol at an early age. Was pursuing a college degree when first symptoms appeared. After hospitalization and a residential program, he was able to complete his Bachelor's degree, and subsequently completed a Master's degree.

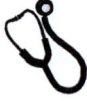

Medical history

No history of head injury, loss of consciousness, seizures, or cardiac problems.

Family history

- Maternal side: substance use
- Paternal side: distant relative with mood disorder

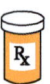

Medication history

- First discharge from residential program: aripiprazole, duloxetine, gabapentin, imipramine, multivitamins, senna
- Second hospitalization (1 month later): imipramine, duloxetine, aripiprazole, gabapentin, multivitamins, oxcarbazepine, quetiapine
- Third discharge from residential program: clozapine, lithium, multivitamins, quetiapine, lamotrigine
- Current medications: clozapine, oxytocin, lamotrigine, armodafinil, metformin, multivitamins

Current history

He currently has a full-time job and meaningful personal relationships. Is compliant with his medications.

PATIENT FILE

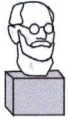
Psychotherapy history
He started psychotherapy when he was 18 for depression and anxiety. Was also in an intensive 4-week residential dialectical behavioral therapy (DBT) program and has continued in outpatient DBT therapy for 7 years. He has also continued in psychotherapy and remains close to his psychopharmacologist.

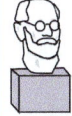
Psychotherapy moment
When treated with oxytocin, he began to talk and make eye contact.

Current Medications
- Clozapine augmented with oxytocin

Attending physician's mental notes (at intervals)
Three years into taking oxytocin, patient reports interesting experience: missed oxytocin for a few days and had less on some days: "I became very flat, no energy. It was hard to be open and spontaneous. I went back to extreme passivity."

Four years later: Oxytocin "calms me down. If my anxiety has my thoughts going, 5–10 minutes later I feel calm and I stop worrying."

Five years into taking oxytocin: Patient reports becoming much more social on oxytocin. He gives good eye contact. Mother reports her son being more playful, charming, and related, on combination of clozapine and oxytocin.

Six years into taking oxytocin: Patient reports "I feel like it works. I feel I need it."

He was always different as a child. Consultants saw him as gifted. He never felt he fit in socially and was often isolated and marginalized until leaving high school. In college he found freedom and "his own people," yet within a short time he was more openly psychotic.

While at college his functioning continued to deteriorate. He had greater and greater social withdrawal and isolation, culminating in a suicide attempt, and hospital admission.

When first seen, the patient seemed to be grossly psychotic and withdrawn. He hardly spoke, was unmotivated, and met the diagnostic criteria for schizoaffective disorder, bipolar type.

Intensive DBT seemed to make no impact and serial treatments with ziprasidone, aripiprazole, and risperidone did not change the presentation of illness. Therefore, we undertook a trial of clozapine.

With clozapine, there was improvement: less overtly anxious, less psychotic, and able to be motivated and be around people more

PATIENT FILE

(although still quite withdrawn). Importantly, from that point on, he maintained absolute sobriety and began going to AA meetings, although he sat alone in the back of the room.

During this period, he did not date but was able to finish schoolwork, with the help of the addition of armodafinil. This was seen as an enormous improvement. His Positive and Negative Symptom Scale (PANSS) scores improved remarkably. However, he was not happy and was always alone.

At this point, since he was withdrawn and isolated and still presented as having negative symptoms of schizophrenia (albeit with high intellectual capacity), lamotrigine was added with minor effect.

At this point, 2 years after initiating clozapine, the patient was now a young man with high intellectual capacity, withdrawn and isolated, still presenting with prominent negative symptoms. He was sober and medication-compliant. Sublingual oxytocin was added to his medication regimen at a dose of 20 IU BID, and titrated a few weeks later to 40 IU BID.

Within 2 weeks, the medical staff, family, and friends noted remarkable changes. He began sitting in the front rows at AA meetings, he began sharing at meetings and helping in setting up the room. He began making friends, and in meeting with his psychiatrist he finally was able to make eye contact and begin talking directly.

Case outcome; use of outcome measures

After stabilizing his psychosis with clozapine and adding oxytocin, the patient had a marked reduction in social anxiety and withdrawal. His psychosocial functioning continued to gradually improve over the subsequent 6 years as he experienced the rewards of engaging in prosocial activities.

Case debrief

This patient with severe, treatment-resistant schizoaffective disorder, bipolar type, had a stabilization of his mood and psychotic symptoms with clozapine, but was left with persistent, disabling negative symptoms. His negative symptoms were markedly reduced with the addition of oxytocin to his medication regimen, in combination with psychotherapy.

Take-home points

- Negative symptoms include blunted affect, alogia (reduction in quantity of words spoken), avolition (reduced goal-directed activity due to decreased motivation), asociality, and anhedonia (reduced experience of pleasure)

PATIENT FILE

- 40–60% of patients with schizophrenia and schizoaffective disorder suffer from negative symptoms that impair functioning and quality of life
- Negative symptoms are difficult to treat; they often do not improve with antipsychotic treatment. They are an unmet psychiatric need for which new treatments are lacking
- Oxytocin and other medications, when combined with psychotherapeutic interventions, hold promise for mitigating the severity of negative symptoms. Patience and perseverance in addressing this disabling condition are required

Performance in practice: confessions of a psychopharmacologist

- Psychopharmacologists can overlook negative symptoms in the flurry to stabilize positive symptoms of psychosis
- Treating positive symptoms, while important, is not enough to habilitate psychosocial functioning and quality of life. Most patients suffering from schizophrenia and schizoaffective disorder need more than just an antipsychotic. In the case of this patient, it took several hospitalizations and a lengthy course of treatment before his negative symptoms were addressed

Tips and pearls

- Be on the lookout to identify and address negative symptoms at the start of treatment. Attend to the patient's level of interaction, interest, and engagement. Inquire into social activities and interests
- Assess medication side effects that may present as or aggravate negative symptoms
- Psychopharmacology should be combined with CBT, cognitive remediation, social skills training, aerobic exercise, and vocational rehabilitation to optimize outcomes and minimize negative symptoms
- Psychosocial interventions – people, place, and purpose – are necessary for the comprehensive habilitation of severe psychotic disorders

Two-minute tutorial

Psychopharmacological options that show limited efficacy for reducing negative symptoms include:

- Antidepressants, including fluoxetine and trazodone
- Ondansetron in doses ranging from 4 to 16 mg daily

PATIENT FILE

- Folate and vitamin B12 in doses of 2 mg and 400 ug respectively. Differences in folate absorption merit consideration of the use of L-methylfolate instead of folic acid
- Clozapine, amisulpride, olanzapine, and cariprazine may be more effective for schizophrenia with prominent negative symptoms
- Intranasal and sublingual oxytocin have shown promise in reducing negative symptoms. Sublingual doses of 20–40 IU BID have shown efficacy in a case series of patients with treatment-resistant schizophrenia treated with clozapine

Secondary negative symptoms may improve with treatment of the underlying condition. Causes of secondary negative symptoms include depression, anxiety, antipsychotic-related sedation, chronic insomnia, substance misuse, chronic insomnia, medical comorbidities, and environmental deprivation.

Electroconvulsive therapy (ECT) and transcranial magnetic stimulation (TMS) may benefit some patients with negative symptoms.

The treatment of schizophrenia and schizoaffective disorder should always include psychosocial and habilitative treatments, including social skills training, cognitive remediation therapy, aerobic exercise, and CBT. These interventions yield moderate effects on negative symptoms, including a reduction of apathy and improved motivation. Family support can also be of benefit for psychoeducation, behavioral problem solving, and crisis management.

Post-test question

What treatment poses the best likelihood of ameliorating the negative symptoms of schizophrenia?

A. Cognitive behavioral therapy (CBT), cognitive remediation, and social skills training
B. Antidepressants
C. A change of antipsychotic
D. Oxytocin
E. A combination of the above

Answer: E

References

1. Bennett, A. & Vila, T. (2010). The role of ondansetron in the treatment of schizophrenia. *British Journal of Psychiatry*, 44, 1301–1306.
2. Carbon, M. & Correll, C. U. (2014). Thinking and acting beyond the positive: the role of the cognitive and negative symptoms in schizophrenia. *CNS Spectrums*, 19(Suppl. 1), 38–52, quiz 35–37, 53. https://doi.org/10.1017/S1092852914000601.

PATIENT FILE

3. Correll, C. U. & Schooler, N. R. (2020) Negative symptoms in schizophrenia: a review and clinical guide for recognition, assessment, and treatment. *Neuropsychiatric Disease and Treatment*, Feb. 21, 16, 519–534. https://doi.org/10.2147/NDT.S225643. PMID: 32110026; PMCID: PMC7041437.
4. Guo, J., Liu, K., Liao, Y., et al. (2024). Efficacy and feasibility of aerobic exercise interventions as an adjunctive treatment for patients with schizophrenia: a meta-analysis. *Schizophrenia*, 10(2). https://doi.org/10.1038/s41537-023-00426-0.
5. Huhn, M., et al. (2019). Comparative efficacy and tolerability of 32 oral antipsychotics for the acute treatment of adults with multi-episode schizophrenia: a systematic review and network meta-analysis. *Lancet*, 394, 939–951.
6. Insel, T. (2022). *Healing: Our Path from Mental Illness to Mental Health*. New York: Penguin.
7. Krause, M., Zhu, Y., Huhn, M., et al. (2018). Antipsychotic drugs for patients with schizophrenia and predominant or prominent negative symptoms: a systematic review and meta-analysis. *European Archives of Psychiatry and Clinical Neuroscience*, 268(7), 625–639. https://doi.org/10.1007/s00406-018-0869-3.
8. Marotta, R., Buono, F., Garakani, A., Collins, E., Cerrito, B., & Rowe, D. (2020). The effects of augmenting clozapine with oxytocin in schizophrenia: an initial case series. *Annals of Clinical Psychiatry*, 32, 90–96.
9. Roffman, J. L., Lamberti, J. S., Achtyes, E., et al. (2013). Randomized multicenter investigation of folate plus vitamin B12 supplementation in schizophrenia. *JAMA Psychiatry*, 70(5), 481–489. https://doi.org/10.1001/jamapsychiatry.2013.900.
10. Singh, S. P., Singh, V., Kar, N., & Chan, K. (2010). Efficacy of antidepressants in treating the negative symptoms of chronic schizophrenia: meta-analysis. *British Journal of Psychiatry*, 197(3), 174–179. https://doi.org/10.1192/bjp.bp.109.067710. Erratum in: *Br J Psychiatry*. 2011 Feb;198:159. PMID: 20807960.
11. Tan, X., Martin, D., Lee, J., & Tor, P. C. (2022). The impact of electroconvulsive therapy on negative symptoms in schizophrenia and their association with clinical outcomes. *Brain Science*, 12, 545. https://doi.org/10.3390/brainsci12050545.
12. Tseng, P. T., Zeng, B. S., Hung, C. M., et al. (2022). Assessment of noninvasive brain stimulation interventions for negative symptoms of schizophrenia: a systematic review and network meta-analysis. *JAMA Psychiatry*, 79, 770–779.

PATIENT FILE

12

Post-psychotic depression: Too good to be true, so it's blue

The Psychopharmacological Dilemma: How is post-psychotic depression treated?

Maanasi Chandarana

Pretest self-assessment question

Which of the following statements is NOT true regarding depression in schizophrenia?

A. Depression can occur at any time in the schizophrenia illness course
B. While receiving treatment with antipsychotic medication, the relative risks of suicide and violence due to concurrent depressive symptomatology are unchanged
C. Behavioral therapies are considered an effective treatment option
D. Depression associated with a patient's auditory hallucinatory experience is not related to the patient's perception of the voice frequency, content, or loudness, but rather to the omnipotence of the voice

Answer: B

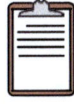

Patient evaluation on intake

The patient is a 65-year-old male with a history of schizophrenia and remote history of alcohol use disorder (AUD). The patient was committed to a forensic state hospital for continued psychiatric assessment, treatment, and care after he was court-adjudicated not guilty by reason of insanity (NGRI) for a felonious charge. While hospitalized, he reported multiple grandiose, persecutory, and somatic-based delusions as well as auditory hallucinations; and he exhibited disordered thought patterns despite maintenance on therapeutic dosing of multiple antipsychotic medications (including clozapine) for adequate treatment trials. Due to his persistent ultra-treatment-resistant psychotic symptomatology, he was referred for electroconvulsive therapy (ECT). During his treatment course with ECT, the patient reported some improvement in his psychotic symptomatology, including less continuous and distressing perceptual disturbances. However, the patient also reported concomitant onset of depressive symptoms, including sadness, guilt, anhedonia, hopelessness, and helplessness.

PATIENT FILE

Psychiatric history
- Mental health history with onset in early adulthood
  - He reported hearing voices and paranoid, grandiose beliefs
  - He exhibited referential and disorganized thoughts
- Behaviorally, the patient reported suicidal ideas and had a history of at least two previous suicide attempts by overdose and self-inflicted laceration to his neck
  - The patient denied physical altercations, interpersonal conflict, and he did not have a history of engaging in violent or assaultive behaviors
- The patient received community-based outpatient and inpatient psychiatric services
  - He was involuntarily psychiatrically hospitalized following suicide attempts
- The patient reported consuming hard liquor and two six-packs of beer daily for decades
  - The patient was admitted to an inpatient rehabilitation center for problematic alcohol use
- The patient was treated with multiple trials of antipsychotic and mood-stabilizer medications as well as a benzodiazepine and beta-blocker medication
  - The patient reported positive treatment response with prior decade-long trial of treatment with clozapine

Social and personal history
- The patient's parents were separated, and he was raised by his stepfather, with whom he said he did not have a good relationship
- He denied experiencing physical and sexual abuse
- Although subjected to disciplinary actions while attending school, he graduated high school
- The patient joined the Armed Services and worked for years as a military mechanic
- Following completion of his military service, he was gainfully employed as a door salesman and electrician, as well as in construction and at restaurants
- He was married three times and fathered two children

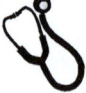

Medical history
- Hypertension
- Hypothyroidism
- Cirrhosis of the liver

PATIENT FILE

- A pre-admission MRI of the patient's brain revealed nonspecific hyperintensity of the putamen
- A post-admission MRI of the patient's brain revealed mild to moderate white matter disease and generalized cerebral atrophy

Family history
- The patient's familial history is notable for possible bipolar disorder in his parents, and bipolar disorder as well as Attention-Deficit/Hyperactivity Disorder (ADHD) in his biological children

Current history
- The patient presented to the evaluation as calm, polite, and cooperative
  - However, the interview was prematurely terminated after the patient voiced sexually inappropriate comments to the admitting psychiatrist
- He was dressed in hospital attire, ungroomed, and disheveled
- His speech rate and rhythm were normal; his speech volume was low
- The patient did not demonstrate psychomotor agitation, retardation, and abnormal involuntary movements
- He exhibited a flattened affective range
- He reported self-inflicted laceration to wrist prior to his hospitalization. He denied experiencing homicidal ideations
- He was described as a poor historian; he denied experiencing auditory hallucinations
- His thought process was fragmented, incoherent, illogical, tangentially to loosely related, and disorganized
- The patient was alert, oriented to person and mostly time, but not place. His recent and remote memory, ability to abstract, and attention were deemed poor
- He demonstrated deficits in his fund of knowledge, cognition, insight, and judgment

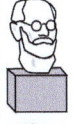

Psychotherapy history
- There is no known psychotherapy history to report

Mechanism of action moment
- Ziprasidone
  - Blocks D_2 receptor
    - Reduces positive symptoms and provides mood stabilization
  - Modulates multiple serotoninergic receptors

PATIENT FILE

- 2A receptor blockade
  - Enhances dopamine release
    - Improved cognitive and affective functioning
- Interaction with 2C and 1A receptor
  - Targets cognitive and affective symptoms
- Interaction with 1D and 5HT7 receptor
  - At higher medication doses and in conjunction with serotonin and norepinephrine receptors, may have treatment effect on affective symptoms
- Lithium carbonate
  - Mechanism of action is complex and not well understood
  - Thought to recruit second messenger signaling pathway including that of cyclic adenosine monophosphate (cAMP) and cyclic guanosine monophosphate (cGMP)
  - Involved in genetic transcription and post-translational modification
    - Competes with other cations involved in signal transduction
  - Decreases the glutamine : gamma aminobutyric acid (GABA) ratio
    - Prevents loss of phosphorylated cAMP Response Element Binding Protein
      - Inhibits glutamate activation of protein kinases
        - Provides neuroprotective effects
- Divalproex
  - Stabilizes neuronal membrane by optimizing K+ efflux and Na+ influx
    - Decreases the glutamate:GABA ratio
      - Decreases glutamate by stimulating glutamine synthetase
      - Increases GABA by increasing GABA levels, GABA release, GABA-B receptor density, and neuronal responsiveness to GABA; and decreases GABA catabolism and turnover
  - Dampens excitatory systems by decreasing aspartate release, cerebrospinal fluid (CSF), somatostatin, and N-methyl-D-aspartate (NMDA)-mediated circuits
  - Increases dopamine turnover
- Hydroxyzine
  - Blocks histamine (H1) receptors
- Duloxetine
  - Blocks serotonin and norepinephrine reuptake pumps facilitating increased serotoninergic and noradrenergic neurotransmission
    - Blockade of norepinephrine reuptake in frontal cortex conceivably increases dopamine neurotransmission in this region

PATIENT FILE

- Potentially desensitizes serotonin 1A and beta-adrenergic receptors
- Weakly blocks dopamine reuptake and increases dopamine neurotransmission
- Haloperidol:
  - Blocks D_2 receptors
    - Reduces positive symptoms and aggressive behaviors
    - In the nigrostriatal pathway, D_2 blockade improves tics and associated symptoms of Tourette's
- Mirtazapine
  - Blocks serotonin 1A, 2C, and 5HT3 receptors
  - Blocks alpha 2 adrenergic presynaptic receptor, facilitating increase in norepinephrine neurotransmission
  - Blocks alpha 2 adrenergic presynaptic serotoninergic neuron receptor, facilitating increase in serotoninergic neurotransmission
  - Blocks H1 histamine receptors
- Clozapine
  - Antagonizes D_2 receptors and serotonin 2A receptors
    - Blocking D_2 receptors reduces positive symptoms of psychosis and provides mood stabilization
    - Blocking serotonin 2A receptors enhances dopamine release in brain regions to minimize motor side effects and improve cognitive and affective symptoms
  - Interacts with 5-HT_{2C} and 5-HT_{1A} which may promote increased efficacy in treatment of cognitive and affective symptoms
- Risperidone
  - Blocks D_2 receptors
    - Reduces positive symptoms and provides mood stabilization
  - Blocks serotonin 2A receptors
    - Enhances dopamine release in brain regions, which reduces motor side effects and enhances cognition and affect
- Olanzapine
  - Blocks D_2 receptor
    - Reduces positive symptoms and provides mood stabilization
  - Blocks multiple serotoninergic receptors
    - 2A receptor blockade
      - Enhances dopamine release
        - Improved cognitive and affective functioning
    - Blockade of serotonin 2C receptor
      - Targets cognitive and affective symptoms
- Sertraline
  - Boosts serotoninergic neurotransmission
  - Desensitizes serotonin 1A receptors
  - Blocks serotonin and dopamine reuptake pumps

PATIENT FILE

Attending physician's mental notes
- The patient was diagnosed with schizophrenia and records reflect his disordered thinking, grandiose beliefs, and inappropriate behaviors with female staff
- At the time of admission to the forensic hospital, he exhibited persistent psychotic symptoms and was a limited historian
- The patient reported therapeutic benefit from treatment prescribed at the referring facility; therefore, those medications were continued:
  - Ziprasidone 20 mg p.o. qHS
  - Lithium carbonate 150 mg p.o. qHS
- Future psychotropic medication consideration includes retrial of clozapine
- Due to the patient's significant memory problems, he may benefit from neurological and neuropsychological evaluation and testing

Further investigation
- Admission labs yielded increased creatinine and blood urea nitrogen (BUN) concentrations in the patient's blood
  - Lithium carbonate was discontinued, and divalproex was added
- To further treat the patient's psychotic symptoms, ziprasidone was discontinued, and olanzapine was ordered
- Therapeutic drug monitoring yielded a supratherapeutic serum divalproex drug level of 114 mcg/mL
  - Divalproex dosing was decreased
- Despite an adequate trial of treatment with olanzapine, the patient reported persistent anxiety symptoms stemming from his somatic preoccupation
  - As the patient also shared his experience of neuropathic lower-extremity pain, prescribed medication trials included with gabapentin, hydroxyzine, and duloxetine

Case outcome
- The patient experienced psychiatric decompensation in the context of concomitant medical infections
  - The patient's paranoid and delusional ideation resulted in his excessive pacing behaviors, fasting, and significant weight loss
  - To further target his symptoms, haloperidol and mirtazapine were added as adjunct therapies to his medication regimen and increased in dosage
- Following recovery from comorbid medical illnesses, the patient continued to report auditory hallucinatory experiences along with delusional ideation, and to exhibit nonlinearly related thoughts

PATIENT FILE

- Pre-treatment lab work as well as an electrocardiogram (EKG) were obtained in anticipation of clozapine treatment
  - The patient's psychiatric history revealed previous positive treatment response with clozapine therapy whilst the patient received community care
- The patient received trials of multiple psychotropic medications, including with haloperidol, mirtazapine, duloxetine, and risperidone without remission of his psychotic symptoms
- Clozapine treatment was initiated; however, the patient developed profound neutropenia (absolute neutrophil count [ANC] of 200 cells/mcL)
  - Clozapine and divalproex were discontinued
  - Olanzapine was continued

Case debrief
- Our patient was diagnosed with schizophrenia and AUD
- He was found NGRI to a felony charge, and he was committed to a state forensic hospital
- The patient reported grandiose, persecutory, and somatic-based delusions, as well as auditory hallucinations, and he exhibited disorganized thinking
- Despite adjustments to the dosing of his prescribed medications, including ziprasidone, lithium, valproate, and olanzapine, the patient reported persistent psychotic and anxiety symptoms
  - Lithium was discontinued in the context of the patient's advanced age and decreased renal function
  - Valproate was reduced as therapeutic drug monitoring yielded supratherapeutic drug levels
- Trials of gabapentin, duloxetine, and hydroxyzine for anxiety were ineffective and were subsequently discontinued
- The patient suffered from a medical illness which led to his psychiatric decompensation, excessive pacing behaviors, decreased oral intake, and weight loss
  - Haloperidol and mirtazapine were added as adjunctive treatments and, ultimately, stopped due to the lack of efficacy
- Although trialed on clozapine, the patient developed neutropenia, and clozapine as well as valproate were discontinued
- The patient received treatment with risperidone and olanzapine but experienced persistent distressing auditory hallucinations and somatic delusions
- To treat his persistent psychotic symptoms, the patient was referred to ECT

PATIENT FILE

- The patient received a course of ECT and, during maintenance phase, the patient reported improved quality, volume, and content of auditory hallucinations
  - However, the patient also reported new onset and predominance of depressive symptoms, including insomnia, anorexia, sadness, guilt, hopelessness, as well as accompanying worry
  - The patient's onset and presentation of depressive symptoms concurrent with improved psychotic symptoms in the preceding months, and absence of a primary affective disorder, were clinically consistent with post-psychotic depression
- The frequency of the patient's ECT was increased; and sertraline was added to his medication regimen
- Ultimately, the patient reported cognitive side effects associated with ECT treatment and declined further treatment with ECT

Take-home points

- Patients diagnosed with schizophrenia who develop comorbid depression are more likely to engage in violent behaviors; to experience legal and substance-related problems; to be victimized; to have thoughts of suicide; to report poorer life satisfaction, mental functioning, family relationships, and medication adherence; and are more likely to relapse
- The prevalence of depression in patients diagnosed with schizophrenia varies widely and ranges from 7% to 75%. The chronicity of schizophrenia, and the variability of depression assessment tools, can influence the prevalence rates. Other clinical factors, such as the diversity in presentations characterized as depression, may also help explain the wide range
  - Depression can present as a symptom, affect, and syndrome
    - An example of a depressive symptom is a distressing, sad mood
    - Affect is a projected mood state based upon an individuals' subjective experience as he or she interacts with his or her internal and external environment
    - Depressive syndrome: constellation of depressive symptoms as well as cognitive and vegetative features (i.e., pessimism, guilt, impaired concentration, lack of confidence, loss of interest or pleasure) and concurrent disturbances in sleep, appetite, and energy level
- Risk factors for depression in schizophrenia include:
  - Age: Increased age is correlated to various psychosocial stressors such as:

PATIENT FILE

- Stressful life events including chronic medical conditions and occupational stress
  - Higher risk of chronic diseases with increasing age is due to financial strain, self-neglect, and long-term use of psychotropic medications
  - Work-related stress often increases because of severe occupational dysfunction and social isolation in schizophrenia
- Longer illness duration has a negative impact on cognitive and social functioning and is associated with self-stigma, poor insight, and demoralization
- Inpatients are more likely to suffer from comorbid depression
  - Hospitalized schizophrenia patients experience severe psychiatric symptoms and relapse, which contribute to increased likelihood of comorbid depression
- Two-thirds to three-fourths of patients experience perceptual disturbances in the form of auditory hallucinations and are moderately distressed to depressed by these symptoms
  - Depression is related to the patient's belief in the power of the voice (but not the voice frequency, content, or loudness)
- Depressive episodes in schizophrenia can:
  - Present through all phases of schizophrenia as an independent and significant symptom dimension
    - Up to 80% of patients experience a clinically significant depressive episode at least once during the early phase of the schizophrenia illness course
  - Be associated with positive symptoms in the acute phase
    - May remit with atypical antipsychotic treatment
  - Overlap with negative symptoms in the post-psychotic or chronic phase
    - Depressive symptoms occurring in the post-psychotic phase are colloquially termed "post-psychotic depression"
- Confounders of depression in schizophrenia include neuroleptic-induced akinesia and akathisia, as well as neuroleptic-induced dysphoria (negative symptoms)
  - Neuroleptic-induced akathisia
    - Akathisia is accompanied by dysphoria and associated with SI and behaviors
  - Neuroleptic-induced akinesia is defined by difficulty initiating or sustaining motor movement
    - Patients can report concurrent sadness, guilt, and shame
  - Neuroleptic-induced dysphoria is theorized as a response to "more than the minimum required" anti-dopaminergic

PATIENT FILE

       medication which exacerbates negative symptomatology of
       schizophrenia
       - Conceivably, this could occur in patients who are vulnerable
         to fluctuant dopamine concentrations, including abundance
         (psychosis) and droughts (negative symptoms) of the
         neurotransmitter
- Differential diagnosis of depression in schizophrenia
  - Includes medical pathology of various organ systems
    - Cardiovascular and pulmonary pathology; immune
      and hematologic dysregulation; cancer; and metabolic,
      neurological, and endocrine disorders
  - Medications
    - Prescription of: beta-blockers, other antihypertensive agents,
      sedative hypnotics, antineoplastics, barbiturates, nonsteroidal
      anti-inflammatory drugs, sulfonamides, and indomethacin
    - Discontinuation of corticosteroids and psychostimulants
  - Acute and chronic, or discontinuation of, use of alcohol,
    cannabis, cocaine, narcotics
  - Discontinuation of nicotine and caffeine
  - Negative symptoms of schizophrenia overlap with depressive
    symptoms in schizophrenia in domains of interest, pleasure,
    energy, or motivation, psychomotor activity, concentration, as
    well as social withdrawal
    - Diminished capacity to experience pleasure (anhedonia) can
      further distinguish negative symptoms from depression
      - Motivational anhedonia (motivation to pursue rewards)
        and consummatory anhedonia (pleasure experienced in
        anticipation of or response to rewards)
        - Consummatory anhedonia and difficulty in anticipating
          future pleasure may be more in keeping with
          depression, whereas motivational anhedonia is
          classified a primary negative symptom
    - Negative symptoms may be distinguishable from depression
      by the presence of a blunted affect
    - Depression is characterized by mood (anxiety, hopelessness,
      and helplessness) and cognitive features including guilt and
      suicidality
    - The Calgary Depression Scale for Schizophrenia (CDSS)
      is widely used to distinguish depression from negative
      symptoms
      - The CDSS emphasizes subjective reports of hopelessness,
        guilt, and SI over agitation, anhedonia, and paranoid
        symptoms, the focus of other depression rating scales

PATIENT FILE

- Demoralization: chronic reactions to disappointment or stress
  - Schizophrenic patients who sense they have less control regarding their illness (i.e., demoralization) are more likely to experience depression
    - Demoralization is important to discern clinically as it is responsive to psychosocial interventions
- "Prodrome of Psychotic Relapse"
  - Prodromal symptoms preceding psychotic decompensation can include dysphoria accompanied by anxiety, withdrawal, guilt, and shame; hypervigilance, perceptual disturbances, or the overinterpretation of perceptions or events
  - These symptoms last days to weeks and supersede prominent and definitive psychotic symptoms
- Depressive episode in schizoaffective disorder
- There are limited options for treating co-occurring depression in schizophrenia
  - There is a dearth of sufficiently powered, randomized controlled trials utilizing antidepressants for the treatment of depression in schizophrenia
  - Studies supporting antidepressant use for treatment of depression in schizophrenia may be confounded by various biases

Performance in practice: confessions of a psychopharmacologist

What are clinical considerations for patients diagnosed with schizophrenia and experiencing co-occurring or post-psychotic depression?

- Although the occurrence of depression in schizophrenia is highly variable, depression is believed to present in first-episode psychosis (FEP) in approximately 80% of cases; in 50% of patients experiencing acute psychosis; and post-psychotic depression has a prevalence rate of about 25–75%
- Depressive symptoms are a harbinger of psychotic decompensation and progression to FEP
- Depressive episodes occurring during the psychotic illness course are associated with poorer outcomes in the domains of safety, mental health relapse and substance use, rehospitalization, medication adherence, social and personal functioning
  - While suffering from depression, patients with schizophrenia may experience increase in suicide and violence risk
    - Clozapine anti-aggressive effect is independent of the psychotropic medication's antipsychotic effect, at an average

PATIENT FILE

serum concentration of 171 ng/dL, and at therapeutic drug levels less than 350 ng/dL
- Clozapine and lithium therapies may decrease suicidality
- Literature supporting the use of antidepressant treatment in first-episode, acute, and chronic phases of psychosis is limited
  - Identifying the stage of the patient's illness may assist with determining potential treatment options
    - While no psychopharmacological agent is demonstrably superior in treating depression occurring at any stage of the schizophrenia illness, depressive symptoms may remit with atypical antipsychotic treatment if associated with acute-phase positive psychotic symptomatology

Tips and pearls

- Depression in schizophrenia is associated with worse outcomes, impaired functioning, personal suffering, higher rates of relapse and rehospitalization, and suicide
  - Themes related to loss, humiliation, entrapment, and defeat may underlie depression in schizophrenia
    - Various authors have proposed that a patient's appraisal of their psychotic episode and diagnosis leads to loss of social goals, roles, and status; is a source of social shame; and represents entrapment and inability to escape their diagnosis
- Depression and schizophrenia have genetic, structural, and symptom overlap
  - Genetic considerations
    - 18% of children born to schizophrenic mothers develop schizophrenia, and 7% develop affective psychosis by 26 years of age
    - An implicated gene in schizophrenia and bipolar disorder is G30/G72 on 13 q
  - Neuroanatomic and neurophysiologic considerations
    - Identified risk factor(s) for development of schizophrenia and depression is volume loss in the prefrontal and temporal cortices, as well as the hippocampus
    - Both depressive and the psychotic symptoms involve dysfunction of central neurotransmitters
      - Implicated neurotransmitters in psychosis are dopamine and glutamate
      - Implicated neurotransmitters include serotonin and noradrenaline in depression
  - Symptom presentation

PATIENT FILE

- Neurotic personality traits and social, interpersonal, and cognitive impairments in childhood and adolescence are precursors to both schizophrenia and depression
- Most patients subsequently diagnosed with schizophrenia and unipolar depression experience a prodromal stage of depressive symptoms and increasing impairment
- Depression in FEP
    - A risk factor for FEP includes childhood trauma
        - 50% of patients experiencing FEP have a history of childhood and physical trauma
    - Psychological underpinnings of depression may be attributed to the personal discrepancy between present circumstance/experience and future goals and self-representation
    - Immune markers under investigation in patients aged 15–25 years of age experiencing FEP are leukocyte elastase, a1-proteinase inhibitor, and S-100
        - Patients with post-psychotic depression had an increase in leukocyte elastase and a1-proteinase inhibitor
            - Higher values were observed in patients with negative affectivity and associated with poorer prognosis (versus patients with positive affectivity and a better prognosis)
    - The years following patients' first psychotic episode are termed post-acute recovery phase
        - Depression during this phase is associated with poor long-term outcomes including increased relapse, suicidality, and poor social and vocational consequences when compared to the sequelae of acute, episodic depression
            - 15% of FEP patients attempt suicide within 3 years of presenting for treatment
    - Post-psychotic depression in FEP is also associated with poor outcomes and impaired social and vocational functioning, as well as increased suicide risk
        - With treatment and improved symptoms and cognition, patients gain insight
            - Increased insight is predictive of depression and suicide in FEP (akin to insight paradox discussed below)
    - Patients experiencing psychosis are believed to only access summaries of autobiographical, episodic events and fewer, specific, detailed memories of positive events while depressed
        - Overgeneralized memory occurs when individuals retrieve a summation versus specific examples of life events and early developmental trauma

- Overgeneralized memory is problematic when imagining specific positive outcomes, prevents access to memories promoting problem solving, and leads to hopelessness
- This phenomenon is observed in individuals diagnosed with unipolar depression, historic depressive episodes, and those who are actively suicidal (irrespective of their history of depression)
  - Psychological approaches to FEP
    - Some authors suggest that self-compassion (i.e., the ability to treat oneself with understanding and kindness during periods of hardship) promotes recovery and growth
      - Self-compassion is believed to decrease ruminative thinking, protect from depression, and reduce psychological harm of stigma in marginalized populations
      - Components of self-compassion
        - Compassionate self-responding: patients are more kind to themselves; recognize that their suffering and imperfection are part of the human experience; and promote a non-judgmental, balanced, and accepting stance toward negative thoughts and emotions
      - Compassion-focused interventions are touted as contributory to improvements in self-compassion, social rank, depression, and shame in the psychosis patient population
      - Uncompassionate self-responding is the term attributed to patients who are highly self-critical of their mistakes and inadequacies, feel alone in their suffering, and overidentify with negative thoughts and emotions such that they are easily overwhelmed by them
        - A study found the presence of an uncompassionate style of relating to oneself, or absence of self-compassion, was a more powerful predictor of depression than the presence of kindness to oneself
    - Mindfulness is defined as "the ability to be aware of and pay attention to what is occurring in the present moment." Can help individuals distance themselves from unhelpful ruminative thought processes surrounding social loss and stigma
      - Can reduce depressive symptoms in FEP
      - Positively associated with satisfaction with life, self-efficacy, and self-esteem in young people at ultra-high risk of psychosis

PATIENT FILE

- Post-psychotic depression can be defined as depression occurring independently of schizophrenia and several months after an acute episode of psychosis
  - Post-psychotic depression was defined in the International Classification of Diseases 10 (ICD–10) as a depressive symptom that "occurs twelve months after psychotic episode while psychotic symptoms are still present but not predominant"
    - Therefore, a patient experiencing post-psychotic depression is one who has suffered from schizophrenia-spectrum illness in the preceding 12 months AND is currently exhibiting depressive symptomatology in addition to persistent hallucinations, thought disorder, or negative symptoms (not attributable to an affective disorder or neuroleptic medication)
  - The Diagnostic Statistical Manual IV (DSM–IV) defines "post psychotic depressive disorder of schizophrenia as a major depressive episode during the residual phase of schizophrenia"
  - Some authors have defined post-psychotic depression as subsequent to remission of acute psychosis and characterized by moderate depression (as reflected in a Beck Depression Inventory [BDI] score of greater than or equal to 15), that is not concomitant with increase in psychotic symptoms, and is preceded by a "subthreshold" or non-depressed phase
  - On average, post-psychotic depressive symptoms occur about 8 months following onset of psychotic symptomatology
- Theoretical etiologies of post-psychotic depression include:
  - "Intrinsic" theory – depression syndrome is an aspect of schizophrenia
  - "Pharmacogenic" theory – depression stems from drug-induced akinetic dysphoria
  - Psychological theory – depression in the context of demoralization from an "uncontrollable" life event (psychosis)
  - Insight paradox – with restoration of some insight, patients' treatment adherence improves and their risk of rehospitalization and psychiatric decompensation decreases
    - However, the patient's improved insight may also contribute to feelings of hopelessness, depression, and suicidality
      - In a recent study, gain in insight was not associated with a worsened depressive state
- Patients who develop post-psychotic depression experience greater loss, humiliation, entrapment, as well as lower self-esteem; and are more self-critical and attribute the cause of psychosis to themselves (self-blame)

PATIENT FILE

- Patients who become depressed believe their future selves are more likely to be defined by "low status roles"; to accept of a less valued social role/goal (termed "down rank"); and to experience internal conflict to change
    - These thoughts of loss, entrapment, and humiliation further depressive symptomatology which contributes to worsening of the thoughts
- Mental health providers may benefit from thoughtful and considered approaches when assessing and diagnosing a patient with schizophrenia with co-occurring depression as depression is present through all phases of schizophrenia as an independent and significant symptom dimension, and there are multiple differential diagnoses and clinical confounders associated with the diagnosis

Two-minute tutorial

- Comorbid depressive symptoms can present in all phases of schizophrenia, and are associated with higher risk of suicide, violence, and polypharmacy; worse psychosocial functioning; and poorer quality of life and functional outcomes
    - Depressive symptoms are noted to be the most common symptom found in patients suffering from schizophrenia
    - Approximately 10% of schizophrenia patients die by suicide
- Depression is linked to an increased risk of transition to first-episode psychosis (FEP), can provoke psychotic decompensation, and can present in post-recovery phases of illness
    - 50% of schizophrenia patients experience depressive symptoms in acute psychotic episode and dysphoria can be a precursor of relapse of psychosis
    - Patients experiencing FEP are more likely to develop post-psychotic depression
- Post-psychotic depression
    - Post-psychotic depression is defined as
        - A depressive symptom that "occurs twelve months after psychotic episode while psychotic symptoms are still present but not predominant" in the ICD–10
        - A "post psychotic depressive disorder of schizophrenia as a major depressive episode during the residual phase of schizophrenia" in the DSM–IV
        - Depression occurring independently of schizophrenia and several months after an acute episode of psychosis

PATIENT FILE

- Post-psychotic depression is not currently represented as a classification, diagnostic criterion, or diagnostic code in the ICD, DSM–5, or the DSM–5–TR
- Prevalence of post-psychotic depression is approximately 25–75%
- Treatment considerations include:
  - No specific antipsychotic medication is noted to be superior in treatment of post-psychotic depression in FEP
    - Atypical antipsychotics are not more effective than typical antipsychotic medications
    - Noradrenergic agents may be more effective than antidepressant medicines, but the data is limited
    - Potential treatments include online therapy (to reduce social isolation) and treatment with n-3 polyunsaturated fatty acids following FEP
  - Antidepressants
    - There is a dearth of sufficiently powered, randomized controlled trials utilizing antidepressants for depression in schizophrenia as well as post-psychotic depression
  - Cognitive behavioral therapy (CBT) for psychosis
    - May assist by targeting or treating the patient's feelings, including their inability to recover (entrapment), difficulty in being well and healthy, and the omnipotence of auditory hallucinations to harm or shame patients
    - CBT for psychosis can reduce distress and worsening of a depressive state
  - Electroconvulsive therapy (ECT)
    - Current literature suggests ECT may have a pro-cognitive effect in patients diagnosed with schizophrenia who experience positive symptomatology
    - ECT is associated with improved patient quality of life across all mental health diagnoses that are primarily indicated for ECT treatment
    - Treatment outcomes associated with application of ECT to depression in schizophrenia are unknown
      - However, theoretically, ECT treatment could potentially improve depressive symptomatology in patients diagnosed with schizophrenia

PATIENT FILE

Post-test question

Which of the following treatment options is validated in the current literature as a viable treatment option for post-psychotic depression?

A. Antidepressant treatment
B. Antipsychotic treatment
C. CBT for psychosis (CBTp)
D. Lithium
E. ECT

Answer: C

References

1. Birchwood, M., Iqbal, Z., Chadwick, P., & Trower, P. (2000). Cognitive approach to depression and suicidal thinking in psychosis. 1. Ontogeny of post-psychotic depression. *British Journal of Psychiatry*, Dec., 177, 516–521. https://doi.org/10.1192/bjp.177.6.516.
2. Birchwood, M., Iqbal, Z., & Upthegrove, R. (2005). Psychological pathways to depression in schizophrenia: studies in acute psychosis, post psychotic depression and auditory hallucinations. *European Archives of Psychiatry and Clinical Neuroscience*, June, 255(3), 202–212. https://doi.org/10.1007/s00406-005-0588-4.
3. Grover, S., Shouan, A., Chakrabarti, S., Sahoo, S., & Mehra, A. (2020). Effectiveness of ECT in management of depression in patients with schizophrenia: an open labelled study. *Schizophrenia Research*, Aug., 222, 530–531. https://doi.org/10.1016/j.schres.2020.05.002.
4. Hafner, H., Maurer, K., Trendler, G., an der Heiden, W., Schmidt, M., & Konnecke, R. (2005). Schizophrenia and depression: challenging the paradigm of two separate diseases – a controlled study of schizophrenia, depression and healthy controls. *Schizophrenia Research*, Sept. 1, 77(1), 11–24. https://doi.org/10.1016/j.schres.2005.01.004.
5. Hardman, J. R., Gleeson, J. F., González-Blanch, C., Alvarez-Jimenez, M., Fraser, M. I., & Yap, K. (2023). The role of insight, social rank, mindfulness and self-compassion in depression following first episode psychosis. *Clinical Psychology and Psychotherapy*, Nov.–Dec., 30(6), 1393–1406. https://doi.org/10.1002/cpp.2881.
6. Iqbal, Z., Birchwood, M., Chadwick, P., & Trower, P. (2000). Cognitive approach to depression and suicidal thinking in psychosis, Part 2. Testing the validity of a social ranking model. *British Journal of Psychiatry*, Dec., 177, 522–528. https://doi.org/10.1192/bjp.177.6.522.

7. Iqbal, Z., Birchwood, M., Hemsley, D., Jackson, C., & Morris, E. (2004). Autobiographical memory and post-psychotic depression in first episode psychosis. *British Journal of Clinical Psychology*, March, 43(Pt. 1), 97–104. https://doi.org/10.1348/014466504772812995.
8. Li, W., Yang, Y., Feng-Rong, A., et al. (2020). Prevalence of comorbid depression in schizophrenia: a meta-analysis of observational studies. *Journal of Affective Disorders*, Aug. 1, 273, 524–531. https://doi.org/10.1016/j.jad.2020.04.056.
9. Neyra Del Rosario, A., Martin, E., Matellan, I., Rodriguez, F., Villodres, M., & Molina, N. (2023). Post-psychotic depression in dual psychosis – efficacy of lurasidone. P.2033 presented at the Barcelona: 36th European College of Neuropsychopharmacology Congress, October 7–10 2023. https://psiquiatria.com/trabajos/usr_9168923575651.pdf.
10. Rahim, T. & Rashid, R. (2017). Comparison of depression symptoms between primary depression and secondary-to-schizophrenia depression. *International Journal of Psychiatry in Clinical Practice*, Nov., 21(4), 314–317. https://doi.org/10.1080/13651501.2017.1324036.
11. Sanchez, I. B., Agudo, A. M., Guerrero-Jimenez, M., et al. (2023). Treatment of post-psychotic depression in first-episode psychosis: a systematic review. *Nordic Journal of Psychiatry*, Feb., 77(2), 109–117. https://doi.org/10.1080/08039488.2022.2067225.
12. Siris, S. (2000). Depression in schizophrenia: perspective in the era of "atypical" antipsychotic agents. *American Journal of Psychiatry*, Sept., 157(9), 1379–1389. https://doi.org/10.1176/appi.ajp.157.9.1379.
13. Stahl, S. M. (2014). *Stahl's Essential Psychopharmacology: Prescriber's Guide*, 5th ed. New York: Cambridge University Press.
14. Tor, P. C., Tan, X. W., Martin, D., & Loo, C. (2021). Comparative outcomes in electroconvulsive therapy (ECT): a naturalistic comparison between outcomes in psychosis, mania, depression, psychotic depression and catatonia. *European Neuropsychopharmacology*, Oct., 51,43–54. https://doi.org/10.1016/j.euroneuro.2021.04.023.
15. Upthegrove, R., Marwaha, S., & Birchwood, M. (2017). Depression and schizophrenia: cause, consequence, or trans-diagnostic issue? *Schizophrenia Bulletin*, March 1, 43(2), 240–244. https://doi.org/10.1093/schbul/sbw097.
16. Zozulya, S., Tikhonov, D., Kaleda, V., & Klyushnik, T. (2022). Dynamics of immune markers in different variants of post-psychotic depression after first-episode psychosis in young adult age. *European Psychiatry*, Sept. 1, 65(Suppl. 1), S366–S367. https://doi.org/10.1192/j.eurpsy.2022.931.

SECTION IV
Iatrogenic Syndromes and Drug-Associated Side Effects

PATIENT FILE

13

Neuroleptic malignant syndrome: Altered and rigid

The Psychopharmocological Dilemma: How do we differentiate between neuroleptic malignant syndrome (NMS) and catatonia?

Ajay Nair, Carolina A. Klein, and Amanie Salem

Pretest self-assessment question
What is the main symptom that differentiates NMS from catatonia?
A. Stupor
B. Rigidity
C. Antipsychotic treatment
D. Autonomic instability

Patient evaluation on intake
- A 19-year-old male who recently has been having less responsiveness and increased muscle rigidity

Psychiatric history
- The patient has no previous psychiatric history noted
- The patient had been admitted to the psychiatric unit involuntarily 2 weeks ago for apparent psychosis, as he had been disorganized and banging on his neighbor's door, stating that his neighbor was "The Antichrist" and that the patient had to "cleanse" his neighbor so he "would be forgiven for his sins"
- Prior to this incident, his parents reported that he had some odd beliefs, but never had anything like this happen to him. He typically would keep to himself and did not like interacting with others much, and was somewhat of a suspicious child, but never really bothered anyone
- A few days before this incident he had started talking a lot, apparently to himself, and discussed "The Antichrist" frequently at home
- He appeared to be up at night during this time, as he could be heard talking and pacing the house at late hours
- On admission to the psychiatric unit 2 weeks ago, he was disorganized and nearly incoherent. He was having religious delusions and was convinced that God was telling him who the devil and his disciples were

PATIENT FILE

- He was started on haloperidol and clozapine, and titrated up to 10 mg BID of haloperidol and 150 mg nightly of clozapine
- Weekend staff noticed that he was nearly unresponsive and was rigid on physical examination, so they called the on-call physician to evaluate

Social and personal history
- He grew up with his parents, his two older sisters and his younger brother in Detroit, Michigan
- He has few friends and tends to keep to himself
- He was a below-average student but graduated high school without needing any accommodations. He has been working at a fast-food restaurant since he was 16 years old, expanding his hours after finishing high school
- He started smoking marijuana recreationally at age 15 and increased to smoking four to seven times a week at age 18.
- He still lives with his family in his childhood home

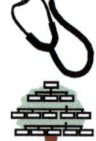
Medical history
- He had surgery for a broken ulna after he fell off a scooter at age 9

Family history
- His father has been diagnosed with alcohol use disorder (AUD), coronary artery disease, and hypertension
- His mother has been diagnosed with hyperlipidemia
- His two older sisters and one younger brother have no medical diagnoses
- He has a maternal uncle who is diagnosed with schizophrenia and takes risperidone

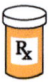
Medication history
- He is currently taking haloperidol 10 mg twice a day and clozapine 150 mg nightly
- Prior to this, he had never taken any prescription medications

Current history
- Staff called with concerns for change in his mental status, requesting an order for a head CT
- He is minimally responsive to questioning, generally staring out into space or answering with frequently unintelligible phrases
- He was noted to be diaphoretic and did not move spontaneously
- On examination he was rigid, with diffusely increased muscle tone

PATIENT FILE

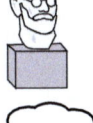

Psychotherapy history
- He has never had psychotherapy

Attending physician's mental notes: initial visit
- He initially presented with what appears to have been a psychotic break and was treated with antipsychotics
- His mental status change was fairly abrupt
- It is important to differentiate whether this mental status change is due to a neurological change, a feature of his psychiatric condition, or a reaction to his medication

Further investigation
What other information would you like to know about the patient's current presentation? What about vital signs and lab results?

- His vital signs were as follows:
  - Temperature: 102.4 degrees Fahrenheit
  - Heart rate: 135
  - Respiratory rate: 32
  - Blood pressure: 164/110
  - SPO_2: 95%
- Pertinent lab findings include:
  - Leukocytosis
  - Anion gap acidosis
  - Creatine phosphokinase (CPK) of 10,340

Case outcome: first interim follow-up visit at 2 hours
- The patient was diagnosed with NMS due to his treatment with antipsychotics, his rapid altered mental status, his muscle rigidity, his autonomic instability, and his lab derangements
- His antipsychotic medications were immediately stopped
- He was transferred to a Critical Care Unit
- He was started on IV fluids to address dehydration and his rising CPK, and placed in a cooling blanket due to his fever
- He was started on diazepam 10 mg IV every 8 hours

Further Investigation
What other pharmacological treatment could be added to help treat his condition?

- Though treatment for NMS is not robustly backed by randomized controlled trials, beyond benzodiazepines, pharmacological

PATIENT FILE

treatment can include dopamine agonists (due to the dopamine blockade being a major factor in the symptoms) or dantrolene (to help treat the muscle rigidity)
- Dantrolene is also used to help with muscle rigidity and breakdown

Mechanism of action moment
- Benzodiazepines are a good treatment, but adding a dopamine agonist may help him through the course of NMS, as D_2 blockade in the hypothalamus is thought to contribute to autonomic instability

Attending physician's mental notes
- Dantrolene can be added to help with his muscle rigidity and help decrease muscle breakdown and the risk of kidney injury
- We will need to see whether non-pharmacological treatment is necessary based on how well we are able to control his symptoms

Case outcome: second interim follow-up visit at 4 hours
- Bromocriptine was started at a dose of 2.5 mg every 6 hours, with instructions to titrate up the dose by 2.5 mg after every two doses to a maximum of 10 mg every 6 hours
- Dantrolene was started at 2.5 mg/kg IV
- The patient's CPK stopped increasing, IV fluids were continued
- His temperature remains at 102.0 degrees Fahrenheit

Further investigation
What additional non-pharmacological interventions could be necessary if the patient does not improve?
- In patients whose cardiopulmonary status cannot be controlled, intubation may be necessary
- Further methods of cooling the body may also be necessary if his temperature is not able to be controlled – such as ice or even an ice bath
- If pharmacological treatment is not effective, electroconvulsive therapy (ECT) is an option

Case outcome: third interim follow-up visit at 12 hours
- His vital signs have started to normalize. His temperature is still elevated at 101.2 degrees Fahrenheit, but showing improvement. His blood pressure has decreased to 145/98. His respiratory rate is 30. His heart rate is 118. His SPO_2 is 97%
- His CPK is 7,300

PATIENT FILE

- He still has a slight anion gap acidosis and leukocytosis, but both also are improving
- He is moving his body spontaneously but is still rigid on examination

Attending physician's mental notes

- Though he is still heavily symptomatic, his symptoms appear under control and are slowly improving
- It is reasonable to remain on the current treatment regimen and follow his course

Case outcome: fourth interim follow-up visit at 24 hours

- Vital signs continue to normalize
  - His temperature is still elevated at 100.6 degrees Fahrenheit, his blood pressure has decreased to 134/90, his respiratory rate is 26, his heart rate is 110, and his SPO_2 is 99%
- He remains confused but is much more responsive to questioning
- He does not appear as diaphoretic
- The Critical Care team is comfortable with him being stepped down to floor status with continuation on his current regimen
- He will improve over the course of the next several days

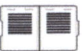

Case debrief

- After initiation on two antipsychotics, the previously antipsychotic-naïve patient developed autonomic instability, encephalopathy and generalized muscle rigidity
- He was managed with a Critical Care admission and by trying to control his autonomic symptoms, aggressive hydration, protection of his cardiopulmonary status, benzodiazepines, dopamine agonists, and dantrolene
- Ultimately, ECT was not necessary due to his response to the pharmacological treatment

Take-home points

- Neuroleptic malignant syndrome is an extremely rare, but life-threatening, condition brought on by treatment with antipsychotic medication
- Treatment should start with immediate cessation of the antipsychotic, hydration, and management of the autonomic instability

PATIENT FILE

- Pharmacological treatments include benzodiazepines and dopamine agonists, as well as dantrolene to treat the muscle rigidity and to prevent muscle breakdown
- If pharmacological treatment is not possible or fails, ECT is another option

Performance in practice: confessions of a psychopharmacologist

What other conditions should be considered in this presentation?

- Catatonia should always be considered in a condition that consists of encephalopathy and muscle rigidity. However, the autonomic instability of neuroleptic malignant syndrome differentiates it from catatonia. A subset of catatonia, usually brought on by continued antipsychotic treatment in the presence of catatonia, is called malignant catatonia. Malignant catatonia looks very similar to NMS, as it also has autonomic instability. Fortunately, its treatment overlaps greatly with NMS, with benzodiazepines or ECT

Why does NMS occur?

- NMS is hypothesized to mainly be due to D_2 blockade in the hypothalamus, which results in autonomic instability. GABA insufficiency in frontal corticostriatal areas has also been implicated, and may be a reason why benzodiazepine treatment is helpful

What are ways that NMS can be avoided?

- Second-generation antipsychotics (SGAs) are less likely than first-generation antipsychotic (FGA) agents to cause NMS. Additionally, high-potency antipsychotics are the most likely to cause NMS
- Slow initiation of antipsychotics can reduce the risk of NMS as well

Tips and pearls

How does the etiology of catatonia differ from the etiology of NMS?

- Catatonia is not very well understood, but GABA imbalances, low dopamine activity, and excessive glutamate have all been identified as potential contributors

How does management of catatonia and of NMS differ?

- Benzodiazepines are a mainstay of management of both NMS and catatonia. NMS also involves the use of muscle relaxers such as dantrolene and/or dopamine agonists such as bromocriptine, but both will need ECT if pharmacological treatments are not working
- Catatonia does not really involve management of any autonomic instability, though this is necessary in malignant catatonia

PATIENT FILE

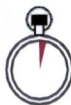

Two-minute tutorial

Neuroleptic malignant syndrome

- NMS is seen in approximately 0.01–0.02% of patients treated with antipsychotics. Two-thirds of cases occur within 2 weeks of starting an antipsychotic
- Typically described symptoms include autonomic instability, including potentially lethal hyperthermia, lead pipe rigidity and generalized tremor, and encephalopathy. Severe cases can have various lab derangements – including metabolic acidosis, leukocytosis, low iron, and elevated catecholamines in the serum – and signs of muscle breakdown (e.g., elevated creatinine phosphokinase and myoglobinuria).
- FGAs, and especially high-potency antipsychotics, are more likely than SGAs to cause NMS. Additionally, NMS induced by SGAs tends to be less severe and have lower mortality rates
- The main pathophysiology of NMS appears to be the D_2 blockade in the hypothalamus, which is thought to underlie the autonomic dysregulation. Decreased GABA activity, particular in frontal corticostriatal tracts, has also been suggested as being involved
- Early diagnosis and treatment are critical, and the first step is discontinuing the offending agent. Benzodiazepines and dopamine agonists are commonly used, with ECT being reserved for more emergent cases or those not responding to pharmacotherapy. Dantrolene has been shown to be helpful in treating muscle rigidity.

Catatonia

- Catatonia requires the presence of at least three of the following symptoms
  - Stupor
  - Catalepsy
  - Waxy flexibility
  - Mutism
  - Negativism
  - Posturing
  - Mannerism
  - Stereotypy
  - Agitation, not influenced by external stimuli
  - Grimacing
  - Echolalia
  - Echopraxia
- Though catatonia can co-occur with various medical conditions, it cannot be diagnosed if it happens only during delirium

PATIENT FILE

- Its prevalence in psychiatric inpatients is approximately 10% and possibly as high as 17%. It is most commonly seen in mood disorders, followed by schizophrenia, and then by general medical or neurological conditions. It is shown in various studies to be underdiagnosed
- Its etiology is not fully understood, but contributions of excessive glutamate activity, low dopamine activity, and imbalance in gamma-aminobutyric acid (GABA) have all been described
- Consideration of catatonia should occur when patients have a notable change in psychomotor function and in responsiveness
- Offending medications should be stopped, including antipsychotic medication, due to the propensity to result in malignant catatonia
- When induced by antipsychotics, the most common symptoms of catatonia are akinesia, stupor, and mutism. Next most commonly seen are waxy flexibility and catalepsy
- Antipsychotic-induced catatonia generally occurs within hours to days of drug exposure
- Treatment is generally done with benzodiazepines or ECT. Typically, a lorazepam challenge is done and if response to lorazepam is seen, treatment is started. If lorazepam is not successful, ECT is then started
  - Doses as high as 24 mg a day of lorazepam can be used in catatonia treatment

Post-test question

What is the main symptom that differentiates NMS from catatonia?

A. Stupor
B. Rigidity
C. Antipsychotic treatment
D. Autonomic instability

Answer: D

References

1. Caroff, S. N., Hurford, I., Lybrand, J., & Campbell, E. C. (2011). Movement disorders induced by antipsychotic drugs: implications of the CATIE Schizophrenia Trial, *Neurologic Clinics*, 29(1), 127–148. https://doi.org/10.1016/j.ncl.2010.10.002.
2. Dhossche, D. M. & Wachtel, L. E. (2016). Catatonia in psychiatric illnesses. In S. H. Fatemi & P. J. Clayton (eds.), *The Medical Basis of Psychiatry*. New York: Springer.

PATIENT FILE

3. Ngo, V., Guerrero, A., Lanum, D., et al. (2019). Emergent treatment of neuroleptic malignant syndrome induced by antipsychotic monotherapy using dantrolene. *Clinical Practice and Cases in Emergency Medicine.* Jan. 4, 3(1), 16–23. https://doi.org/10.5811/cpcem.2018.11.39667. PMID: 30775657; PMCID: PMC6366389.
4. Park, J., Tan, J., Krzeminski, S., Hazeghazam, M., Bandlamuri, M., & Carlson, R. W. (2017). Malignant catatonia warrants early psychiatric – Critical Care collaborative management: two cases and literature review. *Case Reports in Critical Care*, 2017, 1951965. https://doi.org/10.1155/2017/1951965. Epub 2017 Jan 30. PMID: 28250995; PMCID: PMC5303832.
5. Paul, T., Karam, A., Paul, T., Loh, H., & Ferrer, G. F. (2022). A case report on neuroleptic malignant syndrome (NMS): how to approach an early diagnosis. *Cureus*, March 31, 14(3), e23695. https://doi.org/10.7759/cureus.23695. PMID: 35505741; PMCID: PMC9056060.
6. Sienaert, P., van Harten, P., & Rhebergn, D. (2019). The psychopharmacology of catatonia, neuroleptic malignant syndrome, akathisia, tardive dyskinesia, and dystonia. *Handbook of Clinical Neurology*, 165, 415–428. https://doi.org/10.1016/B978-0-444-64012-3.00025-3. PMID: 31727227.

PATIENT FILE

14

Constipation and capacity: The full stop

The Psychopharmacological Dilemma: Treating constipation secondary to antipsychotic medication and finding treatments to target negative symptoms impacting capacity

Seth Judd and Kim-Long Hua-Rupp

Pretest self-assessment question

Which of the following is FDA-approved to treat negative symptoms of a primary psychotic disorder?

A. Clozapine
B. Olanzapine
C. Risperidone
D. Amisulpride
E. None of the above

Patient evaluation on intake

- A 61-year-old non-English-speaking male with past psychiatric history of schizoaffective disorder, depressive type, who was admitted to a forensic hospital under a not guilty by reason of insanity (NGRI) commitment after he was found to have murdered his roommate. He was noncompliant with treatment at the time of the incident offense and was exhibiting marked paranoia toward the victim, who he believed was poisoning him. He had discontinued his psychiatric medication because he believed it was causing him constipation. At the time of this evaluation, the patient was refusing changes to his psychotropic medications and a referral to forensics was placed to assess whether he had the capacity to refuse or consent to psychotropic medication
    ○ Patient has been experiencing paranoia and auditory hallucinations, manifesting as hearing transmissions from the radio. These psychotic symptoms were impacting his ability to communicate. Further, he was experiencing negative psychotic symptoms and symptoms of depression which led to a significant reduction in food and water intake, with persistently very low BMIs. He also exhibited behaviors disturbing to peers in the dining room while talking loudly about getting his food tray
    ○ When interviewed in his room he was lying facing away, was uncooperative and guarded. He maintained poor eye contact with lack of spontaneous speech. He appeared older than his stated

PATIENT FILE

age. Hygiene and grooming were fair. Affect was flat. He was offered interpreter services in his native language but declined and said he would rather speak in English (note: this was very common and the patient would routinely refuse interpreter services)
- He was prescribed risperidone. His treating psychiatrist had recommended starting a second antipsychotic medication, olanzapine. Attempts were made to educate the patient about the benefits, side effects, risks, and alternatives to the recommended treatment plan. However, the patient was unable to consider this change and terminated the interview early

Psychiatric history
- The patient's diagnosis of record is schizoaffective, depressive type
- The patient's psychotic symptoms include:
  - Auditory hallucinations including receiving messages from a radio in his brain resulting in persecutory beliefs about everyday activities, including attending groups
  - Persecutory delusions
  - Distorted reality testing
  - Disorganized thinking
  - Severe negative symptoms including flat affect, poverty of speech, and general lack of drive or motivation to pursue meaningful goals, even in the absence of a depressive episode
- The patient has a history of presenting with the following depressive symptoms:
  - Feelings of hopelessness and helplessness
  - Disturbances in appetite and sleep
  - Suicidal ideation (SI), including history of suicide attempts
  - Anhedonia
  - Avolition
  - Extreme weight loss

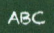

Social and personal history
- Spent a good deal of his childhood as a refugee. Lost both his parents during a civil war. He has one brother and four sisters but has not had contact with them since his incident offense
- Presently has no known family in the United States

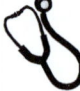

Medical history
- Right nephrectomy
- Diabetes mellitus
- Constipation
- Severely underweight

PATIENT FILE

Family history
- Unknown

Medication history (maximum daily dose listed)
- Patient has had failed multiple trials of antipsychotics and antidepressants including:
  - Aripiprazole (max. daily dose prescribed 30 mg)
  - Doxepin (max. daily dose prescribed 75 mg)
  - Duloxetine (max. daily dose prescribed 60 mg)
  - Haloperidol (max. daily dose prescribed 10 mg)
  - Lithium (max. daily dose prescribed 600 mg)
  - Loxapine (max. daily dose prescribed 250 mg)
  - Mirtazapine (max. daily dose prescribed 15 mg)
  - Olanzapine (max. daily dose prescribed 55 mg)
  - Paroxetine (max. daily dose prescribed 40 mg)
  - Quetiapine (max. daily dose prescribed 800 mg)
  - Risperidone (max. daily dose prescribed 6 mg)
  - Sertraline (max. daily dose prescribed 50 mg)
  - Thiothixene (max. daily dose prescribed 40 mg)
  - Trazodone (max. daily dose prescribed 250 mg)

Current Medications
- Lithium carbonate 600 mg every morning
- Olanzapine 15 mg every morning and 25 mg every evening

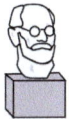

Psychotherapy history
- Limited psychotherapy history as patient's symptoms prevented him from participating in meaningful therapy

Mechanism of action moment
- What is the mechanism of action of olanzapine?
  - Olanzapine is a second-generation antipsychotic. This medication is an antagonist at the 5-HT_{2A} and D_2 receptors, with a higher affinity for the former
  - By blocking D_2 receptors in the mesolimbic pathway, olanzapine can lead to a decrease in positive symptoms, such as hallucinations, delusions, and disorganized speech and behaviors
  - 5-HT receptors are involved in regulating the sensory functions, motility, and secretion of the digestive system, and have been considered as mediators for gut–brain connection

PATIENT FILE

- Additionally, olanzapine blocks peripheral muscarinic M2 and M3 receptors, reducing gastric secretions and inhibiting the motility of GI smooth muscle

Attending physician's mental notes

- Patient has been in and out of forensic hospitals for the past two-plus decades, and has been hospitalized for the past 8 years. Noncompliance with treatment has chronically been a major barrier toward his progress in treatment
- The patient remains highly symptomatic and is refusing changes to his medications to better address his psychotic and depressive symptoms
- In this case, a trained forensic psychiatrist completed the capacity evaluation, but it is important to understand that forensic training is not required to assess capacity, and all psychiatrists should be familiar with assessing capacity
- Legal definitions of capacity can vary based on jurisdiction and legal status. However, there are four general criteria that should be assessed when determining a patient's capacity
  - Patient must be able to communicate a choice regarding treatment
  - Patient must demonstrate an understanding of relevant information regarding the treatment, such as possible benefits and risks
  - Patient must be able to appreciate their situation (i.e., demonstrate insight) and the consequences of accepting or refusing treatment
  - Patient must be able to rationally explain their choice
- The forensic psychiatrist determined the patient lacked capacity as the patient demonstrated no insight into his mental illness. He has not been able to identify his symptoms, the benefits and risks of treatment, or the risks associated with being untreated or undertreated

Further investigation

What else would you like to know? What risk factors are associated with impaired capacity?

- Impaired capacity cannot be assumed in any diagnosis in which intact consciousness is present
- However, any diagnosis that impairs cognition carries a higher risk for impaired capacity, for example:
  - Neurocognitive disorders
  - Medical conditions such as stroke
- Acute psychosis is associated with impairment in at least one of the four criteria in 50% of patients; acute mania has similar risk
- For severe depression, impaired capacity ranges from 20% to 25%
- Lack of insight is the strongest predictor

PATIENT FILE

Case outcome: first interim follow-up visit at 1 year

- Patient's BMI was at 15
- In the past year, he received a trial of risperidone, then loxapine, with little to no benefit. Lurasidone was added and titrated up to 80 mg. No changes in olanzapine or lithium doses were made
- Over this same time period, his psychiatric status has not significantly improved, and he has continued to experience psychotic symptoms, including auditory hallucinations, paranoid delusions, negative symptoms, and disorganized behavior
- He regularly demonstrates irritable mood and has on several occasions engaged in verbal aggression toward staff without provocation
- He continues to show impaired insight into his mental illness, need for care, or risks associated with undertreated or poorly treated psychosis
- A bioethics meeting was held to discuss this patient's case. Recommendations included a trial of clozapine and electroconvulsive therapy (ECT), along with a dietitian referral and modifications to his behavioral plan to closely monitor food intake
- The treatment team was concerned about adding clozapine due to the risk of developing severe constipation. He was being monitored for constipation but was an unreliable historian. For example, he stated he had a bowel movement the day prior, but this was not supported by documentation

Attending physician's mental notes

- Patient has not improved with recent antipsychotic medication changes. He has failed multiple trials of antipsychotic medications over the past three decades
- His negative psychotic symptoms and depressive symptoms continue to significantly impact his ability to function and manage his activities of daily living (ADLs). He is severely restricting his food and water intake, and his current BMI is very low at 15
- Has never been tried on clozapine due to concerns about constipation
- Across studies, clozapine has the highest success rate (40–60%) in treatment-resistant schizophrenia, compared to olanzapine (7–9%) and all other antipsychotics (< 5%)
- Given his current presentation of severe psychosis and low BMI, depriving him of clozapine is more of a health risk and threat to his quality of life than the risks of severe constipation secondary to clozapine
- He should also be strongly considered for ECT in combination with clozapine, as this combination is more effective than clozapine alone

PATIENT FILE

Further investigation

What antipsychotics carry the highest risk for constipation? And what preventative measures could you do before initiating clozapine? What are some of the available adjunct treatments for constipation?

- Clozapine, chlorpromazine, and thioridazine. Also, olanzapine and quetiapine at high doses
  - More than 50% of patients prescribed antipsychotics suffer from constipation
  - Clozapine has a 4.5-fold higher risk of inducing constipation compared to other antipsychotics
- Preventative measures include starting with a secretagogue before initiating the clozapine trial
  - 145 mcg qAM 30 min prior to a meal. If no improvement after 1 week, increase to 290 mcg qAM. Monitor constipation with baseline KUB and levels once clozapine has commenced
- Available adjunct treatments for constipation include the following:
  - Osmotic laxatives: e.g., lactulose, polyethylene glycol
  - Stimulant laxatives: e.g., senna
  - Stool softeners: e.g., docusate sodium
  - *Note: bulk-forming agents are contraindicated*

Case outcome: interim follow-up at 2 years

- Over the past 6 months, patient's psychiatric and physical health have remained poor
- Patient reported depressive symptoms, which are contributing to his anhedonia, avolition, less than optimal appetite, and intermittent passive SI. He stated, "I'm doing bad. I'm dying of constipation," although constipation was being adequately managed at this time. He also reported poor sleep
- Negative symptoms remained present, including alogia, anhedonia, avolition, asociality, and reduced emotional expression
- He continued to endorse hearing messages from a radio in his native language that was coming from his head
- Persistent persecutory delusions and intermittent auditory hallucinations were present
- While he was compliant with medications and showed some improvement in appetite, he did not gain the desired amount of weight to negate the risks of being extremely underweight
  - Lurasidone was increased to 120 mg and a cross-titration of olanzapine to clozapine was started

PATIENT FILE

Attending physician's mental notes: interim follow-up at 2 years

- It is important to distinguish the difference between negative symptoms of a primary psychotic disorder and depressive symptoms of a mood disorder, as this will dictate treatment
- There are five core negative symptoms:
  - Alogia – inability to speak due to a mental deficiency or an episode of dementia
  - Anhedonia – loss of interest in and withdrawal from all regular and pleasurable activities
  - Avolition – lack of interest or engagement in goal-directed behavior
  - Asociality – lack of motivation to engage in social interaction, or a preference for solitary activities
  - Blunted affect – reduced emotional expression
- Depressive symptoms include:
  - Depressed mood
  - Anhedonia
  - Significant appetite or weight changes
  - Psychomotor abnormalities
  - Feelings of worthlessness or guilt
  - Decreased energy
  - Decreased concentration and/or indecisiveness
  - SI
- It can be difficult to distinguish negative symptoms from depressive symptoms as there is significant overlap
  - Anergia, avolition, and anhedonia are common in both
  - Alogia and blunted affect are more specific to negative symptoms
  - SI, decreased mood, and pessimism have higher specificity in depression

Further investigation

What changes to his treatment plan would you recommend to potentially target his depressive and negative symptoms?

- Continue to increase clozapine dose, and a trial of ECT would be most appropriate
  - For major depressive episodes, most studies have found response rates of 80–90%. Of particular note, ECT is a unique treatment in that the greater the level of symptom severity, the more likely the patient will respond to treatment
  - ECT-induced improvement of negative symptoms has led to improvement in global function and cognitive function in patients

PATIENT FILE

Case outcome: interim follow-up at 3 years

- Patient is currently on clozapine 150 mg BID, lithium 600 mg, and lurasidone 120 mg
- Attempts were made to pursue ECT treatment to address his treatment-resistant psychosis. The team was unable to contact a next of kin for medical decision-making and the court dismissed petition for conservatorship. The court then denied hearing for the ECT petition and, as a result, the patient was unable to receive ECT treatment
- Patient continued to exhibit psychotic symptoms. He remained guarded and paranoid with poor eye contact. He was observed responding to stimuli not present
- He continued to be minimally engaged in treatment, attending fewer than 50% of groups, but was medication compliant
- Insight remained impaired
- His negative symptoms continue to impact his functional abilities, such as self-care, interpersonal relationships, and learning and memory
    - Extremely low weight and chronic constipation persisted. In addition to antipsychotic medications, the patient's psychotic thinking and poor compliance with management strategies likely contributed to chronic constipation

Attending physician's mental notes: interim follow-up at 3 years

- Patient was on clozapine 150 mg BID, with a clozapine level of 373
- Typical therapeutic reference ranges for clozapine are 350–600 ng/mL. At this particular forensic hospital, the therapeutic range is 350–1000 ng/mL
- Could consider increasing the dose further if patient is able to tolerate a higher dose
- In this patient it will be particularly important to monitor for worsening constipation
- Also, given his age, will also need to closely monitor for orthostatic hypotension, which can increase his risk for falls
- Records indicated the presence of cognitive deficits, such as learning and memory. Neuropsychological testing would be helpful in determining the patient's baseline cognitive function, although results should be interpreted with caution as individuals with active psychosis may have more difficulty performing cognitive tasks than their peers

PATIENT FILE

Further investigation
Other than ECT, what other treatment recommendations would you make to target negative symptoms of a primary psychotic disorder?
- We would recommend starting cariprazine, with a target dose of 4.5–5 mg per day
    - It is hypothesized that cariprazine's preferential affinity for D_3 over D_2 receptors may contribute to its therapeutic benefits, treating cognitive and negative symptoms. Its moderate affinity for $5-HT_{1A}$ receptors (partial agonist) may also help reduce extrapyramidal symptoms (EPS), which often contribute to masked facies and can be confused with blunted affect
    - A 26-week study showed clinically significant improvement in negative symptoms and functional improvement, with improved scores on the Clinical Global Impressions – Improvement Scale and Personal and Social Performance Scale

Case debrief
- Patient is a male in his 60s with long history of treatment-resistant schizoaffective disorder, depressive type, and has been in and out of forensic hospitals for the past two-plus decades
    - He exhibited a combination of positive and negative symptoms, along with intermittent depressive symptoms including suicidal ideation (SI)
    - Treatment compliance likely related to a number of factors, including severity of symptoms, poor tolerability of treatment, and side effects to antipsychotic medications (e.g., constipation)
    - He lacked insight into his mental illness
    - Negative and depressive symptoms led to poor food intake and patient was severely underweight with low BMI of 15
- The patient was refusing medications change and a forensic consultation was made to assess whether the patient had capacity to consent to or refuse treatment. A forensic psychiatrist determined he lacked capacity due to impaired insight, and he was unable to describe the benefits, risks, and alternatives to antipsychotic medications
- Over the course of the next few years, he was tried on several antipsychotics (olanzapine, risperidone, and lurasidone) without success
- The patient received a trial of clozapine and he was closely monitored for any worsening constipation

PATIENT FILE

- Clozapine only minimally improved his presentation. He continued to exhibit severe psychotic symptoms
- Attempts were made to obtain a court order for ECT treatment but the court denied the petition

Take-home points
- Negative symptoms of a primary psychotic disorder and depression have overlapping symptoms (e.g., anergia, avolition, and anhedonia), which can make distinguishing between the two challenging
  - Alogia and diminished expression tend to be more specific to negative symptoms
  - Depressed mood, SI, and pessimism tend to be more specific with depression
- Assessment of capacity to consent to or refuse treatment does not require forensic training and every psychiatrist should be familiar with evaluating capacity. While legal definitions may vary slightly based on jurisdiction, the evaluator should consider the following criteria:
  - Can the patient communicate a choice?
  - Can the patient demonstrate an understanding of the benefits, risks, and alternatives to proposed treatment?
  - Can the patient appreciate their situation and the consequences of accepting or refusing treatment?
  - Can the patient rationally explain their choice?
- Although impaired capacity cannot be assumed based on diagnosis alone, any diagnosis which impairs cognition increases risk. Lack of insight is the strongest predictor for impaired capacity. Acute psychosis and mania have 50% or greater risk for impaired capacity
- Clozapine has the highest success rate for treatment-resistant schizophrenia (40–60%). Olanzapine has the second-highest success rate but only at 7–9%. All other antipsychotics' success rate is less than 5%
- ECT should be considered for those resistant to clozapine and may have some benefits in reducing negative symptoms
- There are no FDA-approved treatments for negative symptoms. Can consider adding cariprazine to target these symptoms
- Clozapine, chlorpromazine, and thioridazine have the highest rates of constipation
- For patients with history of constipation secondary to antipsychotics, a secretagogue (preventative measure) or laxatives (except bulk-forming agents) can be used

PATIENT FILE

Performance in practice: confessions of a psychopharmacologist

What could have been done better here?

- Patient has a long history of psychotic symptoms and has been institutionalized for a significant portion of his adulthood. Despite this, it appears he was only recently prescribed clozapine due to concerns related to his history of chronic constipation
- This patient could have benefited from an earlier trial of clozapine
- Once a patient has failed two trials of antipsychotic medications, clozapine is recommended as the next antipsychotic, unless a contraindication is present
- Earlier use of clozapine in treatment-resistant schizophrenia has been shown to produce greater benefits in multiple domains
- Underutilization and delayed use of clozapine in this population may lead to unfavorable outcomes

What are possible action items for improvement in practice?

- Become familiar with legal definitions of capacity in your jurisdiction and the four common criteria
- Do not delay starting clozapine in individuals with treatment-resistant psychotic disorders
- Become familiar with treatment options for antipsychotic-induced constipation
  - Use preventative treatments, such as secretagogue, in individuals who are at high risk for developing constipation
- Use interpreter services for patients whose primary language is non-English, even if the patient has some understanding of the English language. This can help improve compliance and provide better psychoeducation when reviewing benefits and risks of treatment

Tips and pearls

- Diagnosis guides treatment and it is important to be able to differentiate between negative symptoms and symptoms of depression. The symptoms that tend to be more specific to negative symptoms are diminished expression and alogia
- There are no FDA-approved treatments for negative symptoms. ECT and some antipsychotics, such as cariprazine, may improve negative symptoms
- For treatment-resistant psychotic disorders, clozapine and ECT should be used earlier in treatment and not be seen as a last resort
- In older patients, clozapine should be titrated slowly to increase tolerability. In patients over 65, there is a higher risk for agranulocytosis, metabolic syndrome, hypersalivation, and sedation

PATIENT FILE

- Constipation is a common occurrence in the elderly
- Clozapine has the highest risk for constipation
- Preventative measures such as a secretagogue should be used in patients at high risk for constipation
- If constipation is present, osmotic laxatives (e.g., lactulose, polyethylene glycol), stimulant laxatives (e.g., senna), or stool softeners (e.g., docusate sodium) can be used to treat this side effect. Bulk-forming agents are contraindicated
- Although this patient was not formally diagnosed with a neurocognitive disorder, cognitive deficits were observed. It is important to remember when prescribing antipsychotic medications with known or suspected dementia to advise patients (and family, caregivers, conservator, etc.) of black-box warning, which indicates increased mortality in elderly patients with dementia-related psychosis

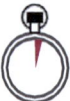

Two-minute tutorial

Negative symptoms

- In schizophrenia, negative symptoms represent an absence or diminution of normal behaviors related to expression (e.g., alogia, decreased affect), motivation (i.e., avolition), or interest (e.g., asociality, anhedonia)
- Negative symptoms can be difficult to recognize, as positive symptoms usually take precedent and are more likely to be the reason for the patient presenting to the clinic or emergency room
- Negative symptoms commonly appear during the prodromal phase and are often present prior to first acute psychotic episode
  - 73% of patients with negative symptoms reported the presence of one of these core symptoms prior to the onset of positive symptoms
  - Can appear during any point in the illness
- Negative symptoms can be measured using the Positive and Negative Syndrome Scale for Schizophrenia (PANSS), Negative Symptoms Assessment 16-item scale (NSA-16), and the Scale for the Assessment of Negative Symptoms (SANS)
- Negative symptoms play a large role in functional outcomes and morbidity, and have a higher burden of illness and are linked to worse outcomes
- Negative symptom neurobiology is hypothesized to arise from hypodopaminergic functioning (as opposed to hyperdopaminergic in positive symptoms)
  - Brain structures involved include the frontal lobe and mesolimbic structures

PATIENT FILE

- Other hypotheses include glutamate deficiency
- D_3 receptors are involved in novel object recognition and social interaction, and therefore are thought to be involved in negative symptoms. In rodents, D_3 receptors mediated effects in cognition and reduced anhedonia
- Current treatment for primary psychotic disorders tend to have limited effects in reducing negative symptoms and there is no FDA-approved medication for such symptoms
- Cariprazine has shown some promise in reducing negative symptoms
  - Cariprazine has high affinity as a partial agonist for D_3 receptors
- ECT may be another option. Studies have shown improvement in negative symptoms, which correlated with overall improvements in function
- Psychosocial interventions should be used alongside antipsychotic medications
  - Skill-based interventions such as cognitive remediation therapy and social skills training
  - Cognitive behavioral therapy (CBT)
  - Family interventions to help provide support for the patient
  - Motivation and Enhancement Training (MOVE)

Post-test question

Which of the following is FDA-approved to treat negative symptoms of a primary psychotic disorder?

A. Clozapine
B. Olanzapine
C. Risperidone
D. Amisulpride
E. None of the above

Answer: E

References

1. American Psychiatric Association. Committee on Electroconvulsive Therapy & Weiner, R. D. (2001). *The Practice of Electroconvulsive Therapy: Recommendations for Treatment, Training, and Privileging: A Task Force Report of the American Psychiatric Association*, 2nd ed. Washington, DC: American Psychiatric Association.
2. Appelbaum, P. S. (2007). Clinical practice: assessment of patients' competence to consent to treatment. *New England Journal of Medicine*, Nov. 1, 357(18), 1834–1840. https://doi.org/10.1056/NEJMcp074045.

PATIENT FILE

3. Chew, M. L., Mulsant, B. H., Pollock, B. G., et al. (2006). A model of anticholinergic activity of atypical antipsychotic medications. *Schizophrenia Research*, 88(1–3), 63–72.
4. Colin, F., Harry G., & Mariam, K. (2017). The recovery of factors associated with decision-making capacity in individuals with psychosis. *BJPsych Open*, 3, 113–119. https://doi.org/10.1192/bjpo.bp.116.004226.
5. Correll, C. U. & Schooler, N. R. (2020). Negative symptoms in schizophrenia: a review and clinical guide for recognition, assessment, and treatment. *Neuropsychiatric Disease and Treatment*, Feb. 21, 16, 519–534. https://doi.org/10.2147/NDT.S225643. PMID: 32110026; PMCID: PMC7041437.
6. John, S., Rowley, J., et al. (2020). Assessing patients' decision-making capacity in the hospital setting: a literature review. *Australian Journal of Rural Health*, April, 28(2), 141–148. https://doi.org/10.1111/ajr.12592 1440–1584. PMID:31960545 lang: eng.
7. Kellner, C. H. (2019). *Handbook of ECT: A Guide to Electroconvulsive Therapy for Practitioners*. New York: Cambridge University Press.
8. Kirrane, A., Majumdar, B., & Richman, A. (2018). Clozapine use in old age psychiatry. *BJPsych Advances*, 24(3), 204–211. https://doi.org/10.1192/bja.2017.26.
9. Krynicki, C. R., Upthegrove, R., Deakin, J. F. W., & Barnes, T. R. E. (2018). The relationship between negative symptoms and depression in schizophrenia: a systematic review. *Acta Psychiatrica Scandinavica*, May, 137(5), 380–390. https://doi.org/10.1111/acps.12873. Epub 2018 March 13.
10. Leucht, S., Corves, C., Arbter, D., Engel, R. R., Li, C., & Davis, J. M. (2009). Second-generation versus first-generation antipsychotic drugs for schizophrenia: a meta-analysis. *Lancet*, Jan. 3, 373(9657), 31–41. https://doi.org/10.1016/S0140-6736(08)61764-X. Epub 2008 Dec. 6. PMID: 19058842.
11. Meyer, J. M. & Stahl, S. M. (2019). *The Clozapine Handbook*. Cambridge University Press.
12. Tan, X., Martin, D., Lee, J., & Tor, P. C. (2022). The impact of electroconvulsive therapy on negative symptoms in schizophrenia and their association with clinical outcomes. *Brain Sciences*, April 25, 12(5), 545. https://doi.org/10.3390/brainsci12050545.
13. Thomas, K. & Saadabadi, A. (2022) Olanzapine [Updated Sept. 8, 2022]. StatPearls [Internet]. Treasure Island, FL: StatPearls Publishing; Jan.– . Available from: www.ncbi.nlm.nih.gov/books/NBK532903.

PATIENT FILE

14. Williams, R., Malla, A., Roy, M. A., et al. (2017). What is the place of clozapine in the treatment of early psychosis in Canada? *Canadian Journal of Psychiatry*, Feb., 62(2), 109–114. https://doi.org/10.1177/0706743716651049. Epub July 9, 2016.
15. Yi,. W., She, S., Zhang, J., et al. (2020). Clozapine use in patients with early-stage schizophrenia in a Chinese psychiatric hospital. *Neuropsychiatric Disease and Treatment*, Nov. 24, 16, 2827–2836. https://doi.org/10.2147/NDT.S261503.

SECTION V
Complex Comorbidities

PATIENT FILE

15

TBI and CTE: Bruised brains

The Psychopharmacological Dilemma: Identifying therapeutic options for treatment-resistant aggression / psychiatric symptoms in a patient with suspected chronic traumatic encephalopathy (CTE) or traumatic brain injury (TBI) and a primary psychotic disorder

Carolina Klein and Hunter Neely

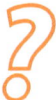

Pretest self-assessment question

What therapeutic intervention is indicated for treatment-resistant psychiatric/aggressive symptoms in a patient with CTE and a comorbid primary psychotic disorder?

A. Clozapine
B. Long-acting injectable (LAI) intramuscular (IM) medications
C. Benzodiazepines
D. Psychotherapy + olanzapine
E. Electroconvulsive therapy (ECT) +/- continued psychopharmacological medications

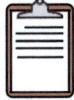

Patient evaluation on intake

- A 25-year-old male presenting with delusions, hallucinations, agitation, affective lability, and neurocognitive impairment
- Patient presented on admission as a mildly disheveled man who appeared his stated age, in his mid-20s
- His mood was euthymic and his affect labile. During his intake interview, his affect ranged from hysterical laughter, to suspicion, to anger, to crying, in rapid progression. He was also noted to be agitated and distractible
- His speech was non-fluent, including frequent stuttering and possible thought blocking. When he was having difficulty with word finding, he tended to get frustrated
- His thinking was concrete and inflexible. He was tangential and would often ramble into irrelevant discussion
- He was highly distractible by external noises in his environment and apparent internal stimuli. At one point during his intake interview, he turned to the side and stated, "Why do you want me dead?"
- He admitted to a history of auditory and visual hallucinations. He denied current suicidal or homicidal ideation

PATIENT FILE

Psychiatric history

- The patient grew up in a chaotic and traumatic home, enduring both physical and sexual abuse by caregivers
- As a child, the patient was diagnosed with Attention-Deficit/Hyperactivity Disorder (ADHD) and has chronically suffered from severe impairments, with behavioral disruption, difficulties with attention and concentration, and poor academic performance
- Reports suggest previous concern for an unspecified learning disability, specifically in math and writing, but he was never formally diagnosed
- As an adult, the patient suffered from psychotic and affective illnesses with refractory aggressiveness. His psychotic and mood symptoms include persecutory delusions (paranoia), auditory and visual hallucinations, irritability, disorganized thought process, and anxiety
- He has a history of multiple head traumas and blackouts since early childhood – such as while playing peewee football as a child; he also hit his head on concrete while playing football as an adolescent. Family reports patient having 10–12 major traumas to the head during his lifetime
- The patient described a history of at least two concussive head injuries, with the most recent occurring 2 years prior to his current psychiatric hospitalization. He reported he was hospitalized and jumped off a bed in a suicide attempt. He landed on his head and lost consciousness. He described a change in his functioning as a result of this injury and reported that he is more disorganized, emotionally labile, and impulsive
- His psychiatric symptoms have remained refractory to medications, leading to repeated admissions to psychiatric facilities in the past decade. He has been placed in numerous residential facilities and has failed every placement because of non-compliance with medications and persistent assaultive behavior
- Patient has a self-reported history of prior methamphetamine use and alcohol use. No recent use in last month. Patient did not state his age at first use of each substance

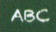

Social and personal history

- Patient reported academic difficulties throughout school
- He described dropping out of school in the eighth grade
- Patient did not report college or continuing education
- No documented work history
- Patient has never been married and does not have any biological children

PATIENT FILE

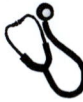

Medical history
- Patient has documented seizure disorder. No mention of age when he experienced his first seizure or the age of the diagnosis
- Patient did not mention current or previous medications to control seizures. Patient cannot recall last seizure

Family history
- No documented family psychiatric, medical, or substance use history in records

Medication history
- Patient has failed multiple trials of various combinations of medications, including antipsychotics, antiepileptic (mood stabilizer) medications, and antidepressants without substantial symptomatic improvement. Despite multiple treatment trials, he has remained psychotic, aggressive, impulsive, and with significant mood fluctuations

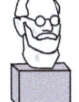

Psychotherapy history
- No history of involvement in psychotherapy

Attending physician's mental notes: initial evaluation
- On initial evaluation, the patient exhibits extreme agitation, emotional lability, disorganized thoughts, internal preoccupation, and isolation
- The differential diagnoses include, but are not limited to: schizophrenia, schizoaffective disorder, bipolar disorder, neurocognitive disorders, psychotic disorder due to underlying medical illness, delirium, substance-induced psychotic disorder, intoxication, malingering
- Given the vast differential diagnoses, further work-up is needed
- Neuropsychological testing referral placed to evaluate his current cognitive deficits and for diagnostic clarification
- Based on the results of neuropsychological testing, my clinical assessment is that the patient's current cognitive presentation appears to reflect some combination of premorbid learning and attention/executive deficits and brain damage secondary to multiple head injuries and possibly substance abuse. His psychotic disorder may also be negatively impacting cognitive functioning. The nature of the behavioral disturbance along with the pattern of cognitive deficits observed on testing is consistent with frontal-subcortical pathology, and in particular implicates dysfunction of the orbitofrontal cortex

PATIENT FILE

- Updated DSM–5–TR diagnoses
  - Major neurocognitive disorder due to traumatic brain injury
    - Neuropsychological testing revealed that patient has multiple, severe cognitive deficits. These include significant impairments in memory and executive functioning (the ability to plan, organize, and sequence information, and use of abstraction)
    - These deficits cause significant impairment in patient's social and occupational functioning and represent a decline from a previously higher level of functioning
    - Although there are likely several contributing factors to the patient's presentation (including substance use and premorbid learning and attentional deficits), the severity of his impairments appears to be due to brain damage secondary to multiple head injuries
  - ADHD, combined presentation
    - Rule out: learning disorder. May translate into specific learning disorders in math and written expression; however, it is also possible that the patient's academic difficulties would be better accounted for by his ADHD, his history of head injury, his psychiatric symptoms, and his trauma. Greater clarity regarding this issue could be addressed in future testing
    Physician prescribed divalproex sodium 1500 mg daily and topiramate 300 mg daily for mood instability, impulsivity, and to raise seizure threshold; olanzapine 10 mg daily for persecutory ideation, mood instability, and impulsivity; and propranolol 20 mg twice daily for aggression and impulsivity

Case outcome: interim follow-up (1.5 months later)

- On the unit, the patient was involved in numerous fist fights with peers, and was frequently agitated, aggressive, and sexually inappropriate with female staff
- He required frequent redirection, and often demonstrated agitation and irritability in response to this redirection
- His ongoing psychiatric symptoms include paranoid delusional thinking, severe irritability, periods of severe depression with suicidal thoughts and gestures, alternating with manic episodes manifested by poor sleep, intrusive behavior, and flight of ideas
- Sometimes, he presented with mixed episodes of depression and mania at the same time

PATIENT FILE

Attending physician's mental notes: 1.5 month follow-up
- In the interim, the patient has had multiple incidents of aggressive, assaultive behavior, many resulting in injuries to peers and staff. He has required seclusion and restraint for threatening and assaulting both staff and peers
- Presence of manic symptoms persist, such as poor sleep, intrusive behavior, flight of ideas, irritability, and aggression. In addition, he experiences periods of depressive symptoms which occur only in the presence of pre-existing psychotic symptoms
- The diagnosis of schizoaffective disorder, bipolar type is proposed
- Further changes made to antipsychotic medications, and mood-stabilizing medications ordered to improve psychosis, affective lability, and aggressive/assaultive behaviors
- The physician prescribes divalproex sodium 1000 mg twice daily for mood lability; citalopram 10 mg daily for mood lability; olanzapine 20 mg daily for psychosis, impulsivity, aggression; and propranolol 20 mg twice daily for impulsive behaviors

Case outcome: interim follow up (1 year later)
- The patient remains easily agitated at less-than-favorable news and reacts disproportionately, including shouting, punching walls, and assaulting people
- During this hospitalization, he exhibited recurrent violent behavior with over 200 incidents of violent acts toward others, requiring 5-point restraints and seclusion. He continues to exhibit aggressive behavior despite the medication change
- Patient is currently prescribed clozapine 450 mg every evening for psychosis; fluphenazine decanoate (a long-acting IM antipsychotic), 100 mg IM every 2 weeks for psychosis; lithium carbonate 900 mg at night for mood stabilization; and valproic acid 500 mg in the morning and 750 mg in the evening for mood stabilization
- The medical records further indicate that the patient has failed multiple trials of antipsychotic medications and other psychotropic medications. Past antipsychotics include aripiprazole, chlorpromazine, fluphenazine, haloperidol, haloperidol decanoate (a long-acting IM antipsychotic), loxapine, olanzapine, quetiapine, and risperidone. He has also failed trials of valproate
- Although compliant with psychotropic medication, he continues to exhibit severe symptoms of psychosis and neurocognitive deficits consistent with a major neurocognitive disorder

PATIENT FILE

Attending physician's mental notes: 1 year follow-up
- Given multiple failed trials of various combinations of psychotropic medications and ongoing violent behavior since admission, an alternative treatment modality should be considered in this patient's case
- Treatment-resistant schizophrenia spectrum disorders are known to respond well to ECT after all medication trials have been exhausted. Given the failed attempt to control this patient's psychotic symptoms and extreme violence with medications, an ECT referral is placed
- There are no apparent contraindications in this patient's case for ECT with comorbid major neurocognitive disorder from repeated prior head injuries. Contraindications would be an active intracranial infection, intracranial malformation, and foreign material surgically implanted in brain. Further work-up would be required in these cases prior to initiating ECT
- Given this patient's pre-existing history of neurocognitive deficits due to repetitive head trauma, baseline cognitive screening (as in the Montreal Cognitive Assessment [MoCA]), in addition to the Mini-Mental State Examination (MMSE), is recommended in order to track potential cognitive improvement or decline in the course of ECT treatments and to be able to compare cognitive functioning as the ECT treatments progress. It is recommended that a cognitive battery screening should be performed each week, on the same day and time as the week prior, and not on the day that ECT is performed to minimize any acute/transient impact ECT may have on cognitive functioning. After a cognitive battery screening is completed each week, the screenings can then be performed once per month for an overall cognitive assessment
- After pre-ECT work-up complete, with medical clearance and cognitive screening performed, ECT treatment is initiated, beginning at three times per week

Case outcome: interim follow-up (1.5 months after ECT initiation)
- 1.5 months following initiation of ECT, the patient's psychotic symptoms have significantly improved and there has been no further documentation of aggression or violence performed by the patient
- The patient was subsequently moved to a different inpatient unit and, soon after, the ECT treatments were discontinued due to concern for worsening cognitive status

PATIENT FILE

- Following discontinuation of ECT, the patient's violence and aggression have returned and his treatment team is considering reinitiation of ECT given this modality's effectiveness in decreasing his violent behavior

Mechanism of action moment

The mechanisms of ECT remain poorly understood; however, it is hypothesized it may exert its benefits through several mechanisms, either independently or in combination. The main theory is that ECT works by inducing neuroplasticity (i.e., neurogenesis, synaptogenesis, angiogenesis, gliogenesis). Somewhat counterintuitively, ECT may also exert its benefits by causing local inflammation in a way that brings about repair (systemic inflammatory processes have been associated with psychopathology, but local inflammatory processes may be beneficial).

Case debrief

- In addition to our patient's initial diagnosis of a major neurocognitive disorder due to repetitive traumatic brain injuries, he was also diagnosed with a psychotic disorder by multiple physicians, specifically documented as schizoaffective disorder, bipolar type
- This patient experienced signs and symptoms of psychosis, mania, depression, impulsivity, aggression, changes in personality, and cognitive impairment due to several potential etiologies
- The limited psychiatric and neurological history of this patient's presentation limits our ability to identify whether the neurocognitive symptoms preceded the psychiatric symptoms or vice versa. This is also further complicated by the vague history of methamphetamine and alcohol use, physical and sexual trauma, reported seizure disorder, and unknown family psychiatric history
- Nevertheless, we are aware of his history of multiple head injuries as reported by his family and himself, with some classified as "concussions," which he first sustained in childhood
- Records indicate that he allegedly observed a noticeable change in his cognitive functioning after closed head injuries, experiencing neurocognitive deficits that were not present, or severe, prior to the head injuries
- Although the patient was unable to explicitly identify when he first began to develop symptoms of neurocognitive deficits, they were reported to become more substantial and impairing as time progressed from the acute injury

PATIENT FILE

- With the accumulation of an increasing number of brain injuries, the patient's neurocognitive symptoms worsened. Specifically, the patient experienced worsening attentional disruption, disorientation/confusion, fluctuating arousal (questionable for delirium), short-term memory impairment, and autobiographical memory impairment / retrograde amnesia. His cognitive symptoms include gross deficits in memory, attention, and concentration
- He also exhibits poor impulse control, intrusiveness, and difficulty maintaining appropriate boundaries, especially with female staff
- The patient's psychotic and mood symptoms include persecutory delusions (paranoia), auditory and visual hallucinations, irritability, disorganized thought process, and anxiety
- In addition, despite compliance with multiple psychotropic medication regimens, this patient exhibited treatment-resistant psychosis and severe aggression and violence toward himself and others, often requiring isolation and restraints
- After years of treatment with multiple antipsychotics, mood stabilizers, and antidepressants, he remained psychiatrically decompensated, with worsening psychosis, cognitive functioning, and aggression over time
- Given the ongoing treatment resistance to multiple trials of medications, an alternative intervention must be considered to treat the symptoms causing impairment, specifically the psychosis and escalating aggression
- This patient has no absolute contraindications for a procedure such as ECT, which has been shown to significantly reduce the psychosis and aggression that are often present with major neurocognitive disorders

ECT as a treatment

- Evidence suggests that, although psychotic disorders may commonly present with neurocognitive impairments similar to major neurocognitive disorders, orientation is usually not affected, nor includes gross abnormalities on cognitive screening instruments
- In addition, the psychotic symptoms associated with a primary psychotic disorder are more likely to remit with the use of multiple antipsychotic agents, such as a D_2-blocking medication
- ECT is an evidence-based treatment used to target treatment-resistant symptoms of psychosis and aggression/violence in those with a major neurocognitive disorder and psychotic disorder alike
- If multiple trials of antipsychotic and mood-stabilizing medications have not improved the impairing aggressive and psychotic/affective

symptoms in a patient, one can consider ECT as the treatment of choice
- ECT is relatively safe for those without contraindicative medical illnesses, who have passed a pre-ECT work-up which assesses for cardiovascular health and safety for inducing seizures, and who are available to have multiple treatments each week
- Neuropsychological testing is recommended prior to initiation of ECT to ensure ability to monitor cognitive functioning during/after ECT, in relation to before ECT. This will allow identification of any cognitive decline directly associated with the ECT treatments themselves
- Regular cognitive screening using a MoCA and MMSE is also recommended: one per week for 3 weeks upon initiation of ECT, and monthly thereafter in order to measure patient's cognitive status from one week to the next
- One should consider any potential reversible medical or neurological condition causing neurocognitive impairments if they do develop in the course of ECT, although the development of memory impairment is common. One can practice administering ECT with lower voltage, alternative electrode placements, etc., when delivering ECT to ensure prevention of inducing cognitive deficits from the procedure itself
- In this case, ECT significantly reduced the psychotic and aggressive/violent behaviors in a patient with comorbid psychotic disorder and major neurocognitive disorder despite years of treatment resistance with multiple psychotropic medications

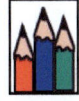

Take-home points
- Psychotic disorders and major neurocognitive disorders may have multiple overlapping symptoms, which can make the diagnosis difficult
- Full assessment of symptom presentation, including a physical examination and thorough history, can inform the provider of the individual's complete symptomatic profile and allow more accurate diagnosis and treatment
- ECT is an evidence-based treatment used to target symptoms resistant to psychopharmacological treatment in psychosis and aggression associated with major neurocognitive disorders and psychotic/affective disorders

PATIENT FILE

Performance in practice: confessions of a psychopharmacologist

- Transient cognitive impairment following ECT procedures is a known potential side effect of the treatment. In order to fully obtain a patient's consent for ECT, one must assess for capacity with each treatment, and this includes explaining the common side effect of transient memory loss. One is expected to explain the indications and contraindications of the procedure, the alternatives, the risks versus benefits, and assess whether the patient can consistently and rationally voice their consent to or not to pursue the procedure
- If a patient is found to lack capacity to consent for treatment, the nearest kin or the person who is the patient's medical power of attorney should be contacted. If there is no designated medical power of attorney, the providers should pursue a court order if they deem the treatment the least restrictive alternative, and appropriate for the care of the individual

Two-minute tutorial

- In major neurocognitive disorders caused by repeated head trauma or TBI, one should consider the distinct disorder commonly referred to as CTE
- CTE has only recently entered the public vocabulary as an association between repeated head trauma and early dementia
- Given that there are no currently agreed-upon diagnostic criteria or neuropathological characterization of CTE at this time, it is considered a preliminary diagnosis
- The primary distinction of CTE versus other major neurocognitive disorders is that, while a preliminary diagnostic class, it is thought to characterize early presentation of mood and behavioral symptoms as well as later progressive cognitive deficits and dementia, but with fewer motor features
- Further research is required to classify the diagnostic criteria, etiology, and disease progression of CTE
- Although it is not currently an official diagnostic disorder in the major neurocognitive disorder category, the constellation of psychiatric and cognitive symptoms and how they specifically develop can help us think through the various neurocognitive disorder constellations

PATIENT FILE

Post-test question

What therapeutic intervention is indicated for treatment-resistant psychiatric/aggressive symptoms in a patient with CTE and a comorbid primary psychotic disorder?

A. Clozapine
B. Long-acting antipsychotic (LAI) IM medications
C. Benzodiazepines
D. Psychotherapy + olanzapine
E. Electroconvulsive therapy (ECT) +/- continued psychopharmacological medications

Answer: E

References

1. American Psychiatric Association. (2022). *Diagnostic and Statistical Manual of Mental Disorders* (5th ed., text rev.). Washington, DC: APA. https://doi.org/10.1176/appi.books.9780890425787.
2. Cano, M. & Camprodon, J. A. (2023). Understanding the mechanisms of action of electroconvulsive therapy: revisiting neuroinflammatory and neuroplasticity hypotheses. *JAMA Psychiatry*, 80(6), 643–644. https://doi.org/10.1001/jamapsychiatry.2023.0728.
3. Golden, C. J. & Zusman, M. R. (2019). Prologue and introduction to CTE and aggression. In *Chronic Traumatic Encephalopathy (CTE)*, Springer Briefs in Psychology. Cham: Springer. https://doi.org/10.1007/978-3-030-23288-7_1.
4. Smith, D. H., Johnson, V. E., Trojanowski, J. Q., & Stewart, W. (2019). Chronic traumatic encephalopathy – confusion and controversies. *Nature Reviews. Neurology*, 15(3), 179–183. https://doi.org/10.1038/s41582-018-0114-8.

PATIENT FILE

16

Addictions: Everyone, everywhere, everything

The Psychopharmacological Dilemma: Finding biological treatment modalities for substance use disorders

Long Hoang and Seth Judd

Pretest self-assessment question
What is a contraindication for naltrexone?
A. Taking an opioid agent
B. Acute kidney injury
C. Metformin
D. Over 65 years old

Patient evaluation on intake
- A 44-year-old male with a long history of schizoaffective disorder, borderline intellectual functioning, antisocial personality disorder, alcohol use disorder (AUD), cocaine use disorder, methamphetamine use disorder, cannabis use disorder, and opioid use disorder, who was transferred to a forensic state hospital for management of psychotic and aggressive behaviors toward himself and others
- His appearance was disheveled. His behavior was cooperative
- His motor activity was normal. His speech was clear, and he was able to provide coherent answers to questions
- His mood was depressed with blunted facial expression
- His thought process was tangential. His thought content included several odd topics such as being involved with demons and devils. However, he did not fixate on this topic or express delusions about these entities
- He denied perceptual disturbance such as auditory hallucination, and he did not appear to be responding to internal stimuli

Psychiatric history
- Psychotic symptoms
  - Auditory hallucinations began at the age of 17 when he was in juvenile detention. His auditory hallucinations are commanding in nature, telling him to hurt himself and others

PATIENT FILE

- He experienced visual hallucinations, seeing demons at the age of 18
- He had delusional thoughts that his mind was transplanted and that he was a robot. He believed that he was a disciple of the devil. He mentioned he was involved with a cult, the devil, and demons
- Depressive symptoms
  - He experienced severe emotional disturbances during his childhood
  - He endorsed feeling depressed, which was frequently followed by a blackout. When he would wake up from the blackout, he would have thoughts of suicide, leading to multiple suicide attempts
  - He also endorsed poor concentration, feeling tired, insomnia, and anhedonia
- Borderline intellectual functioning
  - His intellectual functioning was in the Extremely Low range. His Full-Scale IQ score on the Wechsler Abbreviated Scale of Intelligence (WASI-I) was below 70. His score was consistent with the IQ testing result at another facility
- Antisocial personality disorder
  - He demonstrated symptoms of conduct disorder, such as running away at the age of 12, and engaged in male prostitution to maintain himself. He was caught after he ran away and was placed in juvenile detention. As a juvenile, he obtained charges related to theft/burglary and possession/use of substances
  - As an adult, he demonstrated symptoms of antisocial personality disorder, such as multiple arrest as an adult, hiding weapons or drug use from staff members, impulsivity, using dirty needles for drug use, and inability to maintain employment
- History of suicidal thoughts / suicide attempts / self-inflicting behaviors
  - At age 15 he engaged in self-injurious behaviors (e.g., cutting)
  - He has also attempted to hang himself, shoot himself, or torture himself
- History of multiple hospitalizations
  - History of multiple hospitalizations (at least eight) to psychiatric hospitals, state hospitals, and psychiatric prisons across different states, starting at the age of 15
- History of polysubstance use disorder
  - His history of drug and alcohol abuse started at the age of 11
  - He admitted to using every possible drug, such as speed, methamphetamines, heroin, marijuana, phencyclidine (PCP), ecstasy, and lysergic acid diethylamide (LSD)

PATIENT FILE

- He was preoccupied with getting and using drugs in order to get high. On multiple occasions, he also attempted to choke himself to get high but denied self-harm behaviors. Finally, he would smuggle street drugs into his home unit at the hospital
- He was noncompliant with his medications as well as urine drug tests

Social and personal history
- He was born and raised in a rural town
- His parents divorced when he was 7, and he ran away when he was 12
- He had little contact with his parents as well as with his siblings
- He engaged in male prostitution to provide for himself and obtain drugs, but was arrested and sent to juvenile detention
- He dropped out of school in sixth grade, but eventually received a general educational development (GED) in a correctional facility
- He had multiple arrests with multiple charges
- He has never been married and does not have any children
- He denied any history of physical abuse, sexual abuse, or exposure to violence

Medical history
- Obesity
- Gastroesophageal reflux disease (GERD)
- Viral infection of liver secondary to intravenous (IV) drug use
- Hyperlipidemia
- Lung nodule
- Complex sleep apnea syndrome
- Allergic rhinitis

Family history
- He denied psychiatric family history, but records indicated family history of alcohol and methamphetamine use

Medication history (maximum daily dose listed)
- Aripiprazole 30 mg
- Benztropine mesylate 3 mg
- Bupropion 300 mg
- Citalopram 40 mg
- Clonazepam 2 mg
- Clozapine 450 mg
- Diphenhydramine 50 mg
- Duloxetine 30 mg
- Fluoxetine 20 mg
- Fluphenazine decanoate 125 mg

PATIENT FILE

- Fluphenazine 25 mg
- Haloperidol 30 mg
- Haloperidol decanoate 200 mg
- Haloperidol lactate 40 mg
- Hydroxyzine 350 mg
- Lithium carbonate 1500 mg
- Lithium citrate 40 milliequivalents (meq)
- Lorazepam 2 mg
- Mirtazapine 15 mg
- Naltrexone 100 mg
- Olanzapine 40 mg
- Paliperidone palmitate 234 mg
- Propranolol hcl 30 mg
- Quetiapine furamate 400 mg
- Risperidone 6 mg
- Risperidone microspheres 25 mg
- Sertraline 200 mg
- Topiramate 200 mg
- Trazodone 100 mg
- Venlafaxine 350 mg
- Ziprasidone 200 mg
- Allergies: chlorpromazine, codeine, and trazodone

Current history/medications

- Naltrexone 100 mg for alcohol and opioid use disorders
- Citalopram 20 mg for mood
- Paliperidone palmitate 234 mg intramuscular (IM) qmonth for psychosis
- Haloperidol 15 mg for psychosis and agitation
- Olanzapine 15 mg as needed (PRN) for agitation

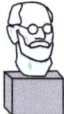

Psychotherapy history

- Due to his low motivation and staying in his bed most of the time, he did not engage in individual therapy or group therapy

Mechanism of action moment

- There are three major classes of opioid receptors:
  - Mu-opioid receptor: regulates analgesia, euphoria, physical dependence, miosis, constipation, vasodilation, and respiratory depression
  - Kappa-opioid receptor: regulates analgesia, diuresis, and dysphoria
  - Delta-opioid receptor: regulates analgesia and constipation

PATIENT FILE

- Naltrexone: opioid receptor antagonist
  - FDA-approved for alcohol dependence, and opioid dependence
  - Pharmacokinetics
    - Extensive first-pass effect
    - Oral administration: half-life ($t_{1/2}$) = 4 hours; intramuscular (IM) injection: $t_{1/2}$ = 5–10 days
    - Primary excretion through urine
  - Target receptors/effect
    - Opioid receptor antagonist with highest affinity for mu receptors:
    - Opioid: prevents exogenous opioids from binding to the receptor, which prevents the pleasurable effects of opioid consumption
    - Alcohol: prevents increased dopaminergic activity after the consumption of alcohol, which reduces the reinforcing effects of alcohol

Attending physician's mental notes

- There is a strong relationship between drug abuse and the onset of psychotic symptoms (see Table 16.1)
  - Recreational substances such as cannabis, cocaine, amphetamine, and hallucinogens have psychotomimetic properties, inducing transient psychotic symptoms
- Drug-induced psychosis is expected to be resolved during an abstinence period
- While, on average, methamphetamine psychosis recovery occurs in about a week, psychotic symptoms can persist for 6 months or longer even in the absence of methamphetamine use. Furthermore, methamphetamine psychosis can convert into a primary psychotic disorder
- Patients with drug-induced psychosis are more likely to abuse more than one drug

Table 16.1 Substance-induced psychoses

Substance	Prevalence of psychosis	Most common psychotic symptoms
Cannabis	0.8%–10%	Paranoia; hallucinations; negative symptoms; feelings of disinhibition or dreaminess; sensations of heightened awareness of music, sounds, and colors or tastes
Cocaine	60%–86.5%	Paranoid delusion, hallucinations, and behavioral abnormalities
Methamphetamine	17%–37.1%	Persecutory delusions, hallucinations, hostility, and conceptual disorganization
Hallucinogens	20.9% for LSD, 18.8% for psilocybe mushrooms	Changes in perception

PATIENT FILE

Further investigation

Given history of noncompliance with medication and reportedly cheeking medications at the jail, what steps can be taken to improve medication compliance?

- Some options to improve medication compliance include:
    - Putting patient on club medications (crushing or opening capsules and mixing in liquid)
    - Switching medications to disintegrated forms
    - Instructing nursing staff to check for cheeking
    - Administering long-acting injection
    - Obtain medication blood levels to monitor compliance

Case outcome

2015–2016

- The patient denied positive symptoms of psychosis, but endorsed prominent negative symptoms including anhedonia, affective flattening, alogia, and avolition
- His presentations remained unchanged. with persistent cravings for drugs, self-harm acts to get "high." He was involved with bringing in and obtaining contraband on the unit, trading medications with peers, and using illicit substances. He had poor insight into his substance use and refused to comply with multiple drug screens
- Patient was started on two medications to target his substance use and addictive behaviors: naltrexone and topiramate. Patient was prescribed up to 100 mg of naltrexone and 200 mg of topiramate. He was also prescribed two antipsychotics: aripiprazole 30 mg and olanzapine 10 mg. To target his depressive symptoms, he was titrated up to 350 mg of venlafaxine

Attending physician's mental notes

2015–2016

- Negative symptoms of a primary psychotic disorder present a clinical challenge as they can appear similar to depressive symptoms in mood disorders
- Negative symptoms include diminished emotional expression, avolition (a decrease in motivated self-initiated purposeful activities), alogia (diminished speech output), anhedonia (the decreased ability to experience pleasure), and asociality (the apparent lack of interest in social interactions)
- Depressive episodes include anhedonia, depressed mood, changes in appetite or weight, sleep disturbances, low energy, low

PATIENT FILE

- concentration, hopelessness/guilt, recurrent SI / suicide attempt, and psychomotor agitation or retardation
- Patients with negative symptoms are more likely to have reduced expression and moderate levels of depression, while patients with depression are more likely to have mostly unimpaired expression and high scores of self-reported depressive symptoms
- Records indicated that patient was affected by his negative and depressive symptoms, significantly contributing to his lack of motivation and effort to progress in treatment. He did not participate in individual therapy and group therapy. He usually refused to get up to discuss his case with treatment team
- To better address these symptoms, will consider switching to another SNRI or SSRI, or ECT

Further investigation

What are some treatment options available to target negative symptoms of a primary psychotic disorder?

- There are no FDA-approved medications for negative symptoms and there are limited treatment options for predominant persistent primary negative symptoms
- Options include reevaluating current antipsychotic regimen and titrate up on dose to reduce secondary negative symptoms
- Overall, SGAs are preferred over first-generation antipsychotics (FGAs), especially cariprazine and amisulpride
- Augmentation with antidepressants can be considered

Case outcome

2018

- He remained inconsistently compliant with his medication, leading to medication adjustment, including a discontinuation of clozapine
- He has a long history of medication noncompliance
- His presentations remained unchanged and he continued to present with depression, infrequent auditory/visual hallucinations, nonlethal self-harm acts, delusions that he must participate in "evil" in order to obtain psychological stability, and negative symptoms
- He continued to display unhealthy coping skills such as attempting self-induced syncope as a way to alleviate emotional distress
- He was prescribed two antipsychotics, 15 mg of haloperidol and 60 mg of ziprasidone, after the discontinuation of clozapine. He was also prescribed 32 milliequivalents (meq) of lithium citrate

PATIENT FILE

for mood stabilization and self-harm/suicidality. He continued to be prescribed 50 mg of naltrexone and 100 mg of topiramate to target his substance use and addictive behaviors. He continued to be prescribed 350 mg of venlafaxine to target his depressive symptoms

Attending physician's mental notes

2018
- There are multiple factors which influence medication compliance
  - Factors that increase compliance: female gender, middle and high socioeconomic status, good doctor–patient relationship, participation in self-help group, motivation for treatment
  - Factors that decrease compliance: male gender, low socioeconomic status, substance use (e.g., excessive alcohol use), unfavored attitude of family members, younger age, poor insight, cognitive impairments, minority ethnicity, low level of education
- Nature of patient's illness can have a strong impact on medication compliance
  - Patients with psychotic symptoms (e.g., feeling persecuted or poisoned) can be hesitant to take medications
  - Patients with grandiose delusions are less likely to be interested in their own treatment
  - Patients with negative symptoms will have low motivation to follow their treatment plan
- Literature shows that habit-based and behavioral-targeted interventions could improve medication adherence. The most effective interventions include face-to-face delivery, delivery by pharmacists, and direct administration to patients
- Psychoeducation appears to encourage medication compliance
- Long-acting injectable (LAI) antipsychotics also improve medication compliance, compared with oral medication

Further investigation

What treatment strategies to improve compliance would be most appropriate for this patient?
- Given this patient has multiple risk factors for decreased compliance, such as substance use, severity of psychotic symptoms, predominant negative symptoms, and cheeking behaviors, a long-acting injectable antipsychotic would be the most appropriate treatment change to improve compliance
- Treating predominant negative symptoms to improve motivation toward his treatment plan is also necessary

PATIENT FILE

- In addition, the patient could benefit from psychoeducation reality testing to improve his insight into need for treatment
- Clozapine was discontinued due to his noncompliance. Clozapine is available as oral tablets, oral disintegrating tablets, and oral suspension. Therefore, to improve compliance with clozapine, either oral disintegrating tablets or oral suspension can be utilized

Case outcome

2019

- He continued to demonstrate negative symptoms by not being motivated to make progress toward his discharge. He remained delusional and continued to be noncompliant with his treatment plan. In addition, he continued to display self-harm behaviors such as auto-asphyxiation using a towel. He did not demonstrate auditory or visual hallucination. However, prominent delusions remained. He continued to believe he was a disciple of the devil and that the devil wanted him to do "dust." He informed staff he recently used methamphetamine he had obtained from a staff member. His insight and judgment remained poor. He stated, "There is nothing wrong with me."
- Paliperidone palmitate was started in 2019 with a loading dose of 234 mg. The monthly dose of paliperidone palmitate was started at 117 mg and then titrated up to 234 mg. In addition, he was prescribed 25 mg of haloperidol for psychosis. He continued to be prescribed 40 mEq of lithium citrate for mood stabilization and suicidality. He was also prescribed 100 mg of sertraline to target his depressive symptoms

Attending physician's mental notes

2019

- The addition of paliperidone palmitate in this patient had little effect on psychosis
- Since the maximum dose of paliperidone palmitate (or, similarly, risperidone microspheres) is equivalent to a daily dose of risperidone 3–6 mg, it's not surprising that this treatment-resistant patient did not adequately respond to this LAI
- Other drawbacks to the use of paliperidone palmitate include the financial burden
- In this patient, other LAIs such as haloperidol decanoate and fluphenazine decanoate should be considered, given their higher daily dose equivalency and cost advantages

PATIENT FILE

Further investigation
Would you consider adding a second LAI? What are the benefits and risks associated with dual LAI treatment?
- Currently, there is no official guideline to address using two LAIs simultaneously. However, this method has been used in clinical practice
- There are a few case reports that demonstrated improvement in psychotic symptoms after a second LAI was added
- It is advised that each LAI should be utilized at the lowest effective dose to decrease side effects and improve toleration
- Given the patient's history of noncompliance with medication and poor response to treatment during periods of compliance, addition of a second LAI should be considered

Case debrief
- Patient's diagnoses include schizoaffective disorder, borderline intellectual functioning, antisocial personality disorder, AUD, cocaine use disorder, methamphetamine use disorder, cannabis use disorder, and opioid use disorder
- He was on multiple classes of medication including antipsychotics (aripiprazole, clozapine, haloperidol, haloperidol decanoate, olanzapine, paliperidone palmitate, perphenazine, quetiapine, risperidone, risperidone microspheres), mood stabilizer (lithium), antidepressants (bupropion, citalopram, doxepin, duloxetine, fluoxetine, mirtazapine, sertraline, venlafaxine) and anxiolytics (clonazepam, diphenhydramine, hydroxyzine, lorazepam)
  - Multiple medications were discontinued due to his noncompliance secondary to multiple factors, such as lack of insight, severe psychotic symptoms, predominant negative symptoms, and severe substance use history
- His symptoms of substance use disorder did not improve even though he had access to substance use disorder groups and was prescribed medications to target his addictive behaviors (e.g., naltrexone and topiramate)
- Negative symptoms of a primary psychotic disorder present as a clinical challenge and can significantly impact motivation and compliance with treatment plan

Take-home points
- Naltrexone is FDA-approved for opioid use disorder and AUD
  - Other agents, such as topiramate or gabapentin, can be used off-label for AUD

PATIENT FILE

- Substance-induced psychosis is common with the use of illicit drugs.
- It is challenging to distinguish negative symptoms from a depressive episode. However, it is necessary to recognize them due to different managements
  - Negative symptoms: antipsychotics (cariprazine, amisulpride), augmentation with antidepressants
  - Depressive symptoms: antidepressants, SGAs, electroconvulsive therapy (ECT), and transcranial magnetic stimulation (TMS)
- Risk factors for medication noncompliance include male gender, low socioeconomic status, substance use (e.g., excessive alcohol use), unfavored attitude of family members, younger age, poor insight, cognitive impairments, minority ethnicity, and low level of education
  - Psychotic symptoms can also worsen compliance
- Clozapine is recommended for treatment-resistant schizophrenia. If treatment compliance is a concern, we can consider clozapine oral disintegrating tablets or oral suspension
- The use of LAIs should be considered early in treatment if patient is noncompliant with antipsychotic medication

Performance in practice: confessions of a psychopharmacologist

Benefits and limitations of LAI

Table 16.2 Dosing conversion between LAI and oral medication

Name	Oral dose	LAI dose
Haloperidol decanoate	Initial LAI dose	20 x oral dose
	Maintenance LAI dose	10–15 x oral dose every 4 weeks
Fluphenazine decanoate	Initial LAI dose	6.25mg every 2 weeks
	10 mg	12.5 every 3 weeks
	20 mg	25 mg every 3 weeks
	30 mg	37.5 every 3–6 weeks
	40 mg	50 mg every 3–6 weeks
Aripiprazole monohydrate	15 mg	300 mg every 4 weeks
	20 mg	400 mg every 4 weeks
Aripiprazole lauroxil	10 mg	441 mg every 4 weeks
	15 mg	662 mg every 4 weeks
	15 mg	882 mg every 6 weeks
	15 mg	1064 mg every 8 weeks
	20mg	882mg every 4 weeks
Paliperidone palmitate	< 3mg	39 mg every 4 weeks
	3 mg	78 mg every 4 weeks
	6 mg	117 mg every 4 weeks
	9 mg	156 mg every 4 weeks
	12 mg	234 mg every 4 weeks
Paliperidone palmitate – 12-week	3 mg	273 mg every 12 weeks
	6 mg	410 mg every 12 weeks
	9 mg	546 mg every 12 weeks
	12 mg	819 mg every 12 weeks

PATIENT FILE

Table 16.2 (cont.)

Name	Oral dose	LAI dose
Paliperidone palmitate – 6-month	9 mg	1092 mg every 6 months
	12 mg	1560 mg every 6 months
Risperidone microspheres	1 mg	12.5 mg every 2 weeks
	2–3 mg	25 mg every 2 weeks
	3–5 mg	37.5 mg every 2 weeks
	4–5 mg	50 mg every 2 weeks
Risperidone subcutaneous	3 mg	90 mg every 4 weeks
	4 mg	120 mg every 4 weeks
Olanzapine LAI	10 mg	**Initial 8 weeks**
		210 mg every 2 weeks or
		405 mg every 4 weeks
		Maintenance
		150 mg every 2 weeks or
		300 mg every 4 weeks
	15 mg	**Initial 8 weeks**
		300 mg every 2 weeks
		Maintenance
		210 mg every 2 weeks or
		405 mg every 4 weeks
	20 mg	**Initial 8 weeks**
		300 mg every 2 weeks
		Maintenance
		300 mg every 2 weeks

- In this case, the LAI used was paliperidone palmitate. It is important to understand its mechanism of action and when it may be appropriate to use instead of risperidone.
    - Risperidone is metabolized into paliperidone (9-hydroxyrisperidone)
    - Dopamine D_2 antagonist: increases dopamine that improves positive symptoms and stabilizes affective symptoms
    - Serotonin $5HT_{2A}$ antagonist: enhances dopamine release in certain brain area
    - Oral paliperidone does not require dose adjustment for patients with hepatic disease, while with oral risperidone it is recommended to reduce the dose
- Limitation of aripiprazole in forensic setting
    - $t_{1/2}$ = 75 hours
    - Due to long half-life and strong binding affinity for D_2 receptor, aripiprazole can hinder the binding of other antipsychotics to those receptors
    - Dopamine partial agonist can worsen psychosis, agitation, aggression, and activation
- Off-label use of topiramate and gabapentin
    - Topiramate: voltage-sensitive sodium channel modulator
        - < 100 mg/day may be effective in treating AUD. Reduce alcohol use in patients with severe AUD

PATIENT FILE

- Topiramate may be useful in treating cocaine use disorder, smoking cessation, and behavioral addictions
  - Preferred choice for patient with seizure disorder
- Gabapentin: glutamate, voltage-gate calcium channel blocker
  - May reduce frequency of heavy drinking days, and an increase in the total percentage of days of abstinence at a high dose of gabapentin

Table 16.3 Other psychopharmacological options to manage substance use disorder

Substance	Medications	FDA approval indication	Mechanism of actions
Alcohol	Acamprosate	Maintenance of alcohol abstinence	Glutamate multimodal, NMDA antagonist, GABA-A allosteric modulator
	Disulfiram	Maintenance of alcohol abstinence	Irreversible inhibition of aldehyde dehydrogenase
	Gabapentin	Off-label use for alcohol dependence	Voltage-gated calcium channel blocker, GABA-A allosteric modulator, alpha-amino-3-hydroxy-5-methyl-4-isoxazolepropionic acid (AMPA)/kainate receptor antagonist, and carbonic anhydrase inhibitor
	Naltrexone	Alcohol dependence Prevention of opioid relapse	Mu-opioid receptor antagonist
	Topiramate	Off-label use for alcohol dependence	Blocks voltage-sensitive sodium channel
Nicotine	Bupropion	Nicotine dependence	Increases dopamine and norepinephrine
	Nicotine replacement therapy	Smoking cessation	Binds selectively to nicotinic-cholinergic receptors
	Varenicline	Nicotine dependence	Acetylcholine receptor antagonist
Opioid	Buprenorphine	Induction and maintenance treatment of opioid dependence	Mu-opioid receptor partial agonist
	Extended-release naltrexone	Opioid dependence	Mu-opioid receptor antagonist
	Lofexidine	Management of opioid withdrawal symptoms	α_{2A}-adrenergic receptor agonist
	Methadone	Opioid dependence Off-label use for neonatal abstinence syndrome	Full agonist at the mu-opioid receptor
	Naloxone	Opioid overdose	Mu-opioid receptor antagonist

Tips and pearls

- Psychopharmacological management (both FDA approved and off-label use) of substance use disorders focuses on AUD, opioid use disorder, and tobacco use disorder
- Dual disorder is common, especially in forensic populations

PATIENT FILE

- It is important to distinguish the differences and similarities between negative symptoms and depressive symptoms due to different psychotropic management
- Medication noncompliance is common. It is necessary to use multiple approaches, such as psychoeducation, targeting depressive and/or negative symptoms, utilizing disintegrating/liquid medication formulation or LAI to improve compliance
- Using dual LAI may not be a common approach, but it is a viable option if clozapine cannot be utilized

Two-minute tutorial

- Substance use disorder is very common in general population. In the forensic setting, a systemic review and meta-analysis found that dual disorder is extremely common, with around half of the prison population with either major depression or non-affective psychosis having comorbid substance use disorder
- Substances such as cannabis, cocaine, amphetamine, and hallucinogens have psychotomimetic properties; therefore, they can induce transient psychotic symptoms
- Cannabis is considered the most widely used recreational drug in the world, and cannabis-induced psychosis (compared to other substances) is associated with the highest risk of the development of schizophrenia. Specifically, heavy, and early (15 years or younger) cannabis use is associated with increased risk of being diagnosed with schizophrenia in the future
- Depending on which substance, pharmacological management will be different
  - AUD: acamprosate, disulfiram, and naltrexone are FDA approved; topiramate and gabapentin are off-label used
  - Tobacco use disorder: bupropion, nicotine replacement therapy, and varenicline are FDA approved
  - Opioid use disorder: buprenorphine, naltrexone ER, lofexidine, methadone, and naloxone are FDA approved
- Chronic psychosis can worsen negative symptoms, which can be difficult to distinguish from depressive symptoms. Reduced expression and moderate level of depression are more likely to be observed in patients with negative symptoms, while unimpaired expression and high level of depression are more likely to be observed in patients with depression. It is essential to consider differences and similarities between negative symptoms and depressive symptoms due to different psychopharmacological approach

PATIENT FILE

- Negative symptoms: SGAs (cariprazine, amisulpride), augmentation with antidepressants
- Depressive symptoms: antidepressants, SGAs, ECT, and TMS
- Management of treatment-resistant schizophrenia can include clozapine. However, if clozapine is not available, and treatment compliance remains an issue, dual LAI regimen can be considered

Post-test question

What is a contraindication for naltrexone?

A. Taking an opioid agent
B. Acute kidney injury
C. Metformin
D. Over 65 years old

Answer: A

References

1. Anton, R. F., Latham, P., & Voronin, K., et al. (2020). Efficacy of gabapentin for the treatment of alcohol use disorder in patients with alcohol withdrawal symptoms: a randomized clinical trial. *JAMA Internal Medicine*, 180(5), 728–736. https://doi.org/10.1001/jamainternmed.2020.0249.
2. Baranyi, G., Fazel, S., Langerfeldt, S. D., & Mundt, A. P. (2022). The prevalence of comorbid serious mental illnesses and substance use disorders in prison populations: a systematic review and meta-analysis. *Lancet Public Health*, June, 7(6), e557–e568. https://doi.org/10.1016/S2468-2667(22)00093-7. PMID: 35660217; PMCID: PMC9178214.
3. Casadio, P., Fernandes, C., Murray, R. M., & Di Forti, M. (2011). Cannabis use in young people: the risk for schizophrenia. *Neuroscience and Biobehavioral Reviews*, 35(8), 1779–1787. https://doi.org/10.1016/j.neubiorev.2011.04.007.
4. Cerveri, G., Gesi, C., & Mencacci, C. (2019). Pharmacological treatment of negative symptoms in schizophrenia: update and proposal of a clinical algorithm. *Neuropsychiatric Disease and Treatment*, June 5, 15, 1525–1535. https://doi.org/10.2147/NDT.S201726. PMID: 31239687; PMCID: PMC6556563.
5. Citrome, L. (2010). Paliperidone palmitate – review of the efficacy, safety and cost of a new second-generation depot antipsychotic medication. *International Journal of Clinical Practice*. Jan., 64(2), 216–239. https://doi.org/10.1111/j.1742-1241.2009.02240.x. Epub Nov. 3, 2009. PMID: 19886879.

PATIENT FILE

6. Conn, V. S. & Ruppar, T. M. (2017). Medication adherence outcomes of 771 intervention trials: systematic review and meta-analysis. *Preventive Medicine*, 99, 269–276.
7. Cuijpers, P., Quero, S., Dowrick, C., & Arroll, B. (2019). Psychological treatment of depression in primary care: recent developments. *Current Psychiatry Reports*, Nov. 23, 21(12), 129. https://doi.org/10.1007/s11920-019-1117-x. PMID: 31760505; PMCID: PMC6875158.
8. Dhaliwal, A., & Gupta, M. (2022). Physiology, Opioid Receptor [Updated July 25, 2022]. StatPearls [Internet]. Treasure Island, FL: StatPearls Publishing; Jan.– . Available from: www.ncbi.nlm.nih.gov/books/NBK546642.
9. Diefenderfer, L. A. (2017). When should you consider combining 2 long-acting injectable antipsychotics? *Current Psychiatry*, 16, 42–46.
10. Fiorentini, A., Cantù, F., Crisanti, C., Cereda, G., Oldani, L., & Brambilla, P. (2021). Substance-induced psychoses: an updated literature review. *Frontiers in Psychiatry*, Dec. 23, 12, 694863. https://doi.org/10.3389/fpsyt.2021.694863. PMID: 35002789; PMCID: PMC8732862.
11. García, S., Martínez-Cengotitabengoa, M., López-Zurbano, S., et al. (2016). Adherence to antipsychotic medication in bipolar disorder and schizophrenic patients: a systematic review. *Journal of Clinical Psychopharmacology*, Aug., 36(4), 355–371. https://doi.org/10.1097/JCP.0000000000000523. PMID: 27307187; PMCID: PMC4932152.
12. Glasner-Edwards, S. & Mooney, L. J. (2014). Methamphetamine psychosis: epidemiology and management. *CNS Drugs*, Dec., 28(12), 1115–1126. https://doi.org/10.1007/s40263-014-0209-8. PMID: 25373627; PMCID: PMC5027896.
13. Greene, M., Yan, T., Chang, E., Hartry, A., Touya, M., & Broder, M. S. (2018). Medication adherence and discontinuation of long-acting injectable versus oral antipsychotics in patients with schizophrenia or bipolar disorder. *Journal of Medical Economics*, Feb., 21(2), 127–134. https://doi.org/10.1080/13696998.2017.1379412. Epub Sept. 29, 2017. PMID: 28895758.
14. Magura, S., Mateu, P. F., Rosenblum, A., Matusow, H., & Fong, C. (2014). Risk factors for medication non-adherence among psychiatric patients with substance misuse histories. *Mental Health and Substance Use*, Nov., 7(4), 381–390. https://doi.org/10.1080/17523281.2013.839574. PMID: 25309623; PMCID: PMC4191826.
15. Manhapra, A., Chakraborty, A., & Arias, A. J. (2019). Topiramate pharmacotherapy for alcohol use disorder and other addictions: a

PATIENT FILE

   narrative review. *Journal of Addiction Medicine*, 13(1), 7–22. https://doi.org/10.1097/ADM.0000000000000443.
16. Mariani, J. J., Pavlicova, M., Basaraba, C., et al. (2021). Pilot randomized placebo-controlled clinical trial of high-dose gabapentin for alcohol use disorder. *Alcoholism: Clinical and Experimental Research*, 45, 1639–1652. https://doi.org/10.1111/acer.14648.
17. Oehl, M., Hummer, M., & Fleischhacker, W. W. (2000). Compliance with antipsychotic treatment. *Acta Psychiatrica Scandinavica*, 407(Suppl.), 83–86. https://doi.org/10.1034/j.1600-0447.2000.00016.x. PMID: 11261648.
18. Rao, K. N, George, J., Sudarshan, C. Y., & Begum, S. (2017). Treatment compliance and noncompliance in psychoses. *Indian Journal of Psychiatry*, Jan.–March, 59(1), 69–76. https://doi.org/10.4103/psychiatry.IndianJPsychiatry_24_17. PMID: 28529363; PMCID: PMC5419016.
19. Richter, J., Hölz, L., Hesse, K., Wildgruber, D., & Klingberg, S. (2019). Measurement of negative and depressive symptoms: discriminatory relevance of affect and expression. *European Psychiatry*, Jan., 55, 23–28. https://doi.org/10.1016/j.eurpsy.2018.09.008. Epub Oct. 29, 2018. PMID: 30384108.
20. Singh, D., & Saadabadi, A. (2022). Naltrexone. June 29. StatPearls [Internet]. Treasure Island (FL): StatPearls Publishing; Jan.– . PMID: 30521232.
21. Stahl, S. M., Grady, M. M., & Muntner, N. (2021). *Stahl's Essential Psychopharmacology, Prescriber's Guide*, 8th ed. Cambridge University Press.
22. Starzer, M. S. K., Nordentoft, M., & Hjorthøj, C. (2018). Rates and predictors of conversion to schizophrenia or bipolar disorder following substance-induced psychosis [published correction appears in *American Journal of Psychiatry*, April 1, 2019, 176(4), 324]. *American Journal of Psychiatry*, 175(4), 343–350. https://doi.org/10.1176/appi.ajp.2017.17020223.
23. Takeuchi, H. & Remington, G. (2013). A systematic review of reported cases involving psychotic symptoms worsened by aripiprazole in schizophrenia or schizoaffective disorder. *Psychopharmacology (Berlin)*. July, 228(2), 175–185. https://doi.org/10.1007/s00213-013-3154-1. Epub June 5, 2013. PMID: 23736279.
24. Veerman, S. R. T., Schulte, P. F. J., & de Haan, L. (2017). Treatment for negative symptoms in schizophrenia: a comprehensive review. *Drugs*, Sept., 77(13), 1423–1459. https://doi.org/10.1007/s40265-017-0789-y. PMID: 28776162.

PATIENT FILE

25. What are dose conversions from oral to injectable for the long-acting injectable (LAI) antipsychotic medications available in the U.S.? [Internet]. SMI Adviser, 2021 [cited Feb. 24, 2023]. Available from: https://smiadviser.org/knowledge_post/what-are-dose-conversions-from-oral-to-injectable-for-the-long-acting-injectable-lai-antipsychotic-medications-available-in-the-u-s.
26. Williams, J. W., Jr., Mulrow, C. D., Chiquette, E., Noël, P. H., Aguilar, C., & Cornell, J. (2000). A systematic review of newer pharmacotherapies for depression in adults: evidence report summary. *Annals of Internal Medicine*, May 2, 132(9), 743–756. https://doi.org/10.7326/0003-4819-132-9-200005020-00011. PMID: 10787370.
27. Xia, J., Merinder, L. B., & Belgamwar, M. R. (2011). Psychoeducation for schizophrenia. *Cochrane Database of Systematic Reviews*, June 15, 2011(6), CD002831. https://doi.org/10.1002/14651858.CD002831.pub2. PMID: 21678337; PMCID: PMC4170907.

17

Personality disorders: Fixing the foundation

The Psychopharmocological Dilemma: Biological treatment options for borderline personality disorder (BPD)

Emilia Laing and Seth Judd

Pretest self-assessment question

Which class of psychotropic medications is FDA approved for borderline personality disorder (BPD)?

A. First- and second-generation antipsychotics (SGAs)
B. Antiepileptics
C. Selective serotonin reuptake inhibitors (SSRIs)
D. Selective norepinephrine reuptake inhibitors (SNRIs)
E. None of the above

Patient evaluation on intake

- Middle-aged female (46 years old) with prior diagnoses of bipolar I disorder, major depression with psychotic features, BPD, and post-traumatic stress disorder (PTSD) who was transferred to a state forensic hospital after unsuccessful attempts to manage her symptoms and behaviors (e.g., suicidal and non-suicidal self-injury) in the community

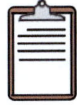

Psychiatric history

- Patient has a history of depression since childhood, self-reported as beginning during late childhood
  - She has a history of childhood sexual abuse
  - She reports first hearing "voices," including command auditory hallucinations (CAH) telling her to kill herself, in her young adulthood after she lost custody of her children
  - Her depression has also been associated with history of persecutory delusions and paranoid ideations
  - She has had numerous hospitalizations for non-suicidal self-injury (NSSI) and suicidal behavior since her 20s
    - Her first hospitalization resulted from cutting herself because she was hearing voices

- The patient has used several methods when attempting suicide, including overdosing on pills, attempting to hang herself, cutting herself, head banging, swallowing foreign bodies, and restricting food intake
- She has received electroconvulsive therapy (ECT) for NSSI and suicidal ideation (SI), with noted improvement in her SIs and hopelessness, and decreased need for PRN medication
- PTSD symptoms include nightmares and flashbacks
- She has a history of substance use and meets criteria for the following substance use disorders: alcohol, cannabis, cocaine, other hallucinogen (ecstasy), and stimulant use disorder (amphetamine-type substance and cocaine)
- She has a history of unstable attachments and reckless sexual behaviors

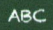

Social and personal history

- Her parents divorced during her early childhood
- She did not graduate from high school but obtained a general educational development (GED) certificate
- She worked for several years as a phlebotomist but had to stop working due to severe depression. Her last period of employment was nearly two decades ago
- She has four children from three different fathers; one son was raised by his grandparents while the three others have been adopted
- She married in her late teens and divorced the same year

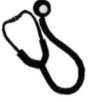

Medical history

- The patient is obese and has hyperlipidemia, hypothyroidism, and gastroesophageal reflux disease (GERD)
- History of traumatic brain injury (TBI) secondary to NSSI, head banging

Family history

- Sister has a history of bipolar disorder (type unspecified) and depression
- Grandparents have diabetes

Medication history

- Amitriptyline 100 mg
- Aripiprazole 30 mg
- Bupropion 450 mg
- Chlorpromazine 600 mg

PATIENT FILE

- Citalopram 40 mg
- Divalproex 3000 mg
- Duloxetine 60 mg
- Fluphenazine decanoate 25 mg intramuscular (IM) once a week
- Haloperidol 30 mg
- Haloperidol decanoate 300 mg IM every 2 weeks
- Lithium 1200 mg
- Lorazepam 6 mg
- Lurasidone 160 mg
- Naltrexone 50 mg
- Olanzapine 30 mg
- Paroxetine 60 mg
- Quetiapine 800 mg
- Sertraline 250 mg
- Temazepam 30 mg
- Topiramate 400 mg
- Trazodone 300 mg
- Valproic acid 500 mg
- Zolpidem 10 mg

Current medications
- Clozapine 375 mg every evening
- Fluoxetine 50 mg every morning
- Melatonin 10 mg every evening
- Mirtazapine 45 mg every evening
- Prazosin 2 mg every evening

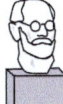

Psychotherapy history
- The patient attends dialectical behavior therapy (DBT) group every Monday, Tuesday, and Wednesday. Recently, DBT has focused on Temperature, Intense exercise, Paced breathing, Progressive muscle relaxation (TIPP); Stop, Take a step back, Observe, and Proceed mindfully (STOP); and Opposite Reaction skills

Mechanism of action moment
- Fluoxetine is the most well-studied antidepressant used in the treatment of BPD
  - Fluoxetine is an SSRI that has 5-HT_{2C}-antagonist actions and weak norepinephrine reuptake inhibition
    - Inhibition of 5-HT_{2C} receptors disinhibits release of norepinephrine and dopamine

PATIENT FILE

- 5-HT$_{2C}$ antagonism has been implicated in fatigue reduction and improvement in concentration and attention
- Since 5-HT$_{2C}$ antagonism is activating in nature, fluoxetine's antagonist actions may make it a less suitable treatment for patients with agitation, insomnia, and anxiety
- The primary indications for ECT are major depression, mania, catatonia, and schizophrenia. Traditionally, ECT has been considered a secondary treatment for patients who fail pharmacotherapy, but it can be considered appropriate initial treatment in certain clinical scenarios, such as life-threatening emergencies
    - The most common indication for ECT is a major depressive episode, with response rates up to 80–90% and remission rates only slightly lower
    - ECT is also highly effective for treating the manic phase of bipolar disorder. It is more rapid than lithium in treating mania
    - Schizophrenia may be the most common indication for ECT worldwide. In the US, ECT has typically been used for schizophrenia with affective features, catatonia, neuroleptic malignant syndrome (NMS), or a history of previous response to ECT. However, recently ECT has been used for medication-refractory illness, regardless of the presence of affective features. ECT combined with antipsychotic medication may synergistically improve psychosis in schizophrenia spectrum disorders
    - ECT is indicated as first-line treatment when there is a need for rapid improvement, such as in patients with catatonia, malnutrition, severe psychosis with agitation, and suicidality. It is also first line in instances when other treatments are riskier, such as in pregnant patients and the elderly. ECT can also be considered first line based on patient preference
- ECT has multiple theorized mechanisms of action. The most well-studied theories include the neurotrophic theory, the classical (monoamine) neurotransmitter theory, the neuroendocrine theory, the anticonvulsant theory, and the connectivity theory
    - **Neurotrophic theory:** Studies have shown that ECT can increase the release of brain-derived neurotrophic factor (BDNF) and increase gray matter volume
    - **Classical neurotransmitter theory:** ECT can alter neurotransmission of dopamine, serotonin, norepinephrine, and other neurotransmitters. Such changes can lead to changes in mood and decrease of psychotic symptoms
    - **Neuroendocrine theory:** This theory suggests that ECT-induced release of hypothalamic or pituitary hormones results in antidepressant effects. ECT results in release of prolactin,

PATIENT FILE

thyroid stimulating hormone (TSH), adrenocorticotropic hormone (ACTH), and endorphins. An antidepressant neuropeptide, "antidepressin," has been theorized to be released from the hypothalamus during the ECT seizure
- **Anticonvulsant theory:** ECT exerts an anticonvulsant effect on the brain. Seizure threshold rises and seizure duration decreases over the course of ECT treatment. This effect has been postulated to be mediated by neurohormones. Gamma-aminobutyric acid (GABA) has also been proposed as a key mediator of ECT's anticonvulsant effect
- **Connectivity theory:** Preliminary data suggests that abnormal baseline neural network connectivity in patients with depression or schizophrenia is re-regulated by ECT

Attending physician's mental notes
- There is significant overlap among mood disorders, PTSD, and BPD
  - BPD is a cluster B personality disorder. BPD patients commonly experience depressive symptoms and often have a history of childhood trauma and emotional neglect. BPD is characterized by a pervasive pattern of symptoms beginning in early adulthood. Symptoms can include instability in personal relationships, self-image, and affects with marked impulsivity. Individuals with BPD experience identity disturbance, recurrent suicidal behavior, marked reactivity of mood, chronic feelings of emptiness, inappropriate anger, and/or transient paranoid ideations or dissociative symptoms
  - Mood disorder, such as major depressive disorder (MDD) and bipolar disorder, often co-occur in individuals with BPD
  - MDD and BPD are characterized by changes in affective states. Both disorders can present with feelings of emptiness and loneliness, suicidal and self-injurious behaviors, and poor self-esteem. BPD can be differentiated from MDD by a chronic or pervasive pattern of affective instability. Those with BPD are more likely to be impulsive and less likely to respond to antidepressants
  - Bipolar disorder and BPD can present with mood swings, impulsive behaviors, suicidal or self-injurious behaviors, irritability, and difficulty maintaining relationships. Differentiation can be made by looking for distinct mood episodes (bipolar disorder) versus chronic, pervasive mood symptoms (BPD). In addition, bipolar disorder, unlike BPD, is characterized by decreased need for sleep and increase in goal-directed activities. Finally, BPD is less likely to respond to mood stabilizers

PATIENT FILE

- PTSD is defined as having experienced a traumatic event. BPD is often linked to childhood trauma and patients with the disorder are at high risk for trauma as adults. Each of these disorders can present with dissociative symptoms, emotional dysregulation, and anger. However, individuals with PTSD tend to have a more negative view of themselves, while BPD has an unstable sense of self. As with the other mentioned disorders co-occurring with BPD, BPD is less likely to respond to antidepressants than PTSD
- First-line pharmacological treatment for mood disorders and PTSD is antidepressants, and this class of psychotropic medication is commonly used in BPD. Although there is no FDA-approved medication for the treatment of BPD, antidepressants can be used to treat the core symptoms, including instability, anxiety, and impulsivity. Other non-FDA-approved treatment options for BPD include antipsychotics and antiepileptics
- Personality disorders frequently coexist with mood disorders, which complicates treatment for these patients. The presence of comorbid mental health diagnoses negatively impacts the outcomes of patients, regardless of whether they receive treatment. For patients specifically with MDD, symptom remission decreases in the presence of a comorbid personality disorder. A concurrent diagnosis of BPD and MDD may increase the severity and duration of MDD. Up to 85% of patients with BPD meet the criteria for MDD, and a diagnosis of BPD is a stronger predictor of MDD persistence than any other risk factor. These patients have lower rates of depression remission than patients with MDD alone. Patients with both BPD and MDD do not respond as well to more traditional treatments such as SSRIs and tricyclic antidepressants (TCAs). Furthermore, depressive symptoms in patients with BPD may not improve without first addressing the personality disorder

Further investigation

What else would you like to know about the patient? Does she have a history of noncompliance with treatment?

- Treatment compliance can be a clinical challenge, especially with individuals who have BPD. BPD patients have high negative attitudes toward medications (60%) and psychotherapy (40%), with the most common reason for medication discontinuation being side effects (> 50%)
- Antipsychotics and other psychotropic medications used for BPD can have significant metabolic side effects. Our patient had been

prescribed first-generation antipsychotics (FGAs), such as haloperidol and fluphenazine, as well as SGAs clozapine and olanzapine
- Of the SGAs, olanzapine and clozapine have the highest association with metabolic disturbances. These medications are strongly associated with weight gain, diabetes mellitus, and hyperlipidemia. These side effects are associated with increased morbidity and mortality, reduced quality of life, and poor drug compliance. Although weight increases most rapidly shortly after starting the medications, studies have shown weight gain may continue long term. Switching to a medication that is less likely to cause weight gain is an option, but patients must be monitored closely for any relapse in symptoms

Case outcome

- 3 years after admission and prior to starting ECT treatment
  - The patient continues to experience desire to harm herself with no improvement in her SIB
    - The patient had 25 reported SIBs earlier in the year
  - She has been recommended to begin ECT due to her prior positive response
    - The patient's interest in ECT was explored to ensure it was not perceived as an extension of self-harm. The patient clearly stated that, apart from a brief period of "memory haze" after treatment, the treatments improved her mood and she no longer had SIs
  - The patient was prescribed clozapine 500 mg every evening for her psychotic symptoms, fluoxetine 40 mg every morning for her depression, lithium 1200 mg every evening for mood stabilization, and prazosin 2 mg every evening for PTSD-related nightmares
    - The patient does not currently have an active involuntary medication order (IMO) if she refuses medication, and she is currently compliant with medication. However, despite her compliance, medication alone failed to treat her severe depressive symptoms and mood instability, anxiety, and impulse control related to her personality disorder

Attending physician's mental notes: first interim progress report

- SI and SIB are some of the hallmarks of BPD, but are also found in MDD and PTSD
  - Treatment of such behaviors is a clinical challenge. The patient has been tried on multiple psychotropic medications and was participating in DBT

PATIENT FILE

- Several structured psychotherapies have yielded positive results in treating such behaviors. These include DBT, dynamic deconstructive therapy, emotion regulation group therapy, and cognitive therapy
- Biological interventions for SI/SIB – other than lithium, ketamine, and ECT – are limited. One review showed promising results with aripiprazole, naltrexone, or SSRIs with or without CBT, while a recent meta-analysis found only antipsychotics, citalopram, and ketamine yielded larger-than-average treatment effects

Further investigation

Would you restart ECT treatment or make other changes/recommendations to the treatment plan?

- Given the patient's history of having a positive response with ECT, adding ECT treatment to her treatment plan would be the next appropriate step
- Check lithium level to ensure compliance and that level is in therapeutic range
- Increase frequency of individual DBT sessions
- Increase dose of fluoxetine or consider switching to an alternative SSRI/SNRI

Case outcome: follow-up 1 year after initiating ECT

- The patient still experiences urges to self-harm but they are more mild and she no longer experiences SIs
  - The patient has not had any self-harm for the past 30 days, is engaging in groups, is fully medication compliant and hasn't requested PRN medications
  - The patient attributes her recent improvement in mood and behavior to ECT and desires for it to be continued until she achieves sustained improvement
- The patient has reconnected with her daughters, who recently were not in touch due to the patient's mood instability
- Over a 15-month period, patient received 47 ECT treatments and was receiving maintenance ECT once a week

Attending physician's mental notes: first interim progress report

- ECT can potentially yield significant decrease in symptoms and greatly improve quality of life
  - Although often seen as a last-resort treatment, 2001 APA Guidelines recommend using ECT earlier in treatment

PATIENT FILE

- ECT is an effective treatment for those with severe, medication-resistant MDD, with rates of remission as high as 75%. However, in patients with a comorbid personality disorder, such as BPD, studies yielded mixed results. Some studies conclude that patients with a cluster B personality disorder (e.g., BPD) have a significantly poorer response to ECT than those with MDD alone, while other studies show equal success or even greater success rates in patients with comorbid personality disorders

Case outcome: follow-up 3 months after patient declined further ECT

- 3-month follow-up after patient declined further ECT treatment
  - The patient has maintained her focus on her goals of achieving discharge, improving her relationships with family, but she continues to be highly critical of herself
  - After several months of stabilization, she has decompensated and once again exhibits regular SIB, including head banging, skin scratching, and punching herself in the face. She states she commonly gets urges to hurt herself but tries to implement her DBT skills when she gets these impulses
  - A little over a week prior to decompensation, ECT treatment was stopped due to patient declining further treatment. She also tested positive for COVID-19 a day before she began engaging in a series of SIBs
    - Her risk status for suicide and SIB have both been labeled as high; she has had 27 reported incidents of SIB this year
    - Treatment team reports recent increase in SIB could be triggered by "separation anxiety." Patient is very close to a peer who is preparing for discharge
    - She states her medication makes her feel "heavy and cloudy" but cannot give specifics

Attending physician's mental note

- During the course of ECT treatment, the patient was determined to have capacity to refuse or consent to ECT treatment. It is important to periodically reassess capacity, as capacity status, especially during periods of decompensation, can change over time
- Fear of abandonment is a core symptom of BPD and can have significant impact on SI, SIB, and therapeutic engagement. For this patient, psychotherapy should specifically target the fears of abandonment

PATIENT FILE

- COVID-19 has been implicated in triggering new mood disorders in patients, such as depression and anxiety. Those with a pre-existing mental health disorder are at increased risk for severe COVID-19, resulting in hospitalization and death
- A retrospective study found an association between COVID-19 infection and NSSI behavior which was due to a variety of factors, such as increased screen time, decreased sleep, and increased anxiety

Further investigation

After reviewing the patient's medication history, are there other psychopharmacological agents that should be considered to target this patient's SI/SIB?

- Ketamine may be an effective psychopharmacological agent for treating such behaviors
- Ketamine can be given IV or intranasally. A recent review indicated most studies used IV ketamine at a dose of 0.5 mg/kg over 40 minutes. The same review also revealed BPD as a covariate did not have a significant impact on the efficacy of this treatment in reducing SI/SIB

Case debrief

- Our patient is diagnosed with MDD with psychotic features, BPD, and PTSD
- The patient had failed multiple trials of psychotropic medications, including antipsychotics, antiepileptics, and antidepressants
  - Non-adherence to medications led to decompensation, with resurgence of auditory hallucinations and SIB
- ECT was recommended and initiated to reduce SI, persecutory and paranoid ideations, to improve impulse control, and to improve overall quality of life
  - The patient received ECT over a 15-month period, which resulted in less use of PRNs, a significant decrease in depressive and psychotic symptoms, and decrease in frequency of SIB and SI

Take-home points

- Patients with personality disorders are 6.5 times more likely to have a comorbid mood disorder than the general population; up to 85% of patients with BPD meet the criteria for MDD
  - A diagnosis of BPD is a stronger predictor of MDD persistence than any other risk factor

PATIENT FILE

- No medication is currently approved for the treatment of BPD, and clinicians should carefully assess the risks and benefits of psychotropic medications before initiating treatment
  - Antipsychotics, antiepileptics, and antidepressants may be effective for various symptoms of BPD, including mood symptoms, anxiety, and impulse control
  - For patients with medication-resistant BPD, ECT can be an effective alternative for treating mood symptoms, SI, or SIB
- DBT is based on cognitive-behavioral principles and is currently the only empirically supported treatment for BPD

Performance in practice: confessions of a psychopharmacologist

- Although there isn't an FDA-approved medication for BPD, medications can still be useful in treating specific symptoms
- Antipsychotics have been shown to improve BPD symptoms of anxiety, impulsivity, and mood dysregulation, with slight variations depending on the specific antipsychotic. The antipsychotics reported as having one or more of these benefits include aripiprazole, clozapine, haloperidol, olanzapine, quetiapine, paliperidone, and ziprasidone
- Antidepressants may be useful in treating the core symptoms of mood instability, anxiety, and impulsivity
  - Duloxetine has been reported to improve clinical status, overall psychopathology, and depression in patients with BPD. It also is selectively effective on impulsivity and affective dysregulation
  - Fluoxetine has been shown to reduce impulsivity, SIB, anger, depressed mood, irritability, anxiety, obsessive–compulsive symptoms, and sensitivity to rejection
  - Fluvoxamine has been reported to reduce rapid mood shifts in BPD
  - Venlafaxine has been reported to reduce somatic symptoms and SIB
- Further studies are warranted to explore the efficacy of antiepileptics in treating symptoms of BPD. The most well-studied epileptics in the treatment of BPD are valproic acid, lamotrigine, carbamazepine, gabapentin, and topiramate
  - Valproic acid may be an effective treatment for impulsive and aggressive symptoms for patients who do not respond to other agents. However, treatment with valproic acid in addition to DBT has not been proven to be more effective than DBT alone
  - Lamotrigine has been shown to reduce aggressive symptoms, affective lability, and impulsivity, though more recent studies have shown that lamotrigine has no effect on patients with BPD

PATIENT FILE

- Topiramate has been shown to successfully treat anger in patients with BPD, as well as assist with weight loss
- Gabapentin has been useful in treating anxiety, affective instability, and depressive symptoms in BPD patients. However, it was often combined with other treatments, thus these findings need to be further evaluated
- Carbamazepine has shown a lack of efficacy in treating BPD symptoms
- The endogenous opioid and reward system is thought to play a role in BPD. Opioid antagonists can potentially reduce BPD-associated symptoms, including SIBs and dissociation. Naltrexone has been studied in BPD and appears to have a biphasic effect. In the acute phase, naltrexone can block the rewarding effects of BPD's self-harm behaviors, and in the chronic phase, it can restore opioid neurotransmission. The benefits of naltrexone appear to be dose-dependent

Tips and pearls

- It is important to understand that, although there are no FDA-approved psychotropic medications for BPD, psychopharmacology is often utilized as an intervention to treat BPD symptoms
- The decision to add a psychotropic medication should be considered on a case-to-case basis. Indications for psychotropic medications include prior response to medication and/or the presence of comorbid psychopathologies (e.g., MDD, PTSD, etc.)
- Education about medications is critical in helping individuals with BPD maintain compliance. A majority of those with BPD have been shown to have negative attitudes toward psychotropic medications, with side effects being the primary concern. Talking to the patient and planning for possible side effects can help reduce their anxiety about potential adverse effects
- Lithium and ECT can significantly reduce SI and SIB
- APA Guidelines recommend ECT should be used earlier in treatment for mood disorders, and not as a last resort

Two-minute tutorial

- BPD is a common psychiatric disorder, with a prevalence in the general population up to 6%, and up to 20% or higher in inpatient settings, including forensic hospitals. BPD is characterized by a pervasive pattern of instability in self-image, affect, interpersonal relationships, and impulsivity

PATIENT FILE

- Treating BPD is a clinical challenge. BPD frequently coexists with other psychiatric conditions, including mood disorders, anxiety disorders, trauma-related disorders, and substance use disorders. Given there is significant overlap of symptoms in BPD and its common comorbidities, recognition and management of comorbidities are essential. Comorbid disorders, such as MDD, may not respond as well to traditional treatments in the presence of BPD
- To date, there is no FDA-approved medication for BPD. However, psychotropic medications, such as antipsychotics, antidepressants, and anticonvulsants, are commonly prescribed
- For antipsychotics, in particular SGAs, metabolic side effects must be closely monitored
  - First line of treatment for metabolic side effects is lifestyle changes. Studies have looked at aripiprazole and metformin to attenuate or reduce weight gain, but results have been modest at best
  - Statins are first-line treatment for hyperlipidemia and can increase high-density lipoprotein (HDL) while lowering total cholesterol, low-density lipoprotein (LDL), and triglycerides
  - First-line treatment for hypertension includes thiazide diuretics, angiotensin-converting enzyme (ACE) inhibitors, angiotensin II receptor blockers (ARBs), and calcium channel blockers (CCBs). However, thiazide diuretics should be used with caution as they can potentially increase blood glucose levels
- Biological treatment options for SI/SIB include lithium, ECT, and ketamine. Studies have looked at other psychotropic medications but have yielded mixed results
- The opioid and reward systems are thought to be linked to the psychopathology of BPD. Naltrexone has been reported to decrease symptoms of BPD, including SIB and dissociative symptoms. The effects of naltrexone appear to be dose-dependent
- ECT is a highly effective but often underutilized treatment that can reduce mood symptoms and improve overall quality of life
  - Major indications for ECT include depression, mania, schizophrenia, and catatonia
- Consider the use of ECT in patients with BPD and active SI/SIB who did not respond to traditional interventions (i.e., psychotherapy and pharmacology)
  - ECT can rapidly treat suicidal drive, and response times are faster than other traditional interventions. Thus, ECT should be considered for high-acuity, high-risk cases

PATIENT FILE

Post-test question

Which class of psychotropic medications is FDA approved for borderline personality disorder (BPD)?

A. First- and second-generation antipsychotics (SGAs)
B. Antiepileptics
C. Selective serotonin reuptake inhibitors (SSRIs)
D. Selective norepinephrine reuptake inhibitors (SNRIs)
E. None of the above

Answer: D

References

1. American Psychiatric Association. Committee on Electroconvulsive Therapy & Weiner, R. D. (2001). *The Practice of Electroconvulsive Therapy: Recommendations for Treatment, Training, and Privileging: A Task Force Report of the American Psychiatric Association*, 2nd ed. Washington, DC: American Psychiatric Association.
2. Ceban, F., Nogo, D., Carvalho, I. P., et al. (2021). Association between mood disorders and risk of COVID-19 infection, hospitalization, and death: a systematic review and meta-analysis. *JAMA Psychiatry*, Oct. 1, 78(10), 1079–1091. https://doi.org/10.1001/jamapsychiatry.2021.1818.
3. Dadiomov, D. & Lee, K. (2019). The effects of ketamine on suicidality across various formulations and study settings. *Mental Health Clinician*, Jan. 4, 9(1), 48–60. https://doi.org/10.9740/mhc.2019.01.048.
4. Dayabandara, M., Hanwella, R., Ratnatunga, S., Seneviratne, S., Suraweera, C., & de Silva, V. A. (2017). Antipsychotic-associated weight gain: management strategies and impact on treatment adherence. *Neuropsychiatric Disorders and Treatment*, Aug. 22, 13, 2231–2241. https://doi.org/10.2147/NDT.S113099.
5. DeJongh, B. M. (2021). Clinical pearls for the monitoring and treatment of antipsychotic induced metabolic syndrome. *Mental Health Clinician*, Nov. 8, 11(6), 311–319. https://doi.org/10.9740/mhc.2021.11.311.
6. Del Casale, A., Bonanni, L., Bargagna, P., et al. (2021). Current clinical psychopharmacology in borderline personality disorder. *Current Neuropharmacology*, 19(10), 1760–1779. https://doi.org/10.2174/1570159X19666210610092958.

PATIENT FILE

7. Fond, G., Nemani, K., Etchecopar-Etchart, D., et al. (2021). Association between mental health disorders and mortality among patients with COVID-19 in 7 countries: a systematic review and meta-analysis. *JAMA Psychiatry.* https://doi.org/10.1001/jamapsychiatry.2021.2274.
8. Huang, X., Harris, L. M., Funsch, K. M. et al. (2022). Efficacy of psychotropic medications on suicide and self-injury: a meta-analysis of randomized controlled trials. *Translational Psychiatry*, 12, 400. https://doi.org/10.1038/s41398-022-02173-9.
9. Kellner, C. H. (2019). *Handbook of ECT: A Guide to Electroconvulsive Therapy for Practitioners.* New York: Cambridge University Press.
10. Lee, J. H., Kung, S., Rasmussen, K. G., & Palmer, B. A. (2019). Effectiveness of electroconvulsive therapy in patients with major depressive disorder and comorbid borderline personality disorder. *Journal of Electroconvulsive Therapy*, March, 35(1), 44–47. https://doi.org/10.1097/YCT.0000000000000533.
11. May, J. M., Richardi, T. M., & Barth, K. S. (2016). Dialectical behavior therapy as treatment for borderline personality disorder. *Mental Health Clinician*, March 8, 6(2), 62–67. https://doi.org/10.9740/mhc.2016.03.62.
12. Mirhaj Mohammadabadi, M. S, Mohammadsadeghi, H., Eftekhar Adrebili, M., et al. (2022). Factors associated with pharmacological and psychotherapy treatments adherence in patients with borderline personality disorder. *Frontiers in Psychiatry*, Dec. 13, 13, 1056050. https://doi.org/10.3389/fpsyt.2022.1056050.
13. Palihawadana, V., Broadbear, J. H., & Rao, S. (2019). Reviewing the clinical significance of "fear of abandonment" in borderline personality disorder. *Australasian Psychiatry*, 27(1), 60–63. https://doi.org/10.1177/1039856218810154.
14. Sarai, S. K., Mekala, H. M., & Lippmann, S. (2018). Lithium suicide prevention: a brief review and reminder. *Innovations in Clinical Neuroscience*, Nov. 1, 15(11–12), 30–32.
15. Stahl, S. M. (2011). Antipsychotic agents. In *Stahl's Essential Psychopharmacology: Prescriber's Guide*, 4th ed. New York: Cambridge University Press, pp. 213–218.
16. Timäus, C., Meiser, M., Wiltfang, J., Bandelow, B., & Wedekind, D. (2021). Efficacy of naltrexone in borderline personality disorder, a retrospective analysis in inpatients. *Human Psychopharmacology*, Nov., 36(6), e2800. https://doi.org/10.1002/hup.2800.

PATIENT FILE

17. Turner, B. J., Austin, S. B., & Chapman, A. L. (2014). Treating nonsuicidal self-injury: a systematic review of psychological and pharmacological interventions. *Canadian Journal of Psychiatry*, Nov., 59(11), 576–585. https://doi.org/10.1177/070674371405901103.
18. Zheng, Y., Xiao, L., Wang, H., Chen, Z., & Wang, G. (2022). A retrospective research on non-suicidal self-injurious behaviors among young patients diagnosed with mood disorders. *Frontiers in Psychiatry*, July 22, 13, 895892. https://doi.org/10.3389/fpsyt.2022.895892.

PATIENT FILE

18

Schizo-obsessive disorder: Repeatedly compelling

The Psychopharmocological Dilemma: Differentiating symptoms of OCD and schizophrenia, and identifying coexistence of both syndromes to determine adequate treatment and estimation of risk and prognosis. Could the treatment of one worsen the other?

Ajay Nair, Amanie Salem, and Carolina A. Klein

Pretest self-assessment question

Which evidence-based treatment of schizophrenia could potentially increase OCD symptoms?

A. Perphenazine
B. Clozapine
C. Loxapine
D. Haloperidol
E. High-dose benzodiazepines

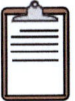

Patient evaluation on intake

- A 43-year-old single male who had been adjudicated not guilty by reason of insanity (NGRI) for charges of statutory burglary, possession of an explosive, and arson, and was previously diagnosed with OCD, schizoid personality disorder, schizoaffective disorder – depressed type, and Attention-Deficit/Hyperactivity Disorder (ADHD), was transferred to Northern Virginia Mental Health Institute

Psychiatric history

- The patient has reported various symptoms of psychosis through his life
  - He reported having visual hallucinations from the age of 4 or 5 until the age of 8 or 10
  - When hospitalized at age 13, he reported auditory and visual hallucinations
  - He reported hearing a "demon" voice throughout adulthood, which gives him commands that he will often follow. This voice appears when he is trying to cope with urges to do something unacceptable
    - He reported the voice telling him that if he did not kill someone, he would have to start a fire, which is why he reports committing arson

PATIENT FILE

- He has had interpersonal difficulties
  - As a child, he was taunted by members of his Boy Scout troop and he was ridiculed by his peers
  - He had conflicts with his father that resulted in thoughts of killing him
- He has some compulsive behaviors
  - As a child, he reported reading his material more than once without the benefit of achieving higher-than-average grades
  - He reported rituals of wiping his finger on trash cans while employed as an adult at Lowe's
  - He reported compulsive inhalation of water in the shower during his hospitalization after his index charges
- He has a history of self-destructive behaviors
  - He has banged and punched his own head, keyed his own car, slammed doors on his fingers, torn his own clothes and ripped paper money
  - He gave himself a concussion once due to a headache lasting a day
- He has a substance use history starting when he was a child
  - He first used alcohol and marijuana at age 12
  - Though he continued occasional use of marijuana during adolescence, his alcohol use increased to four to six beers daily as well as shots of hard liquor
  - He was caught drinking and driving as a 17-year-old in his high school parking lot, he hit his girlfriend under the influence of alcohol at age 20, and he was thrown out of a club for punching a man, under the influence of alcohol, at age 24
  - He had a period as an adult where he was drinking two 24-ounce cans of malt liquor in a sitting three times a week
  - He stopped using marijuana in 2001 because he lost access to his supplier and decided he no longer needed it

Social and personal history

- The patient lived with his parents and brother in a tri-state metro area until his hospitalization after being found NGRI for his offense
- His father emotionally abused him and used excessive force when disciplining him. He continued to have physical altercations with his father into adulthood
- He was closer to his mother than his father
- He witnessed his parents arguing frequently and this affected him
- He was bullied frequently during his childhood and was socially withdrawn

PATIENT FILE

- He participated in his church's youth organization, football in ninth and tenth grade, track and field and weight training
- He graduated high school and withdrew from college after getting two-thirds of the way to an Associate's degree in criminal justice
- He worked for K-Mart for over 5 years as a cashier and a stock clerk
- He worked for Lowe's for 13 years as a loader and cashier, but was terminated in 2007 for putting his hands on a female employee while he was struggling with her for control of a computer keyboard
- He has never been married and has no children
- Two weeks prior to his index offense resulting in his NGRI plea, he was charged with domestic assault and battery of his father

Medical history

- At 18 months he was burned by scalding water and has a large scar on his right forearm
- He has a history of a pilonidal cyst
- He reportedly had a self-inflicted concussion from beating his head
- He has a history of Methicillin-resistant *Staphylococcus aureus* (MRSA) infection
- He is morbidly obese and has been diagnosed with obstructive sleep apnea (OSA)
- He has diabetes mellitus type 2 with peripheral polyneuropathy, as well as hypertension and hyperlipidemia
- He has a history of myocardial infarction (MI)

Family history

- There is no known relevant family history to report

Medication history

- As a child he took carbamazepine, methylphenidate, and dextroamphetamine, unknown doses of all, with unknown efficacy
- Amphetamine salts had been started to address daytime sleepiness and help obsessive–compulsive symptoms, but were soon discontinued due to an EKG showing inferior MI. Though cardiology later ruled out MI, amphetamine salts were never restarted
- He was treated with several antipsychotics, with adequate trials of quetiapine and aripiprazole not decreasing his complaints of voices in his head
- His current regimen is as follows:
  - Risperidone 4 mg nightly for antipsychotic effects
  - Divalproex ER 2500 mg po qHS to target impulse control

PATIENT FILE

Current history
- He thinks he is "being watched" or the "Mafia" may be planning to kill him
- He describes hearing "a demon" in his head that gives him commands
- He is having thoughts that generally are about saying or doing something inappropriate, dangerous, or embarrassing. Examples include thoughts of throwing away items, dropping or breaking items, and, at times, thoughts of harming others and setting things on fire
- He reports behaviors such as dropping things, flipping/twisting items, repeating actions a certain number of times, completing daily activities, and writing in a lengthy, ritualized manner
- He reports some helplessness with regards to some of his thoughts and behaviors, interrupted sleep due to his OSA, decreased energy in the morning, and decreased ability to focus and concentrate. He does not have anhedonia, feelings of worthlessness, or SI

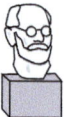

Psychotherapy history
- For the past 10 months he has engaged in a Cognitive Enhancement Therapy (CET) group, where he works on his cognitive functioning in areas of attention, memory, and problem solving
- He has also been engaged in individual cognitive behavioral therapy (CBT)

Mechanism of action moment
- The primary treatment of schizophrenia is the use of antipsychotic medications
  - First-generation antipsychotics (FGAs) primarily focus on D_2 blockade. They also have actions at noradrenergic, histaminergic, and cholinergic sites, which can contribute to associated side effects
- Second-generation antipsychotics (SGAs) combine D_2 blockade with a blockade of serotonergic receptors as well, primarily the $5-HT_{2A}$ receptor

Attending physician's mental notes at initial visit
- This patient describes symptoms of psychosis that started much earlier than typically seen in primary psychotic disorders
- He had conflicted relationships in many spheres of his life, particularly with his father, with whom the conflict has continued into adulthood
- He seems distressed by the symptoms he describes, even reporting helplessness
- He appears overall quite organized in his thought process

PATIENT FILE

Further investigation
Is there anything else you would like to know about the patient? What about his perspective on the voices he hears and the thoughts he has?
- He describes the demon in his head commanding him to do things, but on further exploration, he does not truly believe it is a demon and is able to say that the thoughts are his own and that these thoughts distress him and often lead him to do things that he does not want to do
- He said that he does not feel that any external power is controlling his thoughts or his actions
- He said that his fears that the Mafia is following him or that he is being watched are often assuaged when he thinks about it and realizes that there is no reason for anyone to be watching him. The fears of being watched get exacerbated by his thoughts of doing things that are dangerous

Case outcome: follow-up at 4 weeks
- The patient was started on sertraline 50 mg daily to address intrusive obsessive thoughts and his prior compulsive behaviors. As it was unclear that he was having true psychotic symptoms, his risperidone was tapered to 2 mg daily for a week and then stopped
- He said that he noticed maybe a slight decrease in the intensity and frequency of his intrusive thoughts, but he still had the same ritualized behaviors that were greatly interfering with his life
- Sertraline was increased to 100 mg daily

Case outcome: follow-up at 8 weeks
- He reported about a 25% overall decrease in his intrusive thoughts and in his ritualized behaviors
- Sertraline was further increased to 200 mg daily

Case outcome: follow-up at 14 weeks
- He reported continued improvement, about 60% overall, in both his intrusive thoughts and his ritualized behavior
- He continues to be bothered by both, and though gratified by his symptomatic improvement, continues to hope that further improvement is possible
- He reported feeling good when he was on the risperidone and asks why he had to be taken off the medication

PATIENT FILE

Further investigation

What possible strategies could be used once a patient has an incomplete response to an SSRI for OCD symptoms?

- Change to another SSRI
- Change to clomipramine
- Change to a serotonin–norepinephrine reuptake inhibitor (SNRI; not FDA approved)
- Augment with an antipsychotic

Attending physician's mental notes

- He appears to be responding to the sertraline, but we have reached the FDA maximum dose, and he continues to have symptoms
- Does it make sense to try monotherapy with another agent or to use adjunct treatment when he already has a partial response to monotherapy with sertraline?
- He has tolerated risperidone in the past and says that he felt that it benefited him

Case outcome: follow-up at 20 weeks

- Risperidone 2 mg daily was used as an augmentation of his daily 200 mg dose of sertraline to address residual OCD symptoms
- After 3 weeks on the combination, he reported a significant decrease in his obsessional thoughts and compulsive behaviors and said that he thinks his symptoms are at a manageable level now

Case debrief

- The patient reported symptoms that painted a complicated picture of possible psychosis versus OCD
- On further investigation, it appeared that he did not have true hallucinations and he did not appear to think that he was being controlled by any external power. He identified his thoughts as his own, unwelcome thoughts, and recognized the ritualized behaviors that he was performing due to his thoughts
- He was treated with an SSRI and had a partial response to maximal dose
- Augmentation was then performed with an antipsychotic, which helped to bring his symptoms to a manageable level

Take-home points

- Both OCD and psychosis can present with thoughts compelling people to perform actions that they otherwise would not have

- Obsessive thoughts are often perceived as coming from within the patient's mind and are more likely to be ego-dystonic than psychotic thoughts, which frequently are perceived to be inserted thoughts and are more likely to be ego-syntonic
- First-line treatment for OCD is an SSRI, though clomipramine monotherapy is also FDA approved
- General practice for augmentation is to use an antipsychotic, although augmentation with clomipramine is also done. Newer studies are being undertaken to examine augmentation with stimulants, N-acetyl cysteine, and glutamate antagonists, among other agents

Performance in practice: confessions of a psychopharmacologist

Could this patient be having obsessions and compulsions but still have schizophrenia?

- Though reports of rates of OCD in schizophrenia vary, OCD clearly has a higher prevalence in patients with schizophrenia than in the general population as a whole
- Additionally, many patients with schizophrenia also have obsessive compulsive symptoms, but may not meet criteria for OCD

Could we have tried monotherapy with another agent?

- Often monotherapy with another SSRI or clomipramine is tried after initial treatment has failed
- The combination of partial response to sertraline, previous report of efficacy of risperidone, and potential for psychosis (though appearing unlikely) all led to augmentation with sertraline, but changing to monotherapy with another approved agent is a good strategy as well

What other treatment options could have been considered for OCD?

- Arguably even more important than pharmacotherapy, CBT is indicated for treatment of OCD. Particular focus on exposure and response prevention is recommended
- Procedural treatments have also been studied, including deep brain stimulation (DBS), electroconvulsive therapy (ECT), transcranial magnetic stimulation (TMS), and neurosurgery. These treatments are showing good results, but generally are used for people with severe or treatment-resistant symptoms

PATIENT FILE

Tips and pearls

How can I differentiate psychotic symptoms from obsessions and compulsions?

- It is important to thoroughly evaluate the patient's thoughts and actions
    - Is the patient having true hallucinations, or do they describe their own thoughts?
    - Does the patient describe thoughts as being inserted into their head, or can they identify the thoughts as their own?
    - How much insight does the patient have into the reality of these thoughts?
    - What are the patient's feelings about their thoughts? And what is their affect when describing them? Is there more anxiety or paranoia around the thoughts? Are they trying to ignore or suppress the thoughts, or to neutralize them in any other way?
    - What is the nature of the actions that accompany the thoughts? How much time is spent on the accompanying actions?
- Do not forget to look into other aspects of the mental status examination that may clue you into the diagnosis
    - Is there disorganization in speech or behavior? Are there negative symptoms?
    - What kind of rationale is the patient giving for the behaviors?

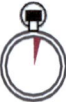

Two-minute tutorial

Obsessive–compulsive disorder

- Patients with OCD have recurrent and persistent intrusive thoughts and they attempt to ignore or suppress them or neutralize them with some other thought or action. They also can have repetitive behaviors or rules they must adhere to that they feel are obligatory in response to an obsession
- These patients more frequently are aware that this is all coming from inside of them, and their thoughts and actions are often ego-dystonic
- Treatment of OCD:
    - OCD treatment should start with CBT with exposure and response prevention
    - Pharmacological treatment starts with FDA-approved medications:
        - Clomipramine
        - Fluoxetine
        - Fluvoxamine
        - Paroxetine
        - Sertraline

PATIENT FILE

- If first-line pharmacological treatment fails, strategies include:
  - Switching to another FDA-approved treatment for monotherapy
  - Augmenting with an antipsychotic
  - Changing to an SNRI
  - Augmenting with another agent, including N-acetyl cysteine or an anti-glutamatergic agent (not as much evidence backing this strategy)
- Severe or treatment-resistant OCD can also be treated by procedural treatments including:
  - Neurosurgery
  - DBS
  - ECT
  - TMS

Schizophrenia

- Patients with schizophrenia have symptoms that may include delusions, hallucinations, disorganized speech, disorganized or catatonic behavior, and negative symptoms. At least two of the five symptoms must be present, and one of the symptoms must be either delusions, hallucinations, or disorganized speech
- Generally, patients with schizophrenia have less insight into their condition than those with OCD, and their thoughts are more likely to be ego-syntonic. They often feel an external source of control and/or the insertion of thoughts into their heads
- Treatment of schizophrenia
  - The primary treatment of schizophrenia is the use of antipsychotic medications
    - FGAs show good efficacy and primarily focus on D_2 blockade. They are more likely to cause side effects including extrapyramidal symptoms (EPS), neuroleptic malignant syndrome (NMS), and tardive dyskinesia. They also have actions at noradrenergic, histaminergic, and cholinergic sites, which can contribute to associated side effects
    - SGAs also show good efficacy. They combine D_2 blockade with a blockade of serotonergic receptors as well, primarily the 5-HT_{2A} receptor
  - Psychotherapeutic techniques continue to be refined and specialized for treatment of schizophrenia
    - Symptom-focused psychotherapy appears to have the best efficacy
  - Procedural techniques, such as repetitive transcranial magnetic stimulation (rTMS) and DBS are increasingly being studied and used

> ○ As awareness about the need for social and community interventions increases, these are increasingly being implemented into treatment of schizophrenia
>
> *Overlap*
> - OCD and schizophrenia are often co-occurring disorders. The prevalence of OCD is greater in people with schizophrenia than it is in the general population as a whole. Furthermore, the co-occurrence of symptoms has led to the study of schizo-obsessive disorder or presentation, which speaks specifically to this population

Post-test question

Which evidence-based treatment of schizophrenia could potentially increase OCD symptoms?

A. Perphenazine
B. Clozapine
C. Loxapine
D. Haloperidol
E. High-dose benzodiazepines

Answer: B

References

1. Carlat, D. (2023). CBT with exposure and response prevention for OCD, The Carlat Report. Available at: www.thecarlatreport.com/articles/4414-cbt-with-exposure-and-response-prevention-for-ocd.
2. Chokhawala, K. & Stevens, L. (2023). Antipsychotic medications [Updated Feb. 26, 2023]. StatPearls [Internet]. Treasure Island (FL): StatPearls Publishing; Jan.– . Available from: www.ncbi.nlm.nih.gov/books/NBK519503.
3. Gaebel, W. & Zielasek, J. (2015). Schizophrenia in 2020: trends in diagnosis and therapy. *Psychiatry and Clinical Neuroscience*, Nov., 69(11), 661–673. https://doi.org/10.1111/pcn.12322. Epub July 1, 2015. PMID: 26011091.
4. Geller, D. A. & March, J. (2012). Practice parameter for the assessment and treatment of children and adolescents with obsessive–compulsive disorder. *Journal of the American Academy of Child and Adolescent Psychiatry*, Jan., 51(1), 98–113. https://doi.org/10.1016/j.jaac.2011.09.019. PMID: 22176943.
5. Goren, J. (2023). Medications to treat OCD: what psychotherapists need to know. The Carlat Report. Available at: www.thecarlatreport.com/articles/4429-medications-to-treat-ocd-what-psychotherapists-need-to-know.

6. Kayser, R. R. (2020). Pharmacotherapy for treatment-resistant obsessive-compulsive disorder. *Journal of Clinical Psychiatry*, Sept. 8, 81(5), 19ac13182. https://doi.org/10.4088/JCP.19ac13182. PMID: 32926602; PMCID: PMC7495343.
7. Poyurovsky, M. (2013). *Schizo-obsessive Disorder*. Cambridge University Press.
8. Poyurovsky, M., Weizman, A., & Weizman, R. (2004). Obsessive–compulsive disorder in schizophrenia. *CNS Drugs*, 18, 989–1010. https://doi.ezproxy.med.nyu.edu/10.2165/00023210-200418140-00004.
9. Recommendations: obsessive–compulsive disorder and body dysmorphic disorder – treatment: guidance. (2005). National Institute for Health and Care Excellence. Available at: www.nice.org.uk/guidance/cg31/chapter/Recommendations.
10. Sandia, I. & Baptista, T. (2020). Ego-dystonia: a review in search of definitions. *Revista Colombiana de Psiquiatría* (English ed.), Dec. 29, S0034-7450(20)30120–7. https://doi.org/10.1016/j.rcp.2020.11.007. Epub ahead of print. PMID: 33735053.
11. Soomro, G. M., Altman, D., Rajagopal, S., & Oakley-Browne, M. (2008). Selective serotonin re-uptake inhibitors (SSRIs) versus placebo for obsessive compulsive disorder (OCD). *Cochrane Database of Systematic Reviews*, 2008(1), CD001765. https://doi.org/10.1002/14651858.CD001765.pub3.

PATIENT FILE

19

Anxiety disorders: Constant worries

The Psychopharmacological Dilemma: What are the clinical considerations and management strategies for comorbid anxiety illnesses or comorbid anxiety and psychiatric disorders?

Maanasi Chandarana

Pretest self-assessment question

Which of the following statements regarding comorbid anxiety disorders are true?

A. Comorbidity of generalized anxiety disorder (GAD) with other anxiety disorders is approximately 50–70%
B. Co-occurrence of two or more anxiety disorders in the same individual tends to be the rule rather than the exception
C. The ventrolateral prefrontal cortex is the neural substrate for catastrophizing and involved in catastrophizing-associated anxiety generation
D. A meta-analysis found that nearly 60% of those with lifetime illicit drug dependence had a comorbid anxiety disorder
E. Rates of comorbid anxiety and personality disorders are believed to range from 15% to 45%

Answer: B

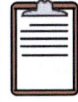

Patient evaluation on intake

The patient is a 55-year-old male with a history of anxiety, Attention-Deficit/Hyperactivity Disorder (ADHD), substance use disorder, and post-traumatic stress disorder (PTSD), who was found incompetent to stand trial (IST) for an incurred felony charge. The patient was subsequently hospitalized at a forensic state hospital for pretrial competency restoration. The patient was restored to legal competence and, after he was court-adjudicated not guilty by reason of insanity (NGRI), again committed to the forensic state hospital for continued psychiatric assessment, treatment, and care. During his hospitalization, he verbalized worry; identified multiple somatic complaints including episodic fainting and dizziness, although not substantiated by objective medical examination; exhibited psychogenic nonepileptic seizures; and stated he was suicidal. The patient often declined further diagnostic assessments and evaluations, and, at times, requested tests and procedures that were not medically indicated.

PATIENT FILE

Psychiatric history
- The patient reported onset of psychiatric symptoms when he was 6 years old; diagnoses of substance-induced mood disorder, other substance use disorder (with antidepressant and benzodiazepine medications), unspecified bipolar and related disorder, unspecified anxiety disorder, unspecified depressive disorder, PTSD, histrionic and borderline personality disorders, cluster B traits, multiple involuntary and voluntary inpatient psychiatric hospitalizations for suicidal ideation (SI), and trauma-associated amnesia; community-based care; and treatment with paroxetine, lorazepam, and divalproex
    - During one of the patient's hospitalizations, he was informed by his clinical team that his experience of psychotic behavior was attributed to supratherapeutic dosing and misuse of paroxetine and lorazepam
        - The patient was advised to not exceed paroxetine 60 mg total daily dosing
    - The patient's described symptomatology included insomnia; loud and pressured speech; dramatic and anxious affect; mood lability; confusion and altered mentation; aggressive, destructive, impulsive, and manipulative behaviors; and his report of various somatic complaints (such as dizziness, lightheadedness, cognitive difficulties, inability to see and read) as well as auditory and visual hallucinations
        - The patient's behaviors to obtain external incentives included:
            - The patient related SI of running into traffic if not admitted to a psychiatric facility
            - The patient was noted to engage in self-injurious behavior (SIB) to gain admission into a psychiatric facility
            - The patient was documented to exhibit psychogenic nonepileptic seizures and fainting spells inconsistent with vasovagal reflex
            - The patient reported various allegations against peers and staff but was observed engaging in provocative behaviors
- Substance use history
    - The patient reported cocaine use and vicarious, intentional, injection of phencyclidine (PCP) by someone else
    - The patient also reported remote alcohol use, with last use 20 years prior

PATIENT FILE

Social and personal history
- The patient was raised by his biological parents and is the third child in terms of birth order
  - At the time of the patient's admission to the forensic hospital, his parents are deceased
- The patient described his childhood as traumatic
  - He reported experiencing historic sexual, physical, and emotional/verbal abuse from his father
    - The patient's family stated they were unaware of these events
  - The patient identified witnessing public rioting at the age of 12 as contributory to his post-traumatic stress disorder (PTSD) diagnosis
  - The patient relayed physical and sexual abuse by his roommate
- The patient graduated high school and dropped out in his freshman year of college due to his PTSD symptomatology
- He shared that he worked as a model, waiter, and for a temporary (temp) agency
  - The patient had not been employed since he was 20 years of age and expressed his preference to remain financially supported through Social Security Disability (SSD) for his diagnosis of PTSD
- The patient denied family contact and having friends
  - He shared he had a close relationship with his various personal attorneys
- The patient denied a marital history
- At times, he resided in shelters and was unhoused until he was placed in an efficiency apartment
- The patient's medical record reflected his pursuit of litigation for housing and discriminatory related issues

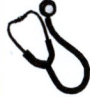

Medical history
- Hyperthyroidism
- Hypertension
- Type 2 diabetes mellitus
- Gastroesophageal reflux disease (GERD)

Family History
- The patient's familial psychiatric history is notable for an undisclosed mental illness in his maternal family, and medical history for cerebrovascular accident (CVA) and cardiac arrhythmia

PATIENT FILE

Current history
- The patient presented to the evaluation as dramatic and demanding
  - The patient attempted to faint multiple times during the evaluation when denied various requests
- He was dressed in carceral attire, and his grooming and hygiene were deemed fair
- His speech rate and volume were elevated, and rhythm was normal
- The patient did not demonstrate psychomotor agitation, retardation, and abnormal involuntary movements
- His affect was labile. He denied experiencing suicidal and homicidal ideations; however, after the evaluation, he was noted to be banging his head against the wall to obtain admission to a different psychiatric facility
- He reported delusional statements with themes related to himself and his peers
- His thought process was linear and goal-directed
- The patient was alert, oriented to person, time, and place. His recent and remote memory, ability to abstract, attention, fund of knowledge, and cognition were deemed fair
- He demonstrated deficits in his insight, judgment, and impulse control

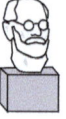

Psychotherapy history
- The patient meets three times a week for 10 months with his psychiatrist for transference-based psychotherapy, with exploration of his worry, somatization, and avoidance
  - The patient exhibits unhealthy, interpersonal coping strategies of projective identification, splitting, and externalization of blame
  - The patient benefits from redirection and confrontation during his sessions due to his reluctance to discuss and process his emotional experiences, overfamiliarity with his therapist, difficulty challenging cognitive distortions, self-regulating, responding healthily to boundary and limit setting, and engaging alternative coping strategies

Mechanism of action moment
- Lorazepam
  - Binds to the benzodiazepine receptor of the gamma aminobutyric acid (GABA)-A ligand-gated chloride channel
    - Enhances inhibitory effects of GABA and foments chloride conductance through GABA channels
  - Inhibitory effect on neurons within the fear circuitry of the amygdala
    - Provides anxiolytic effect

- Inhibition of the cerebral cortex
    - Assists with anti-seizure effect
- Ziprasidone
    - Blocks D_2 receptor
        - Reduces positive symptoms and provides mood stabilization
    - Modulates multiple serotoninergic receptors
        - 2A receptor blockade
            - Enhances dopamine release
                - Improved cognitive and affective functioning
        - Interaction with 2C and 1A receptor
            - Targets cognitive and affective symptoms
        - Interaction with 1D and 5HT7 receptor
            - At higher medication doses and in conjunction with serotonin and norepinephrine receptors, may have treatment effect on affective symptoms
- Buspirone
    - Binds to serotonin 1A receptors
    - Partially agonizes presynaptic somatodendritic serotonin autoreceptors
        - Enhances serotoninergic and antidepressant effect
    - Partial agonism postsynaptically may decrease serotonin activity
        - Facilitates anxiolytic effect
- Topiramate
    - Blocks voltage-gated sodium channels and carbonic anhydrase
    - Has an inhibitory effect on glutamate and potentiates GABA activity
- Paroxetine
    - Blocks the serotonin reuptake pump, as well as marginally blocks norepinephrine reuptake pump
    - Enhances and boosts serotonin and serotoninergic neurotransmission
    - Desensitizes serotonin 1A autoreceptors
    - Has mild anticholinergic effect
- Olanzapine
    - Blocks D_2 receptor
        - Reduces positive symptoms and provides mood stabilization
    - Blocks multiple serotoninergic receptors
        - 2A receptor blockade
            - Enhances dopamine release
                - Improved cognitive and affective functioning
        - Blockade of serotonin 2C receptor
            - Targets cognitive and affective symptoms

PATIENT FILE

Attending physician's mental notes
- The patient relates multiple grandiose statements regarding his personal and friends' fame and notoriety, hyperbolic and dramatic speech, and various demands; he exhibits difficulty with emotional self-regulation and psychosomatically driven behaviors to attain his needs, but does not demonstrate difficulty engaging with reality testing or organized thought patterns, consistent sleep, and sustained energy levels
  - His somatic symptom description and behaviors are not clinically consistent with physical or medical comorbidities and diagnoses
    - The patient was referred to neurology, cardiology, and ophthalmology
      - Pathology of these organ systems explaining his episodic fainting are excluded
  - He describes anxiety attacks of overwhelming and uncontrolled worry, difficulty concentrating, feeling on edge, and somatic complaints of gastrointestinal discomfort (i.e., nausea, diarrhea), dizziness, chest pain, and self-identified nonepileptic psychogenic seizures and vasovagal syncope
  - The patient identifies depressive symptomatology of chronic suicidality, which is fluctuant in nature, but denies current tearfulness, sad mood state, guilt, hopelessness, helplessness, and altered appetite and sleep
    - His interest and hedonism appear preserved and the patient voices future orientation
  - He relays multiple complaints against peers and staff, including physical, verbal, and sexual maltreatment, but denies these allegations upon ensuing fact finding and confrontation
    - Due to concerns regarding his impulsivity and verbalization of maltreatment as well as appraisal that he represents a danger to himself, he is placed on enhanced observation
- He is prescribed lorazepam and paroxetine to assist with his symptom presentation including emotional dysregulation and disinhibition, but the patient's history is notable for historic substance use and misuse and supratherapeutic self-dosing of prescription medications
  - The patient refuses offered as-needed ziprasidone during periods of worsened anxiety and distress, behavioral dyscontrol, as well as externalized, inappropriate, verbally, and physically aggressive behaviors
    - An involuntary medication order (IMO) is administratively sought and approved
      - The patient is prescribed combination therapy of paroxetine, olanzapine, buspirone, and topiramate

PATIENT FILE

Further investigation
- The patient participated in group therapy and was not thought to be at risk for elopement, as appreciated by his treatment team; however, the patient reports various anxieties which underlie his lack of motivation and reluctance to transfer to less restrictive hospital wards and environments
- Despite maintenance on and compliance with his prescribed treatment, the patient has also engaged in multiple behavioral incidents including physically and verbally intimidating acts
  - The patient spat in a staff member's face, choked and pushed staff members, grabbed at and damaged staff clothing, entrapped various staff members in offices and prevented their free movement
  - His behaviors preclude his court-ordered transfer to the community

Case outcome
- The patient's case is followed weekly
- With continued psychopharmacological treatment, therapy, and time, the patient exhibits improved emotional and behavioral regulation, impulsivity, somatization, medication compliance, and engagement with treatment recommendations and providers
  - The patient's clinical team recommends progressive stepwise transition to a less restrictive environment
    - The patient is, ultimately, discharged from the forensic state hospital to an independent living environment with community-based supervision and care

Case debrief
- Our patient was found IST, restored to trial competence, adjudicated NGRI to a felony charge, and he was committed to a state forensic hospital
  - At the time of his post-trial commitment, his psychiatric history was notable for various affective disorders, substance use disorders, prescription medication misuse, as well as characterological traits and pathology
    - The patient's psychotic and manic symptom presentation included loud, pressured speech; combative and agitated affect; paranoid, grandiose delusions; hallucinatory experiences; and bizarre, impulsive behavior
      - Per report, his symptoms did not abate despite multiple trials of antipsychotic, mood-stabilizer, antidepressant, and anxiolytic psychotropic medications

PATIENT FILE

- The patient's history reflected his self-discontinuation of some medications due to his appreciation or misattribution of side effects
    - During his forensic psychiatric hospitalization, the patient relayed overvalued, non-bizarre, non-delusional, beliefs with evidence of intact reality testing
        - His experience of anxiety and perception of stress manifested as psychosomatic symptomatology
            - His report was not corroborated by medical signs and pathology of various organ systems and not attributed to concurrent, comorbid medical diagnoses
        - Performed psychological testing yielded:
            - Average intelligence devoid of cognitive impairment on the Wechsler Abbreviated Scale of Intelligence (WASI-I)
            - Engagement in positive impression management, demonstrable histrionic and anxious personality traits as well as cognitively inflexible anger expression styles on the Personality Assessment Inventory (PAI) and Minnesota Multiphasic Personality Inventory (MMPI)
            - Experience of extreme emotional distress associated with chronic poor self-worth, depression, and anxiety, in addition to somatic symptoms as a way to utilize the sick role and gain support and understanding from others, on the Millon Clinical Multiaxial Inventory-III (MCMI-III) and Rorschach Inkblot Test
            - Absence of features of mental illness feigning and symptom exaggeration on the Structured Interview of Reported Symptoms (SIRS)
- With continued forensic psychiatric hospitalization, treatment with psychotropic medication, and individualized transference-based therapy, and upon transfer to the community setting, the patient's diagnosis is reconciled to include GAD, other specified somatic symptom and related disorder, and borderline personality disorder (BPD)
    - The patient is maintained on combination psychotropic medication regimen of olanzapine, paroxetine, buspirone, topiramate, as well as weekly individualized transference-based psychotherapy
        - With continued treatment and time, the patient exhibits marked improvement in his ability to engage in prosocial behaviors with peers, staff, and his treatment team, in addition to improved impulsivity, affective, mood, and behavioral stability

PATIENT FILE

Take-home points
- The origin, nature, and presentation of anxiety is complex, person specific, and includes overlapping constructs of fear and worry
  - Anxiety, fear, and worry
    - Anxiety and fear can be distinguished by one's orientation to the threat and whether the trigger is nebulous or identifiable
      - Anxiety is distinct from fear as anxiety is in response to a future, ambiguous threat
      - Fear presents when exposed to an imminent, specific threat
    - Anxiety and fear are considered emotional responses to stimuli and/or a mood state
    - Dissimilar to anxiety and fear, worry can be conceptualized as a verbal or thought process predicated upon plausible negative outcomes
  - Etiology of anxiety
    - Clinically, most anxiety disorders have varied contributions from an individual's unique learned and biological history and are influenced by various and repeated experiences over time
      - However, a single event is sufficient to cause situational distress as well as anxiety symptoms, and support a diagnosis of an anxiety disorder
    - Theoretical underpinnings of the origin of anxiety
      - Classical conditioning / direct learning theory: Anxiety or fear is associated with a stimulus or situation upon direct experience or exposure
      - Mowrer's two-factor theory of learning: combines both classical conditioning and operant conditioning, whereby classical conditioning results in fear acquisition, and operant conditioning, particularly negative reinforcement, maintains the anxious state
        - A stimulus induces a fear response via classical conditioning, but personal motivation and behavior to decrease the discomfort or fear reinforce the experience and patterns of thoughts and behaviors
      - Observational learning / indirect learning: Fears are learned vicariously through observing others
      - Negative information transfer: One can learn to be anxious by hearing others talking negatively (or anxiously) about a subject

PATIENT FILE

- Biological preparedness: One develops a phobic response after an aversive interaction with a stimulus
  - The premise of the biological preparedness theory is that people are biologically prepared to learn to fear stimuli that could threaten their survival
- Non-associative pathway: There is no direct, vicarious, or index event, etiology, or learned association commensurate with onset of anxiety and fear
  - The non-associative and biological preparedness paths are believed to have an evolutionary basis or serve an evolutionary purpose
- Theoretical contributions to how one processes and interprets an anxiety-provoking event include:
  - Cognitive theory: Analyzing thought content reveals information about a person's emotional functioning
    - Individuals suffering with anxiety have biased information processing, selectively perceive threats, remain in a hypervigilant state, and overpredict and overanticipate a fear response
    - Clark's model of panic attacks emphasizes the appraisal of a threat as the origin and promoter of developing panic
      - The appraisal is then followed by physical, bodily sensations and mental catastrophizing
    - Beck's theory of anxiety provides that previous, emotionally laden experiences prime anxious beliefs and effect how information is organized in one's memory
  - Biological theory
    - Genetics and temperament
      - General genetic predisposition, in conjunction with environmental factors, contributes to the development of specific disorders
      - Studies have evidenced that individuals at a higher risk of developing an anxiety disorder have a parent with an anxiety disorder
      - Rates of heritability of anxiety spectrum illnesses range from 30% to 40%
      - Genetic contributions to individual personality traits or temperament range from 41% to 61%
      - Some studies suggest behavioral inhibition is a specific risk factor for later development of social anxiety disorder

PATIENT FILE

- - Behavioral inhibition is characterized by the tendency to respond to novel situations with feelings of anxiety, avoidant behaviors, and increased distress
  - Behavioral inhibition is associated with anxiety proneness and anxiety sensitivity
- Integrated theories
  - Triple vulnerability theory: this theory emphasizes the contribution of three vulnerabilities
    - General genetic (or biological) vulnerability: An individual's approach to or withdrawal from certain situations is predicated upon their temperament and personality traits
      - Individual temperament and personality traits are genetically determined to some degree
      - People with anxiety have an overactive behavioral inhibition system in response to novel stimuli; physiologically respond with the fight/flight system in face of fear and panic; and exhibit impulsivity via the behavioral approach system
    - General psychological vulnerability: An individual's psychological vulnerability is due to not feeling in control; attribution of negative events to internal, global, and stable factors; and exposure to parenting styles
    - Specific psychological vulnerability: Specific psychological vulnerability is a learned response to dangerous stimuli and its content is a function of the particular anxiety disorder
      - These vulnerabilities can develop through direct exposure to a dangerous situation, in circumstances that a physiological response is incorrectly associated with a stimulus or situation, and through vicarious conditioning
  - Contemporary learning theory
    - The contemporary learning theory consists of two domains of vulnerabilities (genetic/temperament and learned experiences), coupled with perception of control/predictability of the event, direct or vicarious conditioning, and the unique characteristics of the conditioned stimulus
      - Vulnerabilities within contextual domains (perception of control/predictability of the event, direct or vicarious conditioning, and the unique characteristics of the conditioned stimulus) lead to development of anxiety disorder

PATIENT FILE

- - - Anxiety symptoms are furthered by post-conditioning factors, including "unconditioned stimulus inflation/reevaluation and the presence of inhibitory or excitatory conditioned stimuli"
- Anxiety disorders are classified and distinguished by degree, target of anxiety or fear, or duration
- Anxiety is frequently comorbid with other acute and enduring disorders that have important implications for effective treatment
  - Comorbidity is defined as having co-occurring clinically significant symptoms of both an anxiety disorder and another disorder at some time across the lifespan
  - Although evidence suggests that comorbidity rates decrease after treatment for a primary anxiety disorder, comorbidity rates tend to be substantially higher in those with more severe conditions, and severity serves as a negative prognostic indicator
- Concurrent anxiety disorders: Co-occurrence of two or more anxiety disorders in the same individual tends to be more the rule than the exception
  - Among anxiety disorders, GAD and PTSD were especially likely to co-occur with other disorders
    - GAD
      - The comorbidity of GAD with other anxiety disorders is approximately 66–83%
        - For persons with primary GAD, the most common comorbid anxiety disorders are social and specific phobias, panic disorder, and post-traumatic stress disorder
          - Research into concurrent social phobia with GAD reflects more severe pretreatment symptomatology in both the primary and comorbid conditions
      - Treatment for GAD
        - Each of the proposed treatments for GAD involves self-monitoring symptoms and cues, employment of coping strategies to reduce anxiety, and skill practice
          - Self-monitoring includes identifying negative automatic thoughts, evaluation of anxious beliefs, and restructuring techniques to make ideas adaptive
          - Cognitive therapy includes discourse about one's intolerance of uncertainty, poor problem solving, and avoidance
          - Behavioral exposure/practice

PATIENT FILE

- Some study results suggest that focusing on the GAD-specific elements of cognitive therapy leads to reduction in comorbid anxiety disorders
    - One study reported that participants had more than a 50% decrease in number of comorbid illnesses, which was maintained at follow-up 1 year later
- Anxiety and co-occurring personality disorders
    - Research regarding co-occurring anxiety and personality disorders is inconclusive due to study design but, epidemiologically, rates of comorbid anxiety and personality disorders are believed to range from 35% to 65%
        - About 24% of patients with a diagnosed anxiety disorder are thought to have at least one co-occurring personality disorder, with the most common diagnoses being avoidant, obsessive–compulsive, dependent, and borderline personality disorders
            - Cluster C personality disorders co-occur most often with anxiety disorders
                - Obsessive–compulsive disorder (OCD) is associated with avoidant and obsessive–compulsive personality disorders
            - Higher rates of PTSD are found in those with BPD
        - Patients with social phobia and GAD are more likely to be diagnosed with a co-occurring personality disorder than those with other anxiety disorders
            - Social phobia is found in patients with avoidant personality disorder
            - Panic disorder is associated most highly with borderline, avoidant, and dependent personality disorders
            - Specific phobia is not associated with any personality disorder
    - The relationship between personality disorders and anxiety can be described by three models
        - The linear or causal model provides that either personality disorders are risk factors for anxiety disorders or personality disorders are consequences of anxiety disorders
        - The nonlinear or reciprocal model suggests a bidirectional causal relationship (i.e., that personality disorders influence the development of anxiety disorders, and early anxiety impacts the development of personality disorders)

PATIENT FILE

- The common etiological model theorizes that common etiologies and overlap exist in major psychiatric conditions and personality disorders (formerly Axis I and Axis II criterion, respectively)
  - Prognosis
    - Personality disorders have an adverse impact on anxiety disorder treatment outcomes due to:
      - The patient's difficulty establishing rapport and strong alliance, which is an indicator of treatment outcome
      - Personality disorders may hinder treatment by increasing severity of pathology, generally speaking
      - Individuals with character pathology show impairments in self-insight, which may hinder treatment response
      - Patients who identify fear states of an anxiety disorder as consistent with their self-image or nature may be less likely to seek treatment and have more difficulty engaging in treatments that challenge their identity
- Somatic symptom disorder
  - Somatic symptom and related disorders are characterized by the presence of significantly distressing and impairing somatic symptomatology accompanied by excessive thoughts, feelings, and behaviors related to the somatic and associated health symptoms
    - Somatic symptom and related disorders include the following diagnoses: somatic symptom disorder, illness anxiety disorder, conversion and factitious disorder, psychological factors affecting other medical conditions, and other specified and unspecified somatic symptom and related disorders
    - The Diagnostic and Statistical Manual 5 description of Somatic Symptom and Related Disorder does not require medical inexplicability (and thereby is distinguished from the Diagnostic and Statistical Manual 4 – Text Revision Somatoform Disorders)
  - Patients with somatic symptom disorder exhibit cognitive deficits in: information processing speed, sustained attention, divided attention, working/verbal/visual memories, and phonological verbal fluency
    - These neurocognitive deficits, especially those of divided attention, information processing speed, and working memory are worsened by comorbid depression
      - Anxiety disorders comorbid with somatic symptom disorder were not associated with impaired neurocognition

PATIENT FILE

- However, catastrophizing, resultant to and a manifestation of cognitive inflexibility, is postulated to induce feelings of anxiety and emotional arousal that accompany and are inherent to somatic symptom disorders
    - A study reflects that individuals suffering from this condition may also experience difficulty in the executive domains of planning and mental flexibility
  - The dorsomedial prefrontal cortex (dmPFC) contains Brodmann areas 8 and 9; is implicated in cognitive modulation of emotion; and serves as a conduit between emotional provoking/arousal regions and cognitive control areas of the brain
    - The dmPFC is conceptualized as the neural substrate for catastrophizing in fear-reaction formation, and suspected to be involved in anxiety generation associated with catastrophizing
      - Patients who catastrophize their somatic symptoms experience anxiety, and increased catastrophizing is associated with higher levels of anxiety
      - A study identified that catastrophizing is related to anxiety and mediated by Brodmann 8 in the bilateral dmPFC in patients diagnosed with somatic symptom disorder
        - Although some studies reflect adolescents with GAD having decreased gray matter volume of the dmPFC, and increased gray matter volume of the dmPFC in adolescents with medically inexplicable neurologic functional illness, a study of adults with somatic symptom disorder failed to reveal difference in gray matter volumes of the dmPFC when compared to healthy controls
  - Management of the psychological presentation of somatic symptom and related disorders includes cognitive behavioral therapies (CBTs)
    - Patients with neurocognitive dysfunction may benefit from cognitive rehabilitation treatment (CRT) before implementation or reinitiation of CBT

Performance in practice: confessions of a psychopharmacologist

What are clinical considerations for patients diagnosed with co-occurring anxiety disorders?

- Persons diagnosed with multiple anxiety disorders tend to have more severe symptoms and poor prognosis and outcomes

PATIENT FILE

- Evidence-supported and empirically supported and efficacious treatment for comorbid anxiety disorders, anxiety and personality disorder, anxiety and substance use disorder, and somatic symptom disorders can include various therapies such as CBT, and behavioral and CRT therapies
  - Although current research is inconclusive iregarding whether the primary treatment focus is the primary and/or comorbid disorder, the presence of comorbidity does not diminish benefits of empirically supported treatments
  - Consider adaptation of treatment modality, intervention, and strategy in the presence of complicating or negative prognostic variables and/or lack of response to implemented treatment
    - Case-specific formulations (versus a structured, manualized approach) may better address patients' constellation of symptoms and disorders
- Functional somatic disorders (FSD) are informed by physiological, psychological, and sociocultural factors and defined by patterns of persistent physical symptoms
  - Historical medical diagnoses that are now encapsulated as an FSD include fibromyalgia, chronic pain or fatigue syndromes, and irritable bowel syndrome
    - The constellation of physical symptoms and ailments is associated with significant patient suffering; socioeconomic impact; cost-ineffective and futile diagnostic work-ups, examinations, and procedures; as well as sick leave and long-term disability
  - Physical symptoms may involve one or multiple organ systems
    - Approximately 1.3–2.2% of the general population suffers from multiorgan FSD
  - Nonpharmacological patient education intervention facilitates treatment by empowering and engaging patients in symptom and condition management
  - Pharmacological treatments
    - Low-dose tricyclic antidepressants (TCAs) have been utilized in multiorgan functional somatic disorder
      - However, the use of TCAs is dose limited due to decreased tolerability at higher prescribed dosages
    - Serotonin–norepinephrine reuptake inhibitors (SNRIs) are the most frequently prescribed class of medications
      - Proposed treatment effect is attributed to resolution of concurrent depression that impacts illness perception,

PATIENT FILE

treatment adherence, and behavioral responses to illness; central analgesic effect; reduction in affective arousal and sleep dysfunction; and improved cognitive function
- Current clinical trials are examining the efficacy of treatment with duloxetine 60 mg for comorbid anxiety and depression in patients suffering from multiorgan functional somatic disorder

Tips and pearls

- Anxiety can be coincident with and/or a symptom presentation of a medical or other psychiatric condition, including substance use disorders (SUDs)
  - One study suggested approximately 15% of those with a known anxiety disorder had at least one independent co-occurring SUD, and 17% of those with a known SUD had at least one independent co-occurring anxiety disorder over a single 12-month period
  - A meta-analysis found that nearly 50% of those with lifetime illicit drug dependence had a comorbid anxiety disorder
- Occurrence of comorbid SUD and anxiety disorder is linked to greater symptom severity, impairment, and healthcare utilization; suboptimal outcomes, including non-adherence to treatment, decreased engagement in SUD treatment, greater likelihood of relapse, and poorer functioning after treatment; suicide, homelessness, and reliance on welfare
  - In one study, nearly all individuals who reported two or more comorbidities reported a comorbid anxiety disorder (95.9%)
    - Panic disorder was the most common type of anxiety disorder reported; and PTSD was identified by about 62.0% of participants
    - Posited theories attempting to explain co-occurring anxiety and substance use disorders include:
      - Classic tension-reduction, self-medicating, and stress-dampening: individuals with anxiety disorders will use substances to alleviate, or cope with anxiety
        - Negative reinforcement leads to a pattern of maladaptive substance use and, eventually, an SUD
        - This theory accounts for approximately 75% of cases, in which the anxiety disorder precedes the onset of the SUD
      - Substance-induced anxiety enhancement theory: Withdrawal or intoxication experiences engender anxiety, which leads to the onset of an anxiety disorder over time

- - - This theory accounts for the other 25% of cases – in this model, the SUD precedes the onset of the anxiety disorder
  - Mutual maintenance model of anxiety disorder and SUD comorbidity: there are multiple pathways to the onset of the comorbidity and, once an individual has both problems, the symptoms serve to mutually maintain and exacerbate one another
    - An individual's perception of and sensitivity to anxiety symptoms, coupled with a tendency to fear associated bodily sensations, is linked to both increased anxiety and substance use, suggesting its possible role as a contributing factor
- Epidemiological studies estimate that about 8% of those with co-occurring mental and substance use disorders receive treatment for both problems
  - Comorbidity presents treatment and recovery challenges, with greater success noted with interventions designed to address the complexities of co-occurring issues
  - Treatment approaches designed to address anxiety – substance use comorbidity generally follow one of three treatment formats
    - Sequential: treatments first address the SUD, then move on to the other disorder, in discrete stages
    - Parallel: parallel treatments ensure treatment for both disorders simultaneously
      - Parallel treatment is limited by provision of treatment by various providers, leading to fragmentation of care
    - Integrated: integrated treatment models include creation of a hybrid treatment that treats each disorder independently
      - Care for anxiety – substance use is limited by systemic issues, focus of the extant healthcare system on discrete problems and not the full clinical picture, and lack of development and empirical evaluation of integrated treatments
    - Anxiety – substance use treatments that incorporate elements of cognitive behavioral techniques (i.e., exposure response prevention for obsessive–compulsive disorder, prolonged exposure for PTSD) perform better than those that do not
- Difficulties that limit efficacious treatment include limited access to care services as comorbidity may preclude meeting

PATIENT FILE

  treatment criteria for one condition or the other, limited research regarding treatment options, and clinical disagreement about whether comorbid anxiety and substance use should be treated simultaneously or separately
  - However, treatment of SUDs should always be a clinical priority due to the associated health benefits of reduction or cessation of substance use
- Mental disorders and substance use problems co-occur with great frequency among criminal offenders
  - The lifetime prevalence of co-occurring SUD and anxiety disorders is reported as approximately 84% in prison settings and 74% in forensic psychiatric hospitals
    - Offenders present with higher rates of co-occurring disorders compared to the general population
    - Co-occurring anxiety and substance use disorders are more symptomatic and difficult to treat; associated with higher rates of violence, homicide, and an increased likelihood of incarceration and criminal recidivism; contributory to increased vulnerability to negative outcomes
  - A high rate of comorbidity between substance use and personality disorder is a pertinent issue in clinical practice as co-occurring SUDs and antisocial personality disorder (ASPD) may be less responsive to treatment and more likely to lead to discontinuation of treatment
  - Those who work with people who have a psychiatric disability with co-occurring SUDs must ensure that the substance disorders are addressed to help ensure recovery from the mental illness and to reduce the likelihood of offending

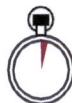

two-minute tutorial

- Anxiety disorders are among the most common mental disorders in adults, with 18.1% meeting criteria for at least one anxiety disorder
  - The 12-month prevalence rate of various anxiety disorders ranges from 0.8 % to 11%, with lifetime prevalence of 16.6%
  - Anxiety disorders, in isolation, are associated with later onset and more likely to remit on their own versus co-occurring disorders
  - Adults with anxiety disorders are often at risk for relationship impairment, physical health concerns, and occupational disability, as well as substance abuse and suicidality
- General clinical and research consensus is that, compared to someone presenting with a single anxiety disorder, those individuals who meet diagnostic criteria for multiple anxiety disorders tend to have more severe symptoms

PATIENT FILE

- Treatment considerations for comorbid disorders
  - Approaches to treating comorbid anxiety disorders have been developed and include transdiagnostic treatments and other treatments designed to address combinations of disorders
    - The premise of the transdiagnostic approach is that anxiety disorders may be interdependent; treatments for specific anxiety disorders are robust; and evaluation and treatment of a diagnosis may lead to identification of other diagnoses
      - Emphasis on commonalities across disorders, which enable patients' perception of control, and on application of techniques learned in treatment can reduce comorbid disorders
        - Effective treatments for various anxiety disorders share common features (e.g., exposure with response prevention, cognitive restructuring, relaxation training)
          - However, exposure treatment may be considered aversive, especially when the approach is described before initiated
          - And those who do not experience a decrease in anxiety during the exposures or between successive exposures doubt the benefit of continued treatment
    - Evidence-supported and empirically supported and efficacious treatment for anxiety disorders includes CBT
      - CBT incorporates physiological, cognitive, and behavioral conceptualizations relevant in the treatment for specific phobia, social phobia, social anxiety disorder, and GAD
      - Although CBT yields strong treatment effects, in the presence of complicating or negative prognostic variables, adaptation of treatment to address specific case formulations may be preferable to a structured, manualized approach
  - Anxiety and personality disorder
    - Clinically, a personality disorder comorbid with an anxiety disorder may serve as a potential prognostic indicator; and therapeutic progress monitoring can assist with identification and implementation of a different treatment strategy if improvement is not made within the period of brief therapy
    - Patients may benefit from a more intensive, longer course of treatment to address characterological traits
  - Overall, the presence of comorbidity does not seem to diminish benefits of empirically supported treatments

PATIENT FILE

- Therapy addresses each of these components with various strategies, including somatic management techniques, cognitive restructuring, and behavioral exposure
  - Therapy treatment factors to consider
    - Therapeutic alliance: the therapeutic alliance can be defined as the bond between therapist and client that engages the client in the therapeutic process
      - It is believed to be a key factor in the effective treatment of anxiety
      - Limitations to the establishment and maintenance of the therapeutic alliance include:
        - A patient's difficulty forming social relationships, which can potentially interfere with the formation of a therapeutic alliance
        - The therapeutic alliance can be damaged due to conducting exposures at a pace the patient feels unprepared for or incapable of handling
        - Damage to the therapeutic alliance may occur if anxiety symptoms do not decrease, abate, or resolve during an in-session exposure
        - Therapeutic alliance ruptures that occur in treatment can be approached via
          - Direct methods, such as providing rationale, exploration of core interpersonal themes, and clarifying any misunderstandings
          - Indirect methods that may involve reframing or changing the task or goal, modeling empathetic characterization, and providing a corrective emotional experience
      - Research on therapeutic alliance and treatment outcomes is in its early stages and findings remain inconclusive
    - Patient motivation: problems with motivation are common in individuals with anxiety disorders; patients often display ambivalence regarding treatment for anxiety, even though they may be aware that excessive anxiety is distressing and interferes in their ability to partake in desirable activities
      - Individuals may hesitate to initiate, or prematurely terminate, treatment for fear of others' negative appraisal of them

PATIENT FILE

- Motivational interviewing can decrease ambivalence to therapy by augmenting intrinsic motivation to change, facilitating open discussion, and resolving ambivalence to change
  ○ Unified or transdiagnostic approaches to treatment may be preferred for individuals who do not fit a specific diagnostic category or who have complicated, comorbid presentations
    - A unified treatment approach emphasizes individualized case conceptualization and targets cognitive-behavioral models of anxiety, including maladaptive cognitive appraisals, poor emotional regulation, emotional avoidance, and maladaptive behavior associated with disordered emotion

Post-test question

Which of the following is NOT a treatment option for somatic and functional somatic disorder?

A. Patient education
B. CRT
C. CBT
D. SSRIs

Answer: D

References

1. de Vroege, L., Timmermans, A., Kop, W. J., & van der Feltz-Cornelis, C. M. (2018). Neurocognitive dysfunctioning and the impact of comorbid depression and anxiety in patients with somatic symptom and related disorders: a cross-sectional clinical study. *Psychological Medicine*, Aug., 48(11), 1803–1813. https://doi.org/10.1017/S0033291717003300.
2. Donovan, A. L. & Bird, S. A. (2019). *Substance Use and the Acute Psychiatric Patient: Emergency Management*. Cham: Springer Nature Switzerland AG.
3. Jespersen, C. P., Pedersen, H. F., Kleinstauber, M., et al. (2024). Efficacy of patient education and duloxetine, alone and in combination, for patients with multisystem functional somatic disorder: study protocol for the EDULOX trial. *Contemporary Clinical Trials*, June., 141, 107524. https://doi.org/10.1016/j.cct.2024.107524.
4. Ogloff, J. R., Talevski, D., Lemphers, A., Wood, M., & Simmons, M. (2015). Co-occurring mental illness, substance use disorders, and antisocial personality disorder among clients of forensic

mental health services. *Psychiatric Rehabilitation Journal*, March, 38(1), 16–23. https://doi.org/10.1037/prj0000088.

5. Pan, X., Ding, W., Sun, X., et al. (2021). Gray matter density of the dorsomedial prefrontal cortex mediates the relationship between castrophizing and anxiety in somatic symptom disorder. *Neuropsychiatric Disease and Treatment*, March 9, 17, 757–764. https://doi.org/10.2147/NDT.S296462.

6. Robinson, L. D. & Deane, F. P. (2022). Substance use disorder and anxiety, depression, eating disorder, PTSD, and phobia comorbidities among individuals attending residential substance use treatment settings. *Journal of Dual Diagnosis*, July–Sept., 18(3), 165–176. https://doi.org/10.1080/15504263.2022.2090648.

7. Stahl, S. M. (2014). *Stahl's Essential Psychopharmacology: Prescriber's Guide*, 5th ed. New York: Cambridge University Press.

8. Storch, E. A. & McKay, D. (2013). *Handbook of Treating Variants and Complications in Anxiety Disorders*. New York: Springer Science+Business Media.

9. Wolitzky-Taylor, K. (2023). Integrated behavioral diagnostic and treatments for comorbid anxiety and substance use disorders: a model for understanding integrated treatment approaches and meta-analysis to evaluate their efficacy. *Drug and Alcohol Dependence*, Dec. 1, 253, 110990. https://doi.org/10.1016/j.drugalcdep.2023.110990.

10. Wolitzky-Taylor, K., Niles, A. N., Ries, R., et al. (2018). Who needs more than standard care? Treatment moderators in a randomized clinical trial comparing addiction treatment alone to addiction treatment plus anxiety disorder treatment for comorbid anxiety and substance use disorders. *Behaviour Research and Therapy*, Aug., 107, 1–9. https://doi.org/10.1016/j.brat.2018.05.005.

PATIENT FILE

20

COVID-19: The new player in town and here to stay

The Psychopharmacological Dilemma: What are the treatment considerations with antipsychotic medications for patients who received the COVID-19 vaccine?

Maanasi Chandarana

Pretest self-assessment question

Which of the following are NOT associated with myocarditis?

A. Clozapine
B. COVID-19 vaccine
C. COVID-19 infection
D. Quetiapine
E. Haloperidol
F. Olanzapine
G. All are associated with myocarditis
H. None is associated with myocarditis

Answer: G

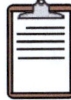

Patient evaluation on intake

The patient is a 45-year-old male with previous diagnoses of schizophrenia, unspecified depressive disorder and substance use disorder (stimulant – methamphetamine-type, cannabis use disorder) who was found incompetent to stand trial (IST). While housed in the correctional setting and awaiting admission to the forensic state hospital, he received treatment with antipsychotic medications for his psychiatric diagnosis. As his symptoms did not remit with antipsychotic medication treatment, the clinician obtained informed consent from the patient for treatment with clozapine. Nine days prior to initiation of clozapine treatment, the patient received the first dose of a COVID-19 vaccine. He was started on clozapine therapy and received a second dose of the COVID-19 vaccine 12 days later. In the ensuing month, the patient was diagnosed with thromboembolism and myocarditis. The etiology of myocarditis was attributed to treatment with clozapine, which was subsequently discontinued. The patient's persistent mental health symptoms interfered with attainment of legal competency while incarcerated, and he was subsequently admitted to a state forensic facility for legal competency restoration.

PATIENT FILE

Psychiatric history

- Mental health history with onset in late adolescence
  - His psychiatric symptoms were first observed by his family who said that the patient was speaking with God
  - He received psychiatric treatment intermittently from when he was 19 years old
    - He was first psychiatrically hospitalized when he was 19 years old; was involuntarily hospitalized for a month at a time on numerous occasions; and treated with multiple antipsychotic medications
    - He was diagnosed with schizophrenia, post-traumatic stress disorder (PTSD), and multiple personality disorder, and demonstrated auditory and visual hallucinations, delusions of grandeur, persecutory delusions, poor self-care and hygiene, blunted affect, and nonlinear thought process per record review
    - He reported 45 previous suicide attempts
    - He was treated with risperidone, aripiprazole, haloperidol, ziprasidone, olanzapine, and clozapine
      - He reported adverse drug reactions during prior medication trials to ziprasidone, quetiapine, olanzapine, lorazepam, and benztropine
      - He was diagnosed with clozapine-associated myocarditis while housed in a correctional setting
    - Following acute inpatient stabilization, the patient decompensated multiple times in the community and had a transient lifestyle preceding forensic hospitalization
  - The patient reported a history of mood symptoms including episodic sad mood, anhedonia, decreased energy; and euphoria, decreased sleep, and increased energy
  - He reported physical abuse including concussion head trauma
- He completed high school and obtained a Bachelor's degree
  - However, he was noted to be an unreliable historian
- The patient has a history of violence with multiple arrests and charges
- The patient was not previously hospitalized in forensic psychiatric facilities

Social and personal history

- Multiple encounters with law enforcement noted, with first documented arrest and incurred charge when he was 15 years of age
- He denied gainful employment and received Social Security benefits for his psychiatric diagnoses
- He reported that he had 200 wives but denied having any children

PATIENT FILE

- Substance use history
  - The patient reported that his drug of choice is cannabis, age of first use as 3 years old, and characterized use as 3–4 marijuana cigarettes/day
  - He relayed methamphetamine use but the age of onset, amount, and frequency of use were unknown
  - He reported previous substance use about 3 months prior to current hospitalization

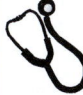

Medical history
- Dyslipidemia
- Hypertension
- COVID-19 vaccine-associated thromboembolism
- Clozapine-associated myocarditis

Family history
- The patient reported a familial history of alcohol use disorder (AUD) and mental illness
  - He said his father was diagnosed with schizophrenia and died by a drug overdose
  - He stated that his mother died by suicide
  - He relayed that his maternal and paternal grandparents were diagnosed with mental illness

Medication history
- He reported treatment with various medication trials, including antipsychotic medication
  - He relayed adverse drug reactions with multiple medications including ziprasidone, olanzapine, quetiapine, lorazepam, and benztropine
  - He was diagnosed with clozapine-associated myocarditis in a correctional facility
- The patient was prescribed haloperidol, diphenhydramine, and sertraline upon admission to the forensic state hospital

Current history
- The patient presented to the evaluation as calm, polite, and cooperative
- His grooming and hygiene were deemed fair
- His speech rate, rhythm, and volume were deemed normal and described as spontaneous and goal directed
  - However, his thought process was noted to be nonlinear when conversing without interruption

PATIENT FILE

- The patient did not demonstrate psychomotor agitation and retardation; but he demonstrated a resting tremor of his upper extremity and suspected oral–buccal–lingual tardive dyskinesia
- He characterized his mood as "good," and demonstrated a stable affect. He denied suicidal thoughts and homicidal ideations
- He reported auditory hallucinations and demonstrated delusions of grandeur; he denied experiencing visual hallucinations
- His thought process was nonlinear at times during the evaluation
- The patient was alert, oriented to person, and place. He asserted that the current year was the previous year. His memory, ability to abstract, fund of knowledge, and attention were deemed fair
- His judgment was deemed poor, and his insight was deemed limited
- His cognitive abilities were deemed intact and akin to his age and educational history

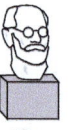

Psychotherapy history

- There is no known psychotherapy history to report

Mechanism of action moment

- Clozapine
  - Antagonizes D_2 receptors and serotonin 2A receptors
    - Blocking D_2 receptors reduces positive symptoms of psychosis and provides mood stabilization
    - Blocking serotonin 2A receptors enhances dopamine release in brain regions to minimize motor side effects and improve cognitive and affective symptoms
  - Interacts with 5-HT_{2C} and 5-HT_{1A} which may promote increased efficacy in treatment of cognitive and affective symptoms
- Haloperidol
  - Blocks D_2 receptors
    - Reduces positive symptoms and aggressive behaviors
    - In the nigrostriatal pathway, D_2 blockade improves tics and associated symptoms of Tourette's
- Diphenhydramine
  - Has anticholinergic properties
    - Decreases excessive acetylcholine activity from dopamine receptor blockade
      - Combats dyskinesia and promotes sedation
  - Blocks histamine (H1) receptors

PATIENT FILE

- Sertraline
  - Boosts serotoninergic neurotransmission
  - Desensitizes serotonin 1A receptors
  - Blocks serotonin and dopamine reuptake pumps
- Risperidone
  - Blocks D_2 receptors
    - Reduces positive symptoms and provides mood stabilization
  - Blocks serotonin 2A receptors
    - Enhances dopamine release in brain regions which reduces motor side effects and enhances cognition and affect

Attending physician's mental notes

- The patient has a history of experiencing psychotic symptoms, including impairment in his thought process, perceptual disturbances of auditory and visual hallucinations, and delusions of grandeur
- His history is notable for substance use, physical abuse resulting in concussions, and multiple contacts with law enforcement
- The patient currently reports auditory hallucinations and delusions of grandeur; he denies depressive symptoms; the patient exhibits a nonlinear thought process during the evaluation
- The patient has the right to refuse medications but provides informed consent for prescribed psychiatric medications
  - Because the patient demonstrates oral–buccal–lingual tardive dyskinesia, haloperidol and diphenhydramine are discontinued, and risperidone is initiated
  - Sertraline is continued
- As-needed medication including chlorpromazine is prescribed to the patient

Further investigation

- The month following his hospitalization, the patient demonstrated persistent symptoms of psychosis, including auditory and visual hallucinations, persecutory and religiously based delusions, and negative symptoms
  - He was observed by the staff responding to internal stimuli
  - His psychotic symptoms precluded his ability to attain competency
- He denied experiencing alterations in his mood symptoms
- He did not request or require treatment with as-needed medications
- He was not placed on enhanced observation or in seclusion and restraints

PATIENT FILE

Attending physician's mental notes
- The patient has a history of experiencing psychotic symptoms, including auditory and visual hallucinations; persecutory, religious, and grandiose delusions; a nonlinear thought process; and mood symptoms
    - He has not demonstrated mood or affective symptoms during his hospitalization but has demonstrated positive and negative symptoms of psychosis
    - The patient's antipsychotic medication, risperidone, was increased to further treat his symptoms
- During his hospitalization, he did not have difficulty following unit rules, behave violently, require as-needed medications, or benefit from placement on enhanced observation, in seclusion, or in restraints
- The patient has the right to refuse medications, has taken prescribed medications volitionally, and has not taken or required as-needed chlorpromazine
- Prescribed psychiatric medications of risperidone and sertraline, and as-needed medication, chlorpromazine, will be continued
- The patient will be monitored and assessed for response to treatment and progress toward competency restoration

Case outcome
- The patient was admitted to a forensic state hospital for legal competency restoration
- The patient reported a history of psychiatric symptoms with onset at 19 years of age and substance use at 3 years of age
- He reported a history of mood symptoms and auditory and visual hallucinations
- The patient was diagnosed with schizophrenia, unspecified depressive disorder, stimulant – methamphetamine-type use disorder, and cannabis use disorder
- The patient was prescribed scheduled psychiatric medications upon admission to our facility
    - The patient has a reported history of multiple adverse drug reactions to multiple antipsychotics
    - He was diagnosed with clozapine-associated myocarditis
    - He exhibited persistent positive and negative psychotic symptoms and oral–buccal–lingual tardive dyskinesia with haloperidol therapy
        - Haloperidol and diphenhydramine were discontinued and treatment with risperidone was initiated
        - Risperidone was increased to maximize therapeutic benefit

- The patient reported a history of mood symptoms and multiple suicide attempts, but he demonstrated and relayed stable mood symptoms at admission and during hospitalization, for which sertraline was continued
- The patient interacted appropriately with his peers and staff and followed unit rules; he was not placed on enhanced observation or in seclusion and restraints; he provided informed consent for treatment with medications and did not demonstrate affective symptoms
- The patient did demonstrate persistent positive and negative psychotic symptoms during his hospitalization
  - His psychotic symptoms precluded his ability to attain legal competency
- The patient's history of psychiatric symptoms and treatment potentially contributed to the patient being an optimal candidate for treatment with clozapine therapy
  - However, he was diagnosed with clozapine-associated myocarditis
  - The patient was prescribed clozapine 9 days after the first administered dose of a COVID-19 vaccine and 12 days before the second administered dose of a COVID-19 vaccine
    - COVID-19 messenger RNA (mRNA) vaccines, COVID-19 infections, and clozapine are associated with adverse side effect of myocarditis

Take-home points

- The worldwide incidence of schizophrenia is approximately 1% of the adult population, and this diagnosis is the tenth leading cause of disability
- Mortality in schizophrenia is 2–3 times higher than in those individuals not diagnosed with this mental illness
- Treatment with clozapine is associated with decreased mortality, suicide, and inpatient hospitalizations, and with improved independence in lifestyle choices and employment when compared to treatment with other antipsychotic medications
  - However, clozapine therapy is associated with serious side effects requiring medical and surgical interventions, including clozapine-associated myocarditis
- The etiology of myocarditis includes infection, drug toxins, and immune dysregulation or disorders of the immune system
  - Symptoms of myocarditis are variable and can range from no reported symptoms (asymptomatic) to nonspecific symptoms including fever, muscle pain, chest pain and/or palpitations, difficulty breathing, and fatigue or malaise

- The sequelae of myocarditis include dilated cardiomyopathy, cardiogenic shock, and death
- Cardiac complications following COVID-19 infection and vaccination include myocarditis
  - Risk of myocarditis is higher following a COVID-19 infection versus COVID-19 vaccination
    - Diagnostically, the symptoms of myocarditis following COVID-19 disease and vaccination are indistinguishable
    - Risk of myocarditis is estimated to be 16 times higher following COVID-19 infection versus vaccination
  - COVID-19 infection
    - Myocardial injury is defined by the presence of an elevated troponin level (greater than or equal to the 99% of the upper limit of the reference range)
    - It is estimated that 13–41% of people diagnosed with severe COVID have cardiovascular complications and, on average, about 20% of cases are associated with myocardial injury
    - Symptoms and signs of COVID-19 infection affecting the cardiovascular system occur at the time of symptom presentation and early in the disease course or late in the disease course
    - Risk factors include older age and comorbid chronic medical conditions of diabetes, hypertension, obesity, and pre-existing cardiovascular disease
    - The pathophysiology of cardiac insult is thought to be secondary to direct viral injury or from the dysregulation of the immune system and ensuing inflammatory cascade induced by the COVID-19 infection
      - The infection is associated with oxidative stress to the microvasculature, direct endothelial and vascular injury, and hypoxemic injury
    - Diagnostic features include clinical symptom presentation and alterations in electrocardiogram (EKG), cardiac magnetic resonance imaging (MRI), transthoracic echocardiogram (TTE) or echocardiogram, cardiac enzymes, and inflammatory biomarkers
      - Exclusion of obstructive coronary artery disease
    - Clinically, cardiac complications associated with COVID-19 infections include thromboembolism, myocardial injury, stress cardiomyopathy, arrhythmia, and sudden death
      - Cardiac arrhythmias are linked with infiltration of inflammatory cells into blood vessels and the cardiac electrical conduction system

PATIENT FILE

- COVID-19 vaccine
  - Myocarditis is associated with administration of mRNA vaccines; most commonly follows receipt of the second vaccine dose; and, demographically, is observed more frequently in males less than 40 years old
    - The Center for Disease Control (CDC) estimates that the incidence of pericarditis and myocarditis in males aged 18–29 years old is 55.3–100.6 per 100,000
    - The increased risk in this patient population may be due to androgenic modulation of inflammatory and genetic factors encoding HLA and cardiac proteins
  - The pathophysiology of cardiac insult may be explained by:
    - Antibodies produced in response to the COVID-19 spike protein subsequently binding to angiotensin-converting enzyme (ACE) receptors of mural cells in the cardiac endothelium, pericytes, which prevent the pericytes from repairing cardiac tissue injuries
      - Young males are suspected of incurring more subtle cardiac injuries which require the action of pericytes
    - Leaked vaccine nanoparticles that enter circulation are endocytosed by cardiac pericytes, myocytes, macrophages, and endothelial cells
    - Recruited neutrophils, that present in response to COVID-19 spike proteins, activate the complement system which induces direct endothelial injury
  - Symptoms present within 3 days following administration of vaccine
    - Symptom report varies from asymptomatic to symptomatic
      - Reported symptoms include subfebrile to febrile temperature, chest pain and/or pressure (in approximately 95% of cases), shortness of breath (in about 20%), weakness, and malaise and fatigue
  - Clinical signs include
    - Elevation in troponins within 48–72 hours
    - Increased inflammatory biomarkers including C-reactive protein (CRP)
    - Changes in performed EKG including nonspecific changes in ST (including ST elevation in 75%) and depression in the PQ intervals
    - TTE demonstrates wall motion abnormalities (approximately 43%), reduced left ventricular ejection fraction of less than 50% (in about 24% of cases), and pulmonary embolus (in around 7%)

- Cardiac MRI findings are similar in both post-COVID-19-infection and post-COVID-19-vaccination myocarditis
  - Subepicardial distribution with basal and inferolateral wall involvement
    - Cardiac MRI in post-COVID-19-vaccination myocarditis shows less septal involvement when compared to COVID-19 infection-associated myocarditis
    - CDC recommendations include delay of about 8 weeks between first and second dose of the COVID-19 vaccine in males less than 40 years old
- Clozapine-associated myocarditis is associated with an IgE-mediated hypersensitivity reaction, genetic or hereditary factors, and the geographic variance in ozone concentration, but not with comorbid medical conditions including nicotine use or diabetes
  - The incidence of clozapine-associated myocarditis varies from 0.05% to 8.5% worldwide
  - The mortality rate of clozapine-associated myocarditis ranges from 21% to 50%
  - In nearly 87% of cases, the onset of symptoms presents within 30 days, and can be as early as 2 weeks, following initiation of treatment with clozapine
  - Risk of myocarditis following initiation of therapy with clozapine treatment may not be dose dependent but may be related to increased dosing earlier in treatment course
    - Myocarditis has occurred in patients receiving 50–600 mg of clozapine daily
  - Reported symptoms parallel those reported following COVID-19 infection and vaccination, and range from nonspecific symptoms of fever, fatigue, muscle aches, chest pain, or palpitations and dyspnea with exertion, to no reported or identified symptoms
  - To diagnose clozapine-associated myocarditis, cardiac and inflammatory biomarkers, cardiac imaging and testing, and consultation with medical providers and cardiac specialists should be obtained
    - Cardiac biomarkers
      - Troponin, brain natriuretic peptide (BNP), CRP
      - In approximately 90% of cases, Troponin T and Troponin I are twice the upper limit of the reference range, and in about 70% of cases, CRP is resulted as greater than 100 mg/L
    - Cardiac studies
      - TTE

PATIENT FILE

- May show impaired ventricular functioning, including decreases in the right and left ventricular ejection fraction, as well as impaired focal wall movement (focal hypokinesis)
- Cardiac MRI
  - Cardiac MRI is thought to be 75% sensitive
  - In myocarditis, nonspecific patterns of edema, late gadolinium enhancement, and noncoronary fibrosis are observed
- Cardiac consultation, medical consultation, surgical consultation are recommended as clinically appropriate and indicated
- Treatment protocol
  - Monitoring for myocarditis should occur when treatment with clozapine therapy is initiated
  - During monitoring, if cardiac troponins are elevated
    - Obtain an EKG, cardiac MRI, TTE, and cardiology consult
      - If there is a decrease of left ventricular ejection fraction noted on TTE, medical protocols for heart failure treatment should be pursued
      - Treatment with clozapine should be stopped
  - If clozapine is discontinued, and to allow cardiac inflammation to subside, an oral rechallenge should not occur for 6 months
  - After 6 months has elapsed, clozapine can be orally rechallenged
    - Cardiac and inflammatory biomarkers, cardiac studies including an EKG and TTE, are obtained prior to rechallenge
    - During this time, the dosing of clozapine should be increased slowly, labs trending cardiac and inflammatory biomarkers should be obtained twice weekly, and a TTE should be obtained every 6 months
  - In cases where the patient has a pre-existing cardiac condition, including hypertension or heart failure without preserved ejection fraction, including left ventricular ejection fraction less than 50%, a beta-blocker and ACE inhibitor (ACEi) or angiotensin receptor blocker (ARB) should be started concomitantly with re-initiation of treatment with clozapine therapy
  - In cases of severe clozapine-associated myocarditis with persistent left ventricular dysfunction and hemodynamic instability, do not rechallenge with clozapine

PATIENT FILE

Performance in practice: confessions of a psychopharmacologist

What are clinical considerations when treating a patient with clozapine-, or post-COVID-19 infection-/vaccination-induced, myocarditis?

- Nonspecific symptoms of myocarditis include chest pain, chest palpitations, chest pressure, dyspnea, exertional dyspnea, malaise and fatigue, fever, and muscle pain
  - Clozapine-induced myocarditis is indistinguishable from post-COVID-19-infection- and post-COVID-19 vaccination-induced myocarditis
    - However, COVID-19 infection-induced myocarditis presents as the initial symptom of the disease or late in disease course and in high-risk populations (i.e., older age groups and those with medical comorbidities of diabetes, hypertension, obesity, and pre-existing cardiovascular disease)
    - And COVID-19 vaccination-induced myocarditis occurs within 3 days of vaccine administration and is more common in males less than 40 years of age after receipt of the second dose of a COVID-19 vaccine series
- The pre-treatment work-up for clozapine treatment includes obtaining an EKG, TTE, and cardiac and inflammatory biomarkers
- The incidence of clozapine-induced myocarditis is 0.05–8.5% worldwide
- In 87% of cases, clozapine-induced myocarditis develops in 2 weeks to 1 month following initiation of treatment
  - Clozapine-induced myocarditis is not dose dependent, but is associated with higher dosing early in treatment course
    - Recommendations include titration of clozapine by 25 mg/day over 4–6 weeks to reach dosing goal
- During their treatment course, and if the patient develops an increase in cardiac troponins, obtain an EKG, cardiac MRI, TTE, and consult medical and cardiology providers
  - If cardiac enzymes are elevated with or without preservation of left ventricular ejection fraction, clozapine therapy should be discontinued
    - An oral rechallenge can occur after 6 months, allowing for cardiac inflammation to subside
      - Clozapine rechallenge occurs slowly and is accompanied by twice-weekly collection of cardiac enzymes and inflammatory biomarkers, as well as semi-annual TTE

PATIENT FILE

- Treatment of myocarditis-associated heart failure includes administration of a beta-blocker and ACEi or ARB and can be initiated upon discovery of decrease in left ventricular ejection fraction and continued with oral rechallenge of clozapine

Tips and pearls

- Myocarditis is a serious complication associated with COVID-19 infections, COVID-19 vaccinations, and treatment with clozapine therapy
  - The presentation of myocarditis from a COVID-19 infection has a bimodal distribution and occurs as the first symptom of the disease or late in the disease course
    - Risk factors including pre-existing cardiac conditions, older age, hypertension, diabetes, and increased BMI
  - Males under the age of 40 years are at increased risk of developing COVID-19 vaccine-associated myocarditis approximately 3 days following administration of the second dose of an mRNA vaccine
    - Current recommendations per the CDC, to reduce the risk of vaccine-associated myocarditis, include waiting 8 weeks between administration of the first and second dose of the vaccine
- While risk factors and associated comorbid conditions can vary based on etiology, clinical symptoms and signs of myocarditis may remain the same or similar regardless of the cause
- Some important facts to keep in mind when evaluating clozapine-associated myocarditis:
  - Incidence is variable yet low
  - In 87% of cases, clozapine-associated myocarditis occurs within 2 weeks to a month following initiation with treatment
  - There does not appear to be any comorbid condition that increases the risk of developing clozapine-associated myocarditis
  - In 90% of cases, Troponin I and Troponin T are two times higher than the upper limit of the reference range, but, in 7% of cases, there may not be an appreciable increase in cardiac troponin
  - Measured CRP can be resulted as 10–20 times the upper limit of the reference range, and in 70% of cases, is greater than 100 mg/L in clozapine-associated myocarditis
  - Although tachycardia can be observed in patients with clozapine-associated myocarditis, an increase in heart rate by 10–15 beats/minute can also be associated with the anticholinergic properties of clozapine

PATIENT FILE

- Even though clozapine-associated myocarditis does not appear to be dose dependent, and the condition has been observed in the dosing range of 50–600 mg, an identified risk factor includes higher dosing of the medication early in the treatment course
  - Recommendations include slow titration of 25 mg/day over 4–6 weeks to reach the target dose
- Current areas of investigation include distinguishing clozapine-associated myocarditis from COVID-19 vaccine-related myocarditis in individuals treated with clozapine therapy

Two-minute tutorial

- Myocarditis is inflammation of the cardiac myocytes and is associated with COVID-19 infection, COVID-19 vaccination, and with clozapine treatment
- Clinical symptoms in myocarditis associated with a COVID-19 infection, treatment with clozapine, and from COVID-19 vaccination are similar, and a patient's symptoms can range from asymptomatic to nonspecific
  - Nonspecific symptoms include chest pain, chest palpitations, chest pressure, dyspnea, exertional dyspnea, malaise and fatigue, fever, and muscle pain
- Diagnostically, obtaining and trending cardiac enzymes, including troponin and BNP; inflammatory biomarkers, including erythrocyte sedimentation rate (ESR) and CRP; cardiac functional and structural tests including EKG, TTE, and cardiac MRI; and appropriate medical and surgical consultation – all can aid with effective diagnosis, treatment, and management
  - Regardless of etiology, myocarditis is associated with elevated cardiac enzymes, elevated inflammatory biomarkers, nonspecific EKG changes, structural and/or functional changes on TTE and cardiac MRI
- Differences in the etiology of myocarditis can be associated with varying onset of symptoms, comorbid medical conditions, and clinical recommendations
  - COVID-19 infection has a bimodal distribution of cardiac complications, with myocardial injury occurring at the time of presenting symptoms and late in the disease course
    - At-risk populations include older patients, and those with pre-existing cardiovascular diseases, diabetes, hypertension, and increased BMI
  - COVID-19 vaccine-associated myocarditis usually presents about 3 days after an mRNA vaccine dose is administered; is most commonly observed with administration of the second

PATIENT FILE

dose of the vaccine; and preferentially affects males who are less than 40 years old
- Clozapine-associated myocarditis can occur over a broad range of prescribed dosing (i.e., is not dose dependent) and is not coincident with other medical comorbidities
  - Clozapine-associated myocarditis may be linked to higher dosing earlier in treatment course
  - Myocarditis usually presents about 2 weeks to 30 days following initiation with clozapine treatment
- Treatment protocol when prescribing clozapine
  - Monitoring for myocarditis should occur when treatment with clozapine therapy is initiated
  - During monitoring, if cardiac troponins are elevated, obtain an EKG, cardiac MRI, TTE, and cardiology consult
    - If there is a decrease of left ventricular ejection fraction noted on TTE, medical protocols for heart failure treatment should be pursued
    - Treatment with clozapine should be stopped
    - After 6 months has elapsed, clozapine can be orally rechallenged
    - Cardiac and inflammatory biomarkers, and cardiac studies including an EKG and TTE are obtained prior to rechallenge
    - Clozapine should be increased slowly, labs trending cardiac and inflammatory biomarkers should be obtained twice weekly, and a TTE should be obtained every 6 months
  - In cases where the patient has a pre-existing cardiac condition, including hypertension or heart failure without preserved ejection fraction, including left ventricular ejection fraction less than 50%, a beta-blocker and ACEi or ARB should be started concomitantly with reinitiation of treatment with clozapine therapy
  - In cases of severe clozapine-associated myocarditis with persistent left ventricular dysfunction and hemodynamic instability, do not rechallenge with clozapine

Post-test question

Which of the following considerations is true regarding treatment with clozapine and post-COVID-19 infection- or vaccination-induced myocarditis?

A. A patient's treatment with clozapine is not changed, as the benefit of treatment with this medication outweighs the risk of psychiatric decompensation with discontinuation of treatment

B. Waiting 6 months before medication rechallenge after obtaining cardiac and inflammatory biomarkers, an EKG, and a TTE
C. Treatment with clozapine is not resumed if a patient has a medical history of cardiac comorbidity and is diagnosed with cardiac complications post-COVID-19 infection or vaccination
D. Treatment for heart failure is not recommended as post-COVID-19 myocarditis is self-limiting
E. The temporal administration of the remainder of COVID-19 vaccine series and boosters remains unchanged

Answer: B

References

1. Bellissima, B. L., Tingle, M. D., Cicovic, A., Alawami, M., & Kenedi, C. (2018). A systematic review of clozapine-induced myocarditis. *International Journal of Cardiology*, May 15, 259, 122–129. https://doi.org/10.1016/j.ijcard.2017.12.102.
2. Dawson, J. L., Clark, S. R., Wilton, L. R., Chiew, K. Y., Procter, N. G., & Bell, J. S. (2022). Clozapine, mRNA COVID-19 vaccination and drug-induced myocarditis. *Australian and New Zealand Journal of Psychiatry*, July, 56(7), 879. https://doi.org/10.1177/00048674211062135.
3. Griffin, J. M., Woznica, E., Gilotra, N. A., & Nucifora, F. C., Jr. (2021). Clozapine-associated myocarditis: a protocol for monitoring upon clozapine initiation and recommendations for how to conduct a clozapine rechallenge. *Journal of Clinical Psychopharmacology*, March–April, 41(2), 180–185. https://doi.org/10.1097/JCP.0000000000001358.
4. Hansbauer, M., Fastantz, E., Lutz, J., & Hasan, A. (2022). Myocarditis after cloazapine initiation and mRNA SARS-CoV-2 vaccination. *Journal of Clinical Psychopharmacology*, Sept.–Oct., 42(5), 502–503. https://doi.org/10.1097/JCP.0000000000001577.
5. Heidecker, B., Dagan, N., Balicer, R., et al. (2022). Myocarditis following COVID-19 vaccine: incidence, presentation, diagnosis, pathophysiology, therapy, and outcomes put into perspective. A clinical consensus document supported by the Heart Failure Association of the European Society of Cardiology (ESC) Working Group on Myocardial and Pericardial Diseases. *European Journal of Heart Failure*, Nov., 24(11), 2000–2018. https://doi.org/10.1002/ejhf.2669.

PATIENT FILE

6. Kadkhoda, K. (2022). Post RNA-based COVID vaccines myocarditis: proposed mechanisms. *Vaccine*, Jan. 24, 40(3), 406–407. https://doi.org/10.1016/j.vaccine.2021.11.093.
7. Knudsen, B. & Prasad, V. (2022). COVID-19 vaccine induced myocarditis in young males: a systematic review. *European Journal of Clinical Investigation*, Dec. 28. https://doi.org/10.111/eci.13947.
8. Mallick, U. (2022). *Cardiovascular Complications of COVID-19: Risk, Pathogenesis and Outcomes*. Cham: Springer Nature Switzerland AG.
9. Samimisedeh, P., Afshar, E. J., Hassani, N. S., & Rastad, H. (2022). Cardiac MRI findings in COVID-19 vaccine-related myocarditis: a pooled analysis of 468 patients. *Journal of Magnetic Resonance Imaging*, Oct., 56(4), 971–982. https://doi.org/10.1002/jmri.28268.
10. Stahl, S. M. (2014). *Stahl's Essential Psychopharmacology: Prescriber's Guide*, 5th ed. New York: Cambridge University Press.

PATIENT FILE

21

Neurological disorders: Near and Fa(h)r

The Psychopharmacological Dilemma: What are treatment options for psychiatric symptoms stemming from a neurological disorder? Is impulsive aggression treated differently in Fahr's disease?

Maanasi Chandarana

Pretest self-assessment question

Fahr's disease is characterized as which of the following?

A. Basal ganglia calcifications due to neuroendocrine pathology and aberrant calcium metabolism
B. A perinatal condition with diffuse intraparenchymal calcifications
C. A syndrome with radiographic imaging of multifocal, curvilinear, calcium accretions of the bilateral basal ganglia, cortex, and cerebellum
D. A constellation of neurological, psychiatric, and cognitive symptoms and idiopathic basal ganglia calcifications

Answer: D

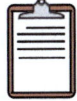

Patient evaluation on intake

The patient is a 25-year-old male with a childhood history of Attention-Deficit/Hyperactivity Disorder (ADHD), oppositional defiant disorder, and pervasive developmental disorder, and previous diagnoses of schizoaffective disorder and intellectual disability, who was found incompetent to stand trial (IST) to felonious charges. The patient received jail-based competency restoration efforts; however, due to his inability to attain legal competency and his persistent violent behaviors, the patient was court-ordered and transferred to a forensic state hospital. After assaulting a police officer upon hospital admission, the patient was transferred to a specialized unit with increased programming, enhanced infrastructure, and security measures reserved for the most unstable and violent patients.

Psychiatric history

- Mental health history with onset in childhood, at approximately 3 years of age
- The patient was first psychiatrically hospitalized when he was 14 years old
- His psychiatric symptoms were described as episodic in nature and characterized as manic and psychotic symptoms including auditory

PATIENT FILE

hallucinations, distractibility, delusions of grandeur, rapid speech, psychomotor agitation, disorganized behaviors, loose associations, flight of ideas, and disorganized thoughts
- Behaviorally, the patient exhibited intrusive, impulsive, and unpredictable acts
  - The patient has a history of self-injurious, physically assaultive, and verbally threatening behavior and interpersonal conflict
    - The patient has a history of head banging
- The patient has an extensive history of violence with multiple arrests, charges, and in-custody offenses
- The patient has been hospitalized in community and forensic psychiatric facilities multiple times
- He was prescribed multiple trials of medications, including antipsychotic, mood-stabilizer, and anticholinergic medications

Social and personal history
- The patient was raised by his older siblings
- He did not graduate high school or obtain a general educational development (GED) certificate
  - The patient reported dropping out of high school secondary to substance use with amphetamines and cannabis
- Multiple encounters with law enforcement noted, which resulted in his placement in juvenile hall
  - The patient was placed in a state-governed facility for intellectually disabled persons
- He was never married and reported that he fathered three children

Medical history
- Seizure disorder
  - The patient was prescribed levetiracetam 500 mg p.o. BID for seizure prophylaxis
- The patient developed lithium carbonate-induced hypothyroidism and gastroesophageal reflux disease (GERD) during his hospitalization
  - He was treated with levothyroxine 88 mcg and omeprazole 20 mg p.o. daily
    - Omeprazole was changed to pantoprazole given the medication's metabolism and resultant 50% reduction of clozapine levels

Family history
- There is no known familial history to report

PATIENT FILE

Medication history
- The patient was prescribed multiple trials of medications, including antipsychotic, mood-stabilizer, and anticholinergic medications

Current history
- The patient presented to the evaluation in restraints and a spit mask after assaulting a police officer
  - He was documented as demonstrating an angry, hostile, and tense demeanor
- His speech rate, rhythm, and volume were normal
- The patient's motor movements were unable to be assessed
- He reported that his mood was "upset." His affect was assessed as mood congruent and reported as irritable, angry, and tense
- He denied suicidal thoughts; he denied experiencing homicidal ideations
- He stated voices instructed him to assault the officer
- His thought process was disorganized
- The patient was alert, and oriented to person, time, place, and situation. His recent and remote memory and attention were deemed fair
- He demonstrated deficits in his fund of knowledge, ability to abstract, and insight

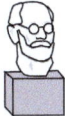

Psychotherapy history
- There is no known psychotherapy history to report

Mechanism of action moment
- Benztropine
  - Decreases acetylcholine activity occurring after dopamine receptor blockade leads to decreased dopamine modulation of acetylcholine
  - Possibly prolongs dopaminergic action at central dopamine receptors by the medication's inhibition of dopamine reuptake and storage
- Paliperidone palmitate
  - Blocks D_2 and serotonin 2A receptors
    - D_2 blockade assists with mood stabilization and positive symptoms of psychosis
    - Serotonin 2A blockade enhances dopamine release, likely offsetting motor side effects from the medication and improving cognitive and affective symptoms

PATIENT FILE

- ○ Antagonism of serotonin 7 may enhance the medication's antidepressant effects
- Clozapine
  - ○ Antagonizes D_2 receptors and serotonin 2A receptors
    - Blocking D_2 receptors reduces positive symptoms of psychosis and provides mood stabilization
    - Blocking serotonin 2A receptors enhances dopamine release in brain regions to minimize motor side effects and improve cognitive and affective symptoms
  - ○ Interacts with 5-HT_{2C} and 5-HT_{1A} which may promote increased efficacy in treatment of cognitive and affective symptoms
- Divalproex
  - ○ Stabilizes neuronal membrane by optimizing K+ efflux and Na+ influx
    - Decreases the glutamate : gamma aminobutyric acid (GABA) ratio
      - Decreases glutamate by stimulating glutamine synthetase
      - Increases GABA by increasing GABA levels, GABA release, $GABA_B$ receptor density, and neuronal responsiveness to GABA; and decreases GABA catabolism and turnover
  - ○ Dampens excitatory systems by decreasing aspartate release, cerebrospinal fluid (CSF) somatostatin, and N-methyl-D-aspartate (NMDA)-mediated circuits
  - ○ Increases dopamine turnover
- Haloperidol decanoate
  - ○ Blocks D_2 receptors
    - Reduces positive symptoms and aggressive behaviors
    - In the nigrostriatal pathway, D_2 blockade improves tics and associated symptoms of Tourette's
- Lithium carbonate
  - ○ Mechanism of action is complex and not well understood
  - ○ Thought to recruit second messenger signaling pathway including that of cAMP and cGMP
  - ○ Involved in genetic transcription and post-translational modification
    - Competes with other cations involved in signal transduction
  - ○ Decreases the glutamine:GABA ratio
    - Prevents loss of phosphorylated cAMP Response Element Binding Protein
      - Inhibits glutamate activation of protein kinases
        - ○ Provides neuroprotective effects

PATIENT FILE

Attending physician's mental notes
- The patient has a history of experiencing psychotic symptoms, including auditory hallucinations, delusions of grandeur, episodic mania, psychomotor agitation, and disorganized thoughts and behaviors
- His psychiatric symptoms limit his functioning and ability to engage in prosocial behaviors, which resulted in his repeated acts of violence, incarcerations, and psychiatric hospitalizations
- Medications prescribed by the referring facility do not appear to be fully targeting his symptoms of behavioral dysregulation. Therefore, haloperidol dosing will be increased from 10 mg by mouth twice a day to 20 mg by mouth twice a day, and the remainder of medications will be continued as prescribed
    - Paliperidone palmitate 234 mg IM q 4 weeks
    - Divalproex 2500 mg p.o. qHS
    - Benztropine 1 mg p.o. BID

Further investigation
- Following admission, the patient demonstrated labile and irritable affect; concrete and tangential thought process; and verbal and physical aggression
    - The dosing of divalproex was reduced to 1500 mg by mouth at bedtime, and lithium carbonate 1050 mg by mouth at bedtime was added
- A few months after he was hospitalized, the patient continued to engage in violent behaviors, despite having the prescribed medications adjusted to dosing which corresponded to therapeutic serum levels of haloperidol, paliperidone palmitate, divalproex, and lithium carbonate
    - Divalproex was increased to 2000 mg p.o. qHS
        - Serum level of 107.3 ug/mL
    - Lithium carbonate was increased to 1200 mg p.o. qHS
        - Serum level of 1.05 mmol/L
    - Haloperidol was continued at 20 mg p.o. BID
        - Serum level 22.5 ng/mL
    - Paliperidone palmitate was continued at 234 mg IM q 4 weeks
        - Serum level of 81.7 ng/mL
    - Benztropine was tapered and discontinued
- In years prior, the patient responded to trials of treatment with clozapine and a rechallenge was considered, recommended, and initiated
    - Clozapine was prescribed

PATIENT FILE

- Dosing of the medication was increased to a maximal total daily dosing of 800 mg while he was concomitantly treated for a latent tuberculosis infection
- Clozapine was, ultimately, decreased to 750 mg following completion of antimicrobial treatment
  - Adjustments to the medication regimen were made by decreasing the dosages of haloperidol, divalproex, and lithium carbonate to accommodate the addition of and treatment with another antipsychotic medication and treatment for latent tuberculosis
    - Dosing of divalproex was changed to 2250 mg p.o. qHS
    - Dosing of haloperidol was adjusted to 25 mg p.o. daily
    - Dosing of lithium carbonate was decreased to 900 mg p.o. daily
  - There were no changes made to the dosing and frequency of administration of paliperidone palmitate 234 mg IM given every 4 weeks
  - Guanfacine was added and increased to 2 mg p.o. daily to treat the patient's ongoing impulsivity
- The patient was noted to have serological testing concerning for a latent tuberculosis infection
  - He was treated with a course of rifampin, isoniazid, and pyridoxine
    - These medications were implicated in the resultant decrease in the patient's serum levels of haloperidol, divalproex, and clozapine
- During his hospitalization, the patient was evaluated by neurology
  - The patient was evaluated for his reported history of Fahr's disease, documented in his juvenile records, and for frequent falls
    - The patient reported falling when moving quickly
    - On physical examination:
      - Cranial nerves II–XII were intact
      - Dystonias, dykinesias, hemiballism, and choreiform movements were not noted
      - The patient's muscle bulk, tone, and strength were deemed normal
      - Deep tendon reflexes were described as trace
      - Sensation to light touch and pain were intact
      - Cerebellar testing was negative
        - Testing assessing Romberg's sign, dysdiadochokinesia, and finger-to-nose testing were unremarkable
    - Neuroimaging demonstrated basal ganglia calcifications

PATIENT FILE

Case outcome

- The patient's case is followed monthly
- Through his hospitalization, the patient engaged in multiple aggressive behaviors that resulted in his placement in seclusion and/or restraints, benefited from treatment with as-needed (PRN) medications, prompted increase in his prescribed medications to therapeutic dosing, and warranted his continued treatment on the specialized unit reserved for the most unstable and violent patients
- The patient's medications and associated serum drug levels were as follows:
  - Clozapine dosed at 750 mg p.o. qHS
    - Level of 955 ng/mL
  - Divalproex dosed at 2250 mg p.o. qHS
    - Level of 97.4 ug/mL
  - Lithium carbonate dosed at 900 mg p.o. qHS
    - Level of 0.79 mmol/L
  - Haloperidol dosed at 25 mg. p.o. qHS
    - Level of 19.3 ng/mL
- The patient's psychosis improved with clozapine therapy; however, he engaged in continued impulsive, violent acts
  - Guanfacine was added to his treatment, which was somewhat beneficial
- The patient exhibited persistent impulsive aggressive behaviors, including verbal aggression / verbal threats, physical aggression, and repetitive self-harm behaviors, through his hospitalization course

Case debrief

- Our patient was diagnosed with Schizoaffective disorder and mild intellectual disability
- Due to his persistent violent behaviors, the patient was transferred from the admission unit at a forensic state hospital to the unit reserved for the most unstable and violent patients
- Despite adjustment in dosing of psychiatric medications, the patient exhibited impulsive aggressive behaviors which posited him as a danger to himself and others, and benefited from multiple psychopharmacological and nonpharmacological therapeutic interventions
  - His psychiatric medication dosages were adjusted in the context of concomitant treatment with medications for latent tuberculosis and GERD

- Per report, the patient was diagnosed with Fahr's disease as a juvenile
  - The patient was evaluated by neurology and did not demonstrate signs of a peripheral nerve, central nervous system, or cerebellar deficit
  - The patient did not report symptoms or demonstrate signs of a movement disorder
  - Requested and resulted neuroimaging showed basal ganglia calcifications
  - Recommendations included continued neurological follow-up, with plan to reassess should the patient develop Parkinsonism or increased stiffness, difficulty walking, and/or additional symptoms

Take-home points

- The lenticulostriatal pathway contains projections from limbic structures (amygdala, nucleus accumbens, and cingulate gyrus) to cortical structures including the thalamus and frontal lobe
  - Pathology of three of the five circuits that connect the lenticular nuclei (putamen and globus pallidus) to the striatum (caudate nucleus and putamen) is implicated in psychiatric conditions
    - The dorsofrontal, orbitofrontal, and anterior cingulate are neuroanatomical regions implicated in schizophrenia, obsessive–compulsive disorder, and depression
    - Variability in symptom presentation may be related to the portion of the striatum affected, with involvement of the dorsal striatum linked to deficits in motor function and cognition, and the ventral striatum related to disorders of motivation
- Fahr's disease is described as pathology of the lenticulostriatal pathway which results in bilateral basal ganglia calcifications
  - In the literature, the condition is classified as a disease when the etiology is idiopathic, versus a syndrome resulting from secondarily impaired calcium metabolism
- Primary or idiopathic disease can be accompanied by genetic aberrations
  - Implicated genes include: Idiopathic Basal Ganglia Calcification (IBGC), Solute Carrier Family 20, member 2 (SLC20A2), Xenotropic and Polytropic Retrovirus Receptor (XPR1), Platelet Derived Growth Factor, subunit B (PDGFB) and Platelet Derived Growth Factor subunit receptor B (PDGFRB), and myogenesis-regulating glycosidase gene (MYORG)
    - The loci for IBGC1 and IBGC2 are found on chromosome 14q48 and 2q37, respectively

PATIENT FILE

- SLC20A2 inheritance pattern is autosomal dominant; the loci is on chromosome 8p11.21; and about 40 pathologic genetic variants have been identified
  - SLC20A2 is expressed in neurons, astrocytes, smooth muscle, and endothelial cells in the globus pallidus of the basal ganglia, substantia nigra, and cerebral cortex
  - SLC20A2 encodes a transmembrane sodium-dependent inorganic phosphate transporter that maintains inorganic phosphate homeostasis required for adenosine triphosphate (ATP) production
  - Mutations result in impaired inorganic phosphate transport
    - Accounts for about 40% of cases with genetic cause of idiopathic Fahr's disease
    - Associated with later age of disease onset and development of movement disorders
      - Approximately 21% of cases are accompanied by Parkinsonism
    - CSF in patients with mutations in SLC20A2 gene have increased inorganic phosphate levels
- XPR1 is located on chromosome 1q25.3, and the pattern of inheritance is autosomal dominant
  - The gene is responsible for phosphate export and homeostasis
  - Genetic anomalies are associated with Fahr's disease, schizophrenia, amyotrophic lateral sclerosis (ALS), frontotemporal degeneration, and Alzheimer's disease
    - Mutations in XPR1 in Fahr's disease are associated with Parkinsonism and cognitive dysfunction in 66.7% of cases
    - Other signs and symptoms include dysarthria, hyperkinetic movement, and cortical calcification
    - Accounts for about 4.3% of cases of Fahr's disease with a genetic aberration
- PDGFB and PDGFRB are implicated in pericyte recruitment, maintenance of the blood–brain barrier, and angiogenesis
  - PDGFB is located on chromosome 22q13.1; the pattern of inheritance is autosomal dominant; the gene encodes a disulfide primer, and is a paracrine growth factor in terms of function
    - PDGFB is expressed in mesenchymal, smooth muscle, and endothelial cells as well as neurons

PATIENT FILE

- Mutations are found in approximately 11–31.4% of cases of Fahr's disease, and genetic aberrances induce calcification of the vascular extracellular space
- Neuroanatomic sites involved include the basal ganglia and cerebellum
- Hyperkinetic movements are observed in about 25% of cases; and other observed patient experiences include cerebellar and psychiatric symptoms and headache
- PDGFRB is located on chromosome 5q33.1; the pattern of inheritance is autosomal dominant; the gene encodes a tyrosine kinase receptor; and the PDGFRB facilitates the recruitment and proliferation of pericytes and smooth muscle cells
  - PDGFRB is expressed in endothelial and vascular smooth muscle cells, neurons, and basal ganglia and dentate nucleus pericytes
  - Mutations are found in about 2–9.5% of cases of Fahr's disease and are associated with calcium deposition in vessel walls
  - The genetic anomaly is associated with earlier age of onset
  - Symptom presentation can include headaches, cognitive impairment, and depression
- MYORG is a novel gene implicated in Fahr's disease
  - The inheritance pattern is autosomal recessive; the gene encodes glycosyl hydrolase enzymes; and the gene is expressed in the cerebellum
  - Few studies have been published; areas affected include the basal ganglia and cerebellum; the identified average age of onset is about 52 years; and reported symptoms include motor impairment and dysarthria
- In 50% of cases, a genetic locus or genetic contribution is not identified
- The age of onset is 30 to 40 years of age, the disease course is progressive, and the prevalence is 3.3 to 4.5/100,000
  - Neurological deterioration occurs over two decades following the onset of symptoms
- Fahr's disease manifests as a constellation of neurological, cognitive, and psychiatric symptoms
  - Parkinsonism (52.3%), cognitive dysfunction (40.9%), and psychiatric (38.6%) are the most commonly exhibited symptoms

PATIENT FILE

- Earlier disease onset is associated with psychiatric and cognitive symptoms versus later onset of disease which is associated with movement disorders
- Neurological symptoms are heterogeneous and include headaches, seizures, cerebellar symptoms, and involuntary movements
  - Seizures and extrapyramidal symptoms (EPS) occur in approximately 22% and 56%, respectively
  - Abnormal movements include: Parkinsonism (85%), chorea (19%), dystonia (8–19%), tremor (8%), athetosis (5%), and orofacial dyskinesia (3%)
- Cognitive symptoms may manifest as a subcortical dementia with frontotemporal pattern and deficits in motor speed, executive functioning, and visuospatial skills, and memory impairments
- Psychiatrically, Fahr's disease can be accompanied by mood disorders including depression, mania, and anxiety; psychotic symptoms; substance use disorders; and personality changes
  - In 40% of cases, the patient's initial symptoms are psychiatric
  - Psychiatric symptoms may be clinically explained by extensive intracranial calcification and subarachnoid dilatation
  - The most common psychiatric symptoms include mood symptoms of depression and mania, with symptoms of depression occurring more frequently
    - Symptoms of obsessive–compulsive disorder (OCD) are present in about 30% of cases
  - Psychotic symptoms include auditory hallucinations, complex visual hallucinations, persecutory delusions, referential thinking, and catatonia
- Objective findings include lab and imaging testing results
  - Labs do not demonstrate abnormalities in parathyroid hormone (PTH), calcium, phosphate, and alkaline phosphatase
  - Pathology
    - Grossly, frontotemporal, cerebral cortex, and caudate nucleus atrophy may be observed; along with the presence of gray discoloration and gritty accumulations surrounding the periventricular region, including the globus pallidus, putamen, and anterior thalamus
    - Microscopically, neurofibrillary tangles and neuronal drop-out may be identified in the nucleus basalis of Meynert
      - Neuronal plaques are not present
      - Intravascular calcium deposits may be observed

- Inflammatory reaction surrounding the calcium deposit and consisting of reactive microglia and astrocytes may be identified
- Other findings include gliosis and white matter demyelination
  - Imaging
    - CT is used to identify and diagnose calcium deposits which present as hyperdense lesions on imaging, whereas MRI findings clinically correlate to functional impairment
      - Findings on CT include calcium deposition within the lentiform, caudate, and thalamic nuclei; subcortical white matter and centrum semiovale; cerebellum including the vermis; and the pons and medulla of the midbrain
        - Visually, the deposits appear as hyperdense, extensive, coarse conglomerations which may be distinguishable from physiological processes by the involvement of the putamen and dentate nucleus
        - Disease course severity, symptoms, and age correspond to the burden of calcifications, as demonstrated by involvement of the lentiform and caudate nucleus as well as the entirety of the basal ganglia
        - CT can be utilized to radiographically distinguish calcium from iron deposits in neurodegeneration with brain iron accumulation (NBIA)
      - Approximately 1% of younger patients and 20% of older patients' imaging studies reveal bilateral basal ganglia calcification in the absence of a diagnosis of Fahr's disease
        - Physiological calcium deposits are smaller, visually faint, symmetric, and limited to the globus pallidus
        - In 70%, autopsy reveals calcium deposits in the globus pallidus, dentate nucleus, and tail of the hippocampus without a corresponding diagnosis of Fahr's disease
- Treatment is symptom focused and consists of addressing psychiatric and neurological manifestations of the disease
  - Psychiatric treatment includes the use of antidepressants, antipsychotics, and mood-stabilizer medications
    - The use of lithium may be limited to individuals without comorbid medical conditions associated with dehydration or renal disease
    - Electroconvulsive therapy (ECT) has been utilized in cases of treatment-refractory psychiatric symptoms

- ECT may exacerbate delirium in susceptible patients (for example, those with subcortical dementia)
- Basal ganglia calcifications may be associated with increased intracranial pressures and may limit the use of ECT
    - Neurological treatment includes the use of antiepileptics and treatment for Parkinsonism
        - Parkinsonism due to basal ganglia calcification may respond to a trial of levodopa
    - Targeted therapies
        - Bisphosphonates decreased osteoclast function and may improve calcium homeostasis
        - Vitamin D deficiency is found in some patients with mutations in SLC20A2
            - Supplementation facilitates vitamin D promotor region binding and upregulation of mRNA production
    - Current recommendations also include treatment of secondary causes of basal ganglia calcifications
- Secondary basal ganglia calcification is associated with various neuroendocrine, infectious, toxic and immunologic, and other disorders
    - Neuroendocrine
        - Hypoparathyroidism
            - Associated findings include anomalies in laboratory, radiographic, and neurologic findings
                - Labs may reveal a decreased PTH, hypocalcemia, and hyperphosphatemia
                - Symptoms of hypocalcemia include parathesia and cramps, carpal and pedal muscle spasticity, neuromuscular irritability, seizures, and EKG abnormalities
                - Radiographically, bilateral symmetric calcifications of the basal ganglia, corona radiata, subcortical white matter, and cerebellum may be visualized
                - Neurologically, patients may report frequent falls, loss of consciousness, and cognitive decline; and demonstrate seizures, postural and gait instability, a resting tremor, and Parkinsonism
    - Infection
        - Infections associated with calcification of the basal ganglia include brucellosis, Acquired Immunodeficiency Syndrome (AIDS), and perinatal and congenital infections

> **PATIENT FILE**

- Brucellosis rarely demonstrates basal ganglia calcifications on imaging
  - When it does occur, it is associated with the development of neurobrucellosis which occurs in 5–10% of cases and affects the peripheral and central nervous system
- AIDS is commonly associated with intracranial calcium deposition
  - Pathologic calcification occurs in the basal ganglia, putamen, globus pallidus, and blood vessels
- Congenital/perinatal infections include the TORCH infections, toxoplasmosis, rubella, cytomegalovirus (CMV), and herpes pathogens
  - Calcifications in these conditions are diffuse and within the brain parenchyma
- Toxic and immunological etiologies
  - Lead and carbon monoxide poisoning
    - Radiographic findings include intracranial calcification, including that of the basal ganglia
      - Specifically, with lead poisoning, the calcium accretions are multifocal, curvilinear in shape, and involve bilateral basal ganglia, cortex, and cerebellum
  - Systemic lupus erythematosus (SLE)
    - 30% of patients with SLE develop neurolupus with brain calcifications
      - On CT, imaging findings include diffuse basal ganglia, centrum semiovale, cerebellum, and cerebral cortex calcification in neurolupus
- Other disorders
  - Pseudohypoparathyroidism is distinguished from hypoparathyroidism by the finding of normal or normal–high levels of PTH
    - Pseudohypoparathyroidism and hypoparathyroidism laboratory findings both include hypocalcemia and hyperphosphatemia
  - Cockayne syndrome is a childhood leukodystrophy characterized by hyporeflexia, hyper-reflexia and spasticity, abnormal gait and ataxia, tremor, seizures, hearing and vision loss, and behavioral changes
    - The CT radiological findings are variable with differing subtypes of the syndrome, and include calcification of the basal ganglia, putamen, and cerebral cortex

PATIENT FILE

- Aicardi–Goutières syndrome is a familial progressive encephalopathy and leukodystrophy that clinically presents as early-onset seizures; other signs include microcephaly and cerebral atrophy as well as calcification of basal ganglia
  - Calcifications, when present, are punctate lesions deep in the periventricular white matter and involve the putamen, pallidus, and thalamus
- Mitochondrial disorders – specifically, 13% of cases of Mitochondrial Encephalopathy with Lactic Acidosis (MELAS) and Myoclonic Epilepsy with Ragged Red Fibers (MERRF) findings include basal ganglia calcification
- Coats disease is described as abnormal retinal vessel development, and basal ganglia and deep white matter calcifications may be present
- Neurodegenerative disorders – specifically, NBIA and neuroferritinopathies lead to excess iron storage with resultant inflammation, cystic degeneration, and dystrophic calcification of the putamen or basal ganglia

Performance in practice: confessions of a psychopharmacologist

What are clinical considerations when treating a patient diagnosed with Fahr's disease?

- Fahr's disease is a progressive condition with Parkinsonian, psychiatric, and cognitive symptom presentations
  - Symptom-based treatment includes use of antidepressants and mood-stabilizer medications to target affective symptoms; antipsychotics to treat psychotic symptoms; antiepileptics for seizure prophylaxis; and levodopa for Parkinsonism
  - Clozapine can reduce impulsive, aggressive symptoms independent of the presence of comorbid psychotic symptoms and cognitive impairment
  - ECT can be indicated for treatment-refractory psychiatric disorders, management of agitation in neurocognitive disorders, and neuroleptic malignant syndrome (NMS)
    - ECT can exacerbate delirium in patients with subcortical dementia
    - Basal ganglia calcifications can induce increased intracranial pressure limiting the application of ECT
  - Additional treatment includes targeted therapies with bisphosphonate agents and vitamin D repletion (in patients with mutations in SLC20A2), as well as diagnosis and management of secondary basal ganglia calcification

PATIENT FILE

Tips and pearls
- Fahr's disease is idiopathic or secondary basal ganglia calcification that results in neuropsychiatric symptoms, seizures, and movement disorders
- The age of onset is 30 to 40 years, neurological deterioration occurs over two decades following the onset of symptoms, and the disease course is progressive
  - Earlier disease onset is associated with psychiatric and cognitive symptoms, and later disease onset is associated with movement disorders
  - The most common demonstrable features of Fahr's disease are Parkinsonism (52.3%), cognitive dysfunction (40.9%), and psychiatric (38.6%) symptoms
    - Neurological symptomatology includes movement disorders and, when present, occurs with the following relative rates: Parkinsonism (85%), chorea (19%), dystonia (8–19%), tremor (8%), athetosis (5%), and orofacial dyskinesia (3%)
    - Cognitive symptoms may manifest as a subcortical dementia with frontotemporal pattern and deficits in motor speed, executive functioning, and visuospatial skills, and memory impairments
  - In about 40% of cases, the patient's initial symptoms are psychiatric
    - Psychiatric symptoms include mood symptoms (depression > mania) including anxiety, and psychotic symptoms (auditory hallucinations, complex visual hallucinations, persecutory delusions, referential thinking, and catatonia)
- A diagnosis of Fahr's disease may be considered once disorders of calcium–phosphate metabolism, autoimmune, parathyroid pathology, infection, and toxic exposure are excluded
  - In 20% of cases of basal ganglia calcifications, the calcification is physiological, and may not be pathological
    - CT findings in Fahr's disease include involvement of the lentiform, caudate, and thalamic nuclei; subcortical white matter and centrum semiovale; cerebellum including the vermis; and the pons and medulla of the midbrain
      - The deposits appear as hyperdense, extensive, coarse conglomerations
      - They may be distinguishable from physiological processes by the involvement of the putamen and dentate nucleus
      - Physiological calcifications of the basal ganglia are smaller, visually faint, symmetrical, and limited to the globus pallidus

- If supported by family history, genetic studies may reveal a genetic etiology of the disease
  - In 50% of cases, a genetic aberration is not identified
- Treatment primarily consists of symptom management and targets associated movement disorders and neurological and psychiatric symptoms
  - Symptom-based treatment includes use of antidepressants, antipsychotics, antiepileptics, and anti-Parkinsonism, as well as mood-stabilizer medications
    - Parkinsonism due to basal ganglia calcification may respond to a trial of levodopa
    - Patients with Fahr's disease are more susceptible to EPS and developing NMS
    - ECT has been utilized in cases of treatment-refractory psychiatric symptoms but may exacerbate delirium and be of limited use in patients with increased intracranial pressure
    - Targeted therapy includes prescription of bisphosphonate agents and vitamin D repletion

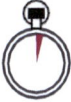

Two-minute tutorial

- Fahr's disease can manifest with symptoms that include:
  - Psychiatric symptoms include those of mood – most frequently depression, followed by mania, and anxiety, including OCD, as well as psychosis and catatonia
  - Neurological symptoms include headache, seizures, cerebellar symptoms, and movement disorders
  - Cognitive symptoms include subcortical dementia with possible frontotemporal distribution
- The etiology of Fahr's disease is idiopathic or from abnormal calcium metabolism
  - Imaging studies and laboratory testing can aid diagnosis of Fahr's disease and distinguish idiopathic basal ganglia calcifications from secondary basal ganglia calcifications
    - Labs in idiopathic Fahr's disease demonstrate normal PTH, calcium, phosphate, and alkaline phosphatase levels
- Current treatment options focus on symptom management with the burden of treatment targeting mood, psychotic, epileptic, and movement disorder symptoms
  - Other therapies include bisphosphonates and vitamin D repletion to improve calcium homeostasis and, in nutritionally deficient states, upregulate mRNA production, respectively

PATIENT FILE

Post-test question

Which of the following are NOT viable treatments for the constellation of symptom presentations in Fahr's disease?

A. Guanfacine
B. Levetiracetam
C. Clozapine
D. ECT
E. Levodopa

Answer: A

References

1. Donzuso, G., Mostile, G., Nicoletti, A., & Zappia, M. (2019). Basal ganglia calcifications (Fahr's syndrome): related conditions and clinical features. *Neurological Science*, Nov., 40(11), 2251–2263. https://doi.org/10.1007/s10072-019-03998-x.
2. Ghormode, D., Maheshwari, U., Kate, N., & Grover, S. (2011). Fahr's disease and psychiatric syndromes: a case series. *Indian Journal of Psychiatry*, July–Dec., 20(2), 136–138. https://doi.org/10.4103/0972-6748.102527.
3. Lauterbach, E. C., Cummings, J. L., Duffy, J., et al. (1998). Neuropsychiatric correlates and treatment of lenticulostriatal diseases: a review of the literature and overview of research opportunities in Huntington's, Wilson's, and Fahr's diseases. A report of the ANPA Committee on Research. *Journal of Neuropsychiatry and Clinical Neurosciences*, Summer, 10(3), 249–266. https://doi.org/10.1176/jnp.10.3.249.
4. Peters, M. E., Brouwer, E. J., Bartstra, J. W., et al. (2020). Mechanisms of calcification in Fahr disease and exposure of potential therapeutic targets. *Neurology: Clinical Practice*, Oct., 10(5), 449–457. https://doi.org/10.1212/CPJ.0000000000000782.
5. Rosenblatt, A. & Leroi, I. (2000). Neuropsychiatry of Huntington's disease and other basal ganglia disorders. *Psychosomatics*, Jan.–Feb., 41(1), 24–30. https://doi.org/10.1016/S0033-3182(00)71170-4.
6. Stahl, S. M. (2014). *Stahl's Essential Psychopharmacology: Prescriber's Guide*, 5th ed. New York: Cambridge University Press.

SECTION VI
Specialty Forensic Populations

PATIENT FILE

22

Incompetent to stand trial (IST) Murphy Conservatorship (MurCON): Conserved or convicted?

The Psychopharmacological Dilemma: What are the clinical considerations for an individual who is found incompetent to stand trial, unrestorable to trial competence, and civilly committed or conserved?

Maanasi Chandarana

Pretest self-assessment question

Which of the following factors are NOT associated with an "unlikely to be restored to legal adjudicative competence" finding?

A. Female gender
B. Mental health diagnoses including a substance use disorder
C. Age of 65 years or older
D. Previous treatment with antipsychotic medication
E. History of psychiatric hospitalizations

Answer: A

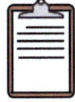

Patient evaluation on intake

The patient is a 52-year-old male with previous diagnoses of schizophrenia and substance use disorder (cannabis, opioid – heroin type, stimulant – methamphetamine, crack, and cocaine type) who was found incompetent to stand trial (IST) to an incurred felony charge. The patient was subsequently hospitalized at a forensic state hospital for pretrial competency restoration. The patient was unable to regain his legal competency abilities, civilly committed, and assigned a Conservator by the court. Due to his persistent violent behaviors and felony assault of a hospital staff member, the patient received a course of electroconvulsive therapy (ECT) and was transferred from one forensic hospital to another forensic state hospital. The patient was admitted to a specialized unit with increased programming, enhanced infrastructure, and security measures reserved for the most unstable and violent patients .

Psychiatric history

- Mental health history with onset in childhood
  - He was described as physically and sexually inappropriate with peers and family members

PATIENT FILE

  - Described in the medical record with onset of these behaviors occurring when the patient was 6 years old
- He was diagnosed with schizophrenia and reported non-command and command auditory hallucinations (CAH), persecutory delusions, delusions of grandeur, and hyper-religious beliefs and thoughts
  - Mental health providers noted that he also exhibited negative symptoms, deficits in his executive functioning, and cognitive rigidity
- The patient has an extensive history of violence with multiple arrests, charges, and one in-custody offense
- The patient has been hospitalized in community and forensic psychiatric facilities multiple times
- He was prescribed multiple trials of medications including antipsychotics and mood-stabilizer medication
- The patient received court-ordered ECT for persistent aggression and violence

Social and personal history
- The patient is the oldest child of his immediate family, and he has two younger brothers
- He stated that he experienced physical abuse and that both of his parents drank alcohol
- The patient, per report, verbally threatened his mother and physically assaulted his father
  - He was involuntarily psychiatrically hospitalized after the incident with his mother
  - His father obtained a restraining order against the patient for 3 years
- He had learning and behavioral difficulties in school which prompted his placement in special education classes
- He graduated high school but did not obtain a general educational development (GED) certificate, an advanced degree, or receive additional education in a specific trade or craft
- The patient had difficulty maintaining consistent employment due to his unpredictable behaviors
  - He reported that he panhandled and worked in transient positions, including painting
- The patient stated that he had one relationship with a female partner and fathered a child
  - His partner and the patient separated when their child was 2 years old, and his partner obtained a restraining order against the patient

- The patient reported that the mother of his child updated him about his child over the years
- Multiple encounters with law enforcement noted with first documented arrest and incurred charge when he was 20 years of age
- Substance use history
  - The patient reported using alcohol and cannabis when he was 14 years old and illicit substances when he was 20 years old
    - He relayed using cocaine, crack cocaine, intravenous heroin, and huffing paint
    - He said he used lysergic acid diethylamide (LSD) and phencyclidine (PCP) once
    - The patient reported that he used opioids and amphetamines for 7 years. He identified his drug of choice as crystal methamphetamine, preferred route as snorting, and last use 2 years prior to his hospitalization within the state forensic hospital system
  - He reported substance use treatment via drug rehabilitation programs, which were unsuccessful
  - The patient said that members of a church attempted to assist him with his substance use
    - When the patient refused their offer to help him, he reported that he was "excommunicated" from the church

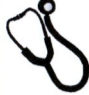

Medical history

- Seizure disorder
- History of head trauma following multiple head injuries, including the patient's fall downstairs as a toddler, and a motor vehicle accident, during which the patient, when riding a bicycle, was dragged underneath a car for about 25–40 feet, when he was 7 years old
- History of atypical mesothelial proliferation resulting in adhesion pleurodesis and lobectomy

Family history

- The patient stated that his father drank excessive amounts of alcohol
- There is no known familial medical history to report

Treatment history

- The patient was prescribed trials of medications including multiple antipsychotics and treated with 30 sessions of ECT for treatment-refractory psychotic symptoms, affective symptoms, and aggressive and violent behaviors

PATIENT FILE

Current history
- The patient presented to the evaluation as calm, polite, and cooperative
- He was dressed in hospital attire, and his grooming and hygiene were deemed fair
- His speech rate, rhythm, and volume were normal
- The patient did not demonstrate psychomotor agitation, retardation, and abnormal involuntary movements
- He reported that his mood was sad, and his affect appeared constricted. He denied suicidal thoughts. He denied experiencing homicidal ideations
- He denied experiencing hallucinations and did not demonstrate delusional thought content, thought insertion, and thought extraction
- His thought process was linear and goal directed
- The patient was alert, and oriented to person, time, and place. His recent and remote memory, ability to abstract, attention, fund of knowledge, and cognition were deemed fair
- He demonstrated deficits in his insight and judgment

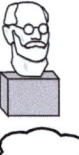

Psychotherapy history
- There is no known psychotherapy history to report

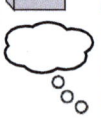

Attending physician's mental notes
- The patient has a history of experiencing psychotic symptoms, including non-command and command auditory hallucinations; persecutory delusions that his food was poisoned, manipulated, or contaminated; delusions of grandeur; negative symptoms of avolition, amotivation, alogia, and flattened affect; and ideas of reference
- He also demonstrates deficits in executive functioning, insight, and judgment which limit his ability to engage in prosocial behaviors and contribute to his impulsive and aggressive behaviors
- The patient demonstrates behaviors that deviate from sociocultural norms in the domains of cognition, affectivity, interpersonal functioning, and impulse control
- Medications prescribed by the referring facility appear to be targeting his symptoms of affective and behavioral dysregulation. The patient is currently prescribed three antipsychotic medications. Therefore, olanzapine will be discontinued, and the following medications will be continued:
  - clozapine 800 mg p.o. qHS
  - Haloperidol decanoate 200 mg IM every 2 weeks

PATIENT FILE

Further investigation

- The patient presented to his first monthly treatment team meeting with elevated mood state and overproductive speech
  - Prior to his transfer, he received treatment with divalproex and lithium carbonate, which were both discontinued in preparation for treatment with ECT at the referring state forensic hospital
  - Divalproex extended release was started and titrated to 2500 mg by mouth at bedtime, and haloperidol decanoate dosing was increased to 225 mg IM every 2 weeks
- About 2 months after his admission, to further treat the patient's symptoms of mania, lithium carbonate was also restarted and increased to 1200 mg by mouth at bedtime
  - The patient was receiving multiple as-needed medications in the months following his admission, and he physically struck another patient without provocation
  - A serum clozapine level resulted as 1213 ng/mL, for which the dosing was decreased to 600 mg by mouth nightly
  - A few weeks later, while the patient was taking 600 mg of clozapine by mouth every night, his level was 256 ng/mL
    - The dose of his clozapine was increased again to 700 mg p.o. at bedtime
  - The patient's level of haloperidol resulted as 10.9 ng/mL, and the attending physician increased the dosing of haloperidol decanoate to 300 mg IM every 2 weeks
- Three months after the patient was admitted, his clozapine level was documented as 609 ng/mL, and clozapine dosing was increased to 750 mg nightly
- The following month, the attending physician noted that the patient's serum divalproex level was subtherapeutic, so the formulation of divalproex was changed to liquid (delayed release) and increased to 2000 mg twice a day
  - The patient was placed on more thorough mouth checks after he was found to be cheeking medications

Mechanism of action moment

- Clozapine
  - Antagonizes D_2 receptors and serotonin 2A receptors
    - Blocking D_2 receptors reduces positive symptoms of psychosis and provides mood stabilization
    - Blocking serotonin 2A receptors enhances dopamine release in brain regions to minimize motor side effects and improve cognitive and affective symptoms

PATIENT FILE

- Interacts with 5-HT$_{2C}$ and 5-HT$_{1A}$ which may promote increased efficacy in treatment of cognitive and affective symptoms
- Divalproex
  - Stabilizes neuronal membrane by optimizing K+ efflux and Na+ influx
    - Decreases the glutamate : gamma aminobutyric acid (GABA) ratio
      - Decreases glutamate by stimulating glutamine synthetase
      - Increases GABA by increasing GABA levels, GABA release, GABA$_B$ receptor density, and neuronal responsiveness to GABA; and decreases GABA catabolism and turnover
  - Dampens excitatory systems by decreasing aspartate release, cerebrospinal fluid (CSF) somatostatin, and N-methyl-D-aspartate (NMDA)-mediated circuits
  - Increases dopamine turnover
- Haloperidol decanoate
  - Blocks D$_2$ receptors
    - Reduces positive symptoms and aggressive behaviors
    - In the nigrostriatal pathway, D$_2$ blockade improves tics and associated symptoms of Tourette's
- Lithium carbonate
  - Mechanism of action is complex and not well understood
  - Thought to recruit second messenger signaling pathway including that of cyclic adenosine monophosphate (cAMP) and cyclic guanosine monophosphate (cGMP)
  - Involved in genetic transcription and post-translational modification
    - Competes with other cations involved in signal transduction
  - Decreases the glutamine:GABA ratio
    - Prevents loss of phosphorylated cAMP Response Element Binding Protein
      - Inhibits glutamate activation of protein kinases
        - Provides neuroprotective effects

Case outcome

- The patient's case is followed monthly
- Over the ensuing months, the patient's blood level of medications, corresponding to therapeutic dosing, fluctuated and were indicative of sporadic compliance with medication
  - Regardless of the suboptimal compliance and therapeutic effect of the prescribed medication, the patient was not involved in physical altercations with other hospital patients and staff after 5 months of hospitalization

- However, the patient experienced breakthrough seizures and extrapyramidal symptoms (EPS), for which levetiracetam was added to his medication regimen for seizure prophylaxis, and amantadine was added for abnormal involuntary movements
- Routine electrocardiogram (EKG) testing revealed nonspecific T wave changes and right bundle branch block
  - The patient remained asymptomatic and, initially, refused a repeat EKG
  - A few months later, the patient provided consent for another EKG which was unchanged
- During his hospitalization, the patient's medications were adjusted monthly to attempt to attain therapeutic dosing while considering and offsetting side effects from prescribed treatment
  - The patient suffered from multiple falls which were attributed to orthostasis in the context of clozapine treatment
    - Fludrocortisone was prescribed to treat the patient's orthostatic hypotension
  - Amantadine dosing was increased, and physical therapy was prescribed to maximize the patient's mobility
  - Dosing of clozapine and haloperidol decanoate were adjusted; dosing of divalproex and lithium carbonate was not changed; and therapeutic drug monitoring was routinely ordered
  - Clozapine decreased to 700 mg p.o. qHS
    - Level fluctuated from 256 ng/mL to 1213 ng/mL; most recently 524 ng/mL
  - Haloperidol decanoate decreased to 250 mg IM every 2 weeks
    - Levels fluctuated from 7.9 ng/mL to 14.7 ng/mL; most recently 7.9 ng/mL
  - Divalproex remained dosed at 2000 mg p.o. BID
    - Levels fluctuated from 39.3 ug/mL to 106.4 ug/mL; most recently 59.9 ug/mL
  - Lithium carbonate remained dosed at 1200 mg. p.o. qHS
    - Level of 0.94 mmol/L
- Through his hospitalization, the patient received continuous treatment on the specialized unit reserved for the most unstable and violent patients
- The patient's impulsivity and behaviors improved following treatment with ECT at the referring facility and a few months following hospitalization to the receiving facility, regardless of fluctuations in serum levels of clozapine, haloperidol, and divalproex

PATIENT FILE

Case debrief
- Our patient was diagnosed with schizophrenia versus schizoaffective disorder and substance use disorder
- He was found IST to a felony; his legal competency abilities were not restored; and he was subsequently conserved
- Due to his persistent violent behaviors, including the incurrence of an in-hospital felonious charge, the patient received a course of ECT and was transferred from one forensic hospital to the unit reserved for the most unstable and violent patients of another forensic state hospital
- Despite adjustments to the dosing of his prescribed medications, including clozapine, divalproex, and haloperidol decanoate, the patient's serum drug levels fluctuated. However, the patient did not exhibit further impulsive aggressive behaviors which posited him as a danger to himself and others following treatment with ECT and within a few months of transferring to another forensic hospital

Take-home points
- Competency to stand trial is a legal construct informed and shaped by national and state landmark cases and case law
  - *Dusky* v. *US (1960)*: established what legal abilities a person must demonstrate to ensure preservation of his or her constitutional rights when proceeding to trial
    - *Dusky* defined competency as: "whether he has sufficient present ability to consult with his lawyer with a reasonable degree of rational understanding and whether he has a rational and factual understanding of the proceedings against him"
    - Differing statutory requirements identify the permissible amount of time that can elapse before an individual is evaluated for competency; that is needed for competency restoration; and for maximum commitment to restore one's competence
      - Individual state laws may also outline provision of involuntary medication, in what setting competency restoration can occur, and how progress towards restoration is reported to the court
    - Identifying an actionable methodology to assess a person's legal competency to stand trial not only ensures a just judicial procedure, but also has implications in balancing liberty interests, the timeliness, efficiency, and effectiveness of mental health treatment, and public safety

PATIENT FILE

- ○ Restoration to competency includes assessing an individual's legal competency, treating underlying psychiatric illness precluding competency with medications, and interventions that buttress an individual's knowledge, ability to communicate, and decision making as related to trial competence
    - Psychiatric, social, educational, and legal factors associated with an increased likelihood of being found IST include previous psychiatric hospitalization, diagnosis with a psychotic disorder, previous arrest, lack of gainful employment, incomplete high school education
    - In forensic settings, substance use, personality, and psychotic disorders are the most prevalent diagnoses in those patients found IST
        - Between 1999 and 2014, the census of patients forensically hospitalized for competency restoration increased by 76%
    - A primary method by which competency is restored includes treating an underlying psychiatric illness with medication
        - Approximately 75–90% of individuals' adjudicative abilities are restored within 6 months
        - About 50–75% of patients with mental illness do not take their prescribed medications consistently
        - In 1975, the United States Supreme Court ruled that the issue of competency can be raised at any time during the legal proceedings and after competency has previously been restored (*Drope* v. *Missouri*, 1975)
    - Time to restoration can be highly variable and range from 20 days to 1.5 years
- In cases in which there is no substantial likelihood, or it is unlikely, that a patient's competency can be restored, criminal proceedings may be dismissed and pursued later
    - ○ Factors which may be associated with the inability for a person to attain competency in the foreseeable future include psychiatric history, mental health diagnoses, treatment with psychotropic medication, primary language, age, and gender
        - Associated mental health factors:
            - Diagnoses: developmental, cognitive, substance use, personality, and psychotic disorders
            - Previous mental health history and psychiatric hospitalization
            - Treatment with psychiatric medications, especially if treatment was involuntary or nonvoluntary

> **PATIENT FILE**

- Non-English primary language
- Those individuals older than 65 years of age
  - In 32% of cases involving patients 65 years of age or older who are found IST, the person is not able to be restored to competency (versus 15% of those 65 years of age or younger)
- Male gender more than female gender
  - The patient may have various statutorily defined dispositions including civil commitment
    - As of 2012, 30 states statutorily define a maximum commitment date, and 10 states do not have a definitive maximum commitment date, by which an individual can be restored to competency
    - ten states permit civil commitment if a person's legal competency cannot be restored for the foreseeable future
  - *Jackson v. Indiana* (1972) further identified due process rights afforded to those individuals found IST when the court ruled that the length of time a patient committed for competency restoration must bear a "reasonable relation" to the purpose of commitment
    - In cases where there is no substantial likelihood of restoring the patient's legal competency, civil commitment is not necessarily justifiable
  - The premises establishing legal competency and civil commitment differ
    - Some states require that a person is at risk of imminent harm to themselves and/or others, or that the person is gravely disabled, to warrant civil commitment
    - Legal incompetency to stand trial does not require a finding of dangerousness to self or others or a finding of grave disability, although those with psychiatric illness that posit the individual at risk to harm self or others, or grave disability, can preclude competency
  - In California, the Lanterman–Petris–Short (LPS) Act of 1967 defined grave disability as "a condition in which a person, as a result of a mental health disorder, is unable to provide for his or her basic personal needs for food, clothing, or shelter"
    - A person whose legal adjudicative abilities were not restored and is gravely disabled can be committed pursuant to the LPS Act for 1 year
      - An individual who is imminently dangerous to themselves or others can be involuntarily psychiatrically hospitalized but cannot be civilly committed per the LPS Act in the absence of a finding of grave disability

- A Murphy Conservatorship (MurCON) differs from the LPS Act in that the foundation of the civil commitment rests upon the finding of dangerousness
    - An individual whose controlling offense, for which he or she was found IST, includes a "felony involving death, great bodily harm, or a serious threat to the wellbeing of another person" can be civilly committed for 1 year without a finding of grave disability
    - To initiate or renew a MurCON, the person must represent a substantial risk of physical harm to others by reason of mental disease, disorder, or defect
    - The standard of proof must be beyond a reasonable doubt
- Ethical and legal considerations of this conservation model include clinical difficulty, reliability, and accuracy of predicting dangerousness; absence of adjudication prior to conservation; and perceived differences in the purpose of hospitalization

Performance in practice: confessions of a psychopharmacologist

What are clinical considerations for patients deemed IST and unlikely to be restored to legal competence?

- Legal incompetence to stand trial does not require a finding of dangerousness to self or others or a finding of grave disability
- 75–90% of patients found IST can be restored to legal competence within 6 months by treatment of the patient's mental health condition with psychotropic medication
    - Clozapine is a potential treatment option for patients with treatment-resistant illness (approximately 30–60% efficacious)
        - About 40–70% of patients' symptoms are ultra treatment-resistant and will not respond to treatment with clozapine
- ECT reduces the burden of psychiatric symptoms and aggression; is associated with improved insight; and can assist with competency restoration, including in ultra treatment-resistant cases
- A patient's demographics (gender, age) and mental health history, including previous treatment with psychiatric medications, hospitalizations, diagnoses, may preclude restoration to adjudicative competence
    - Approximately 10 states permit civil commitment if a person's legal competency cannot be restored for the foreseeable future
- Familiarity with local hospital policy and state and federal law governing civil commitment can aid the practitioner in determining an approach in cases where the patient cannot be legally restored

PATIENT FILE

Tips and pearls

- This case involves the application of ECT in a forensic setting for a patient found IST to a felonious charge whose trial competency was not restored for the foreseeable future
  - Due to his ongoing violent behaviors, the patient was conserved and assigned a court-appointed Conservator
  - The patient's aggressive and violent behaviors responded to ECT and, following his transfer to a sister forensic state facility, he did not engage in continued acts of violence a few months following hospitalization at the receiving facility
- ECT is associated with various physiological, neuroendocrine, neurotransmitter, and anti-inflammatory responses
  - Different systems that are the subject of ongoing research and implicated following ECT treatment include:
    - Physiologically, ECT increases blood flow, glucose metabolism, and oxygen consumption in the ictal phase and decreases blood flow and glucose metabolism in the post-ictal phase in the frontal and temporal cortices
      - It is postulated that the positive treatment effects of ECT occur in the post-ictal phase and with repeated ECT procedures
        - Increase in neuronal density has been observed in the hippocampus and amygdala with subsequent ECT treatment
    - Neuroendocrine: hypothalamic–pituitary axis (HPA) and hypothalamic–pituitary thyroid axis
      - Modulation of the HPA control system decreases cortisol-induced hyperactivity
        - HPA overactivity is associated with decreased brain volumes, cognitive effects, astrocyte proliferation, and decreased brain-derived neurotrophic factor (BDNF)
      - ECT potentially influences the concentration of thyroid-releasing hormone (TRH) and thyroid stimulating hormone (TSH)
    - Inflammatory: peripheral and central lymphocytes and macrophages and immune mediators
      - ECT alters the function of interleukins and tumor necrosis factor
      - ECT decreases activity of microglia and astrocytes
    - Neurotransmitters and associated receptors: glutamate, GABA, dopamine, serotonin, and alpha adrenergic and dopamine receptors

PATIENT FILE

- ECT influences glutamate concentrations associated with angiogenesis and increased neurogenesis
- ECT increases the concentration of GABA and serotonin
  - Increases in the concentration of serotonin lead to production of BDNF which promotes neurogenesis
- ECT modulates dopamine in the hippocampus and alters dopamine receptors by promoting D_1 receptor transcription and ligand binding and decreasing D_2 receptor binding
- ECT reduces noradrenaline affinity for binding to the alpha-2-adrenergic receptor

• ECT is an established treatment modality for schizophrenia that was first used in 1938
  - Studies suggest that 10–30% of patients diagnosed with schizophrenia have treatment-resistant symptoms which are minimally responsive to treatment with antipsychotic medications
    - Treatment of schizophrenia with clozapine therapy is successful in about 30–60% of cases
      - It is postulated that adjunctive bilateral ECT in addition to clozapine treatment may be more effective than clozapine therapy alone
      - It is noted that combination therapy with ECT and an antipsychotic medication induced greater and more rapid treatment effect for aggression in schizophrenia by improving symptoms of hostility and persecutory delusions versus treatment with an antipsychotic alone
  - Despite clozapine's established use in treatment-refractory cases and for psychotic and non-psychotic aggression, approximately 40–70% of patients experience ultra treatment-resistant symptoms, which marginally respond to the medication
    - However, application of ECT with about 16–20 sessions was associated with clinical improvement in these cases
    - The anti-aggressive effects of ECT may last up to 6 months following the last treatment session
  - Therapy with ECT is associated with improvement in positive symptoms of psychosis including delusions and hallucinations, as well as anxiety, aggression, and hostility
    - The Cochrane review suggests that ECT can rapidly improve global functioning and reduce psychotic symptoms in patients
    - ECT is associated with improvement in cognition in the domains of visuospatial processing and executive functioning

PATIENT FILE

- The therapeutic effect on negative symptoms is currently unknown or unclear
  ○ The American Psychiatric Association recommends utilizing ECT for psychosis exacerbations in schizophrenia, and suggests that treatment with ECT should be approached similarly to medical interventions with parallel risk:benefit ratios
  ○ ECT can possibly reduce healthcare costs by decreasing extended forensic hospital stays
    - ECT reduces the burden of psychiatric symptoms and aggression; is associated with improved insight; and can assist with competency restoration
- Despite its uses, clinical indications, relatively safe side effect profile, and efficacy, treatment with ECT is not widely utilized or available in forensic settings
  ○ Identified organizational and medical provider factors contributing to the underutilization of ECT include unfamiliarity with rules, policies, and directives delineating site-specific practices, and physicians' professional training and experience
  ○ Other barriers to ECT treatment include those in the domains of legal, ethical, patient, and public constraints
    - Legal concepts that limit the use of ECT include the patient's right to refuse treatment, voluntariness, and informed consent
      - Right to refuse treatment
        ○ Patients may refuse treatment with ECT in California, New York, Massachusetts, North Carolina, and Wisconsin
      - Voluntariness
        ○ A patient's decision can be considered involuntary when the patient does not volitionally provide consent, versus when a patient cannot make a choice and, thus, is nonvoluntary
        ○ Public, personal, and professional perception may contribute to a sense that involuntary or nonvoluntary treatment with ECT is akin to punishment
      - Informed consent
        ○ Cognitive processes associated with providing informed consent include those of information processing, memory, and insight
        ○ Approximately 1–3% of patients receiving ECT in the United States and Europe lack decision-making capacity

PATIENT FILE

- Worldwide studies and case reports suggest that the patient's decision-making capacity and satisfaction improve when receiving ECT
- There was no described difference in the patient's sense of satisfaction as defined by their treatment outcome and experience regardless of whether they consented to treatment with ECT
* Historically, courts have granted ECT treatment when the following is established:
  - ECT is a reasonable and necessary treatment option proven by clear and convincing evidence and less intrusive therapies have failed
  - The patient does not have decision-making capacity regarding ECT treatment
    - Court approval could plausibly be sought in cases that a patient is unwilling to provide consent and is at risk of harming himself or herself and/or others
      * This is considered compulsory treatment, which grants the State police powers to approve "necessary, reasonable," treatment, "proportional" to the risks posed by the intervention
      * Compulsory ECT treatment is rarely indicated
    - Court may approve treatment when the patient is unable to participate in the consent process regardless of the patient's willingness
  - The benefit of ECT therapy outweighs the risk associated with this intervention
    - The risk associated with ECT is low when compared to the risk of mortality resulting from suboptimally treated, or untreated, psychiatric illnesses
- Ethical considerations
  * Autonomy is preserving a patient's agency to make choices and decisions
    - ECT may re-establish healthier thoughts and behaviors as well as legal adjudicative abilities
  * Beneficence is the professional obligation to promote health and wellness
    - ECT is a cost-effective, low-risk, potentially lifesaving, first-line treatment in severely mentally ill and medically frail patients
    - ECT has no absolute contraindications

PATIENT FILE

- ECT may reduce the risk of long-term disability, premature death, and suffering in severe psychotic or suicidal depression
- Nonmaleficence is the duty to prevent harm
  - Treatment with ECT is well tolerated and associated side effects are described as mild, self-limited, and symptomatically treated
- Justice is the equitable treatment of all individuals
  - ECT offers a less restrictive treatment modality that mitigates the risk of harm to the patient and society by decreasing the burden of psychiatric illness and shortening the length of hospitalization
    - Some patients may experience personal uncertainty or discomfort when deciding to pursue ECT
      - A side effect associated with ECT includes memory loss which resolves in a few days to weeks
        - The likelihood of developing cognitive side effects from ECT decreases with right unilateral electrode placement and application of ultra-brief pulse stimuli techniques, without compromising efficacy
    - Public scrutiny and stigma associated with ECT treatment still limit its use

Two-minute tutorial

- ECT has multiple applications since its inception
  - ECT has been utilized as a treatment option for both psychiatric and neurological conditions
    - ECT has, reportedly, been applied to cases of aggression in Alzheimer's dementia, Parkinson's disease, dyskinesias, epilepsy, and toxic and metabolic encephalopathies
  - ECT's psychiatric indications include catatonia, NMS, treatment-refractory suicidality and depression, as well as psychosis accompanying bipolar and affective disorders and schizophrenia
  - Other applications include treatment-refractory OCD and Tourette's syndrome
- Treatment of schizophrenia with clozapine therapy is successful in about 30–60% of cases
  - Approximately 40–70% of patients experience ultra treatment-resistant symptoms which marginally respond to clozapine even though the medication's use is established in treatment-refractory cases and psychotic and non-psychotic aggression

PATIENT FILE

- However, application of about 16–20 ECT sessions in these cases was associated with clinical improvement
- Despite the safety profile, efficaciousness, low risk-to-benefit ratio, and clinical indication, the use of ECT as a viable treatment option remains limited
  - Factors influencing the widespread use of ECT include a patient's willingness to consent, right to refuse treatment, and decision-making capacity; the courts' legal and statutory limitations and characterization of ECT as a treatment of last resort; and professional and public attitudes toward ECT as a valid therapeutic intervention
- When compared to its availability and application in the private sector, the use of ECT is limited in forensic settings
  - Following its use from 1930 to 1960, ECT regulations limited its use
    - State laws that addressed the age a patient could receive ECT, the methodology of obtaining and documenting informed consent, physician eligibility requirements, mandates informing administrative reporting, and conditions for treatment in those patients who lack capacity to consent
  - In 1988, Appelbaum and Grisso's conceptualization of informed consent included the ability to appreciate a situation, circumstance, and resultant outcome; to understand information relevant to making a decision; to reason, rationalize, or manipulate information; and to communicate a decision
    - However, there is a lack of standardized assessments that identify the presence or absence of decision-making capacity for ECT treatment
  - When a patient lacks decision-making capacity, a surrogate decision maker may be chosen, designated, or assigned
    - The role of a surrogate is to make a treatment decision based upon a patient's known preferences, a substituted judgment standard which is informed by knowledge of the patient, or the best-interest standard (the decision made in the patient's best interest)
    - Although a surrogate decision maker may be identified, their ability to provide consent for nonvoluntary ECT can be limited by the court
      - Under the premise of a proactive *parens patriae*, the state and court may protect those deemed unable to care for themselves
      - The courts may require their approval or authorization for a surrogate to provide consent for treatment

PATIENT FILE

- Other court-imposed limitations that potentially affect delivery of ECT treatment include the appreciation of ECT as different than that of emergency medical treatment; as a treatment of last resort; or as requiring a higher standard of proof (clear and convincing) for authorization
- Treatment with ECT has been demonstrated to improve decision-making capacity and restore legal competency abilities
  - The state has a vested interest in prosecuting and restoring incompetent defendants, which is fomented by the severity of their criminal charges
- When considering ECT intervention, balancing ethical duties and principles of autonomy, nonmaleficence, justice, and beneficence may better promote delivery of patient care and preserve patients' rights
- The American Psychiatric Association cites Section 3 of the American Medical Association Code of Ethics in a description of considering the benefit-to-risk ratios of ECT, and advises that "A physician shall respect the law and also recognize a responsibility to seek changes in those requirements which are contrary to the best interests of the patient"

Post-test question

Which of the following statements about competency restoration are NOT true?

A. The *Dusky* v. *US* ruling established the legal abilities required to proceed to trial

B. The legal abilities enumerated by the *Dusky* ruling include an individual's ability to understand the nature of the criminal proceedings and rationally work with their attorney in the conduct of a defense

C. Legal competency requires a finding of grave disability and/or dangerousness to others

D. 75–90% of patients found IST can be restored to legal competence within 6 months by treating the patient's mental health condition with psychotropic medication

E. ECT reduces the burden of psychiatric symptoms and aggression; is associated with improved insight; and can assist with competency restoration including in ultra treatment-resistant cases

Answer: C

References

1. Appelbaum, P. S. & Grisso, T. (1988). Assessing patients' capacities to consent to treatment. *New England Journal of Medicine*, 319(25), 1635–8. https://doi.org/10.1056/NEJM198812223192504. Erratum in: N Engl J Med 1989 Mar 16;320(11):748. PMID: 3200278.
2. Cabeldue, M., Green, D., McGrath, R. E., & Belfi, B. (2021). Factors related to repeat forensic hospital admissions for restoration of competency to stand trial. *Journal of Forensic Psychology Practice*, 21(2), 91–117. https://doi.org/10.1080/24732850.2020.1834834.
3. Callahan, L. & Pinals, D. A. (2020). Challenges to reforming the competence to stand trial and competence restoration system. *Psychiatric Services*, April 2, 71(7), 691–697. https://doi.org/10.1176/appi.ps.201900483.
4. Dare, F. Y. & Rasmussen, K. G. (2015). Court-approved electroconvulsive therapy in patients unable to provide their own consent: a case series. *Journal of ECT*, Sept., 31(3), 147–149. https://doi.org/10.1097/YCT.0000000000000189.
5. Heilbrun, K., Giallella, C., Wright, H. J., et al. (2019). Treatment for restoration of competence to stand trial: critical analysis and policy recommendations. *Psychology, Public Policy, and Law*, 25(4), 266–283. https://doi.org/10.1037/law0000210.
6. Hirose, S., Ashby, C. R., Jr., & Mills, M. J. (2001). Effectiveness of ECT combined with risperidone against aggression in schizophrenia. *Journal of ECT*, March, 17(1): 22–26. https://doi.org/10.1097/00124509-200103000-00005.
7. Iltis, A. S., Fortier, R., Ontjes, N., & McCall, W. V. (2023). Ethics considerations in laws restricting incapacitated patients' access to ECT. *Journal of the American Academy of Psychiatry Law*, 51(1), 47–55. https://doi.org/10.29158/JAAPL.220029-21.
8. Kristensen, D., Brandt-Christensen, M., Ockelmann, H. H., & Jorgensen, M. B. (2012). The use of electroconvulsive therapy in a cohort of forensic psychiatric patients with schizophrenia. *Criminal Behaviour and Mental Health*, April, 22(2), 148–156. https://doi.org/10.1002/cbm.826.
9. Livingston, R., Wu, C., Mu, K., & Coffey, M. J. (2018). Regulation of electroconvulsive therapy: a systematic review of US state laws. *Journal of ECT*, March, 34(1), 60–68. https://doi.org/10.1097/YCT.0000000000000460.
10. Morris, D. R. (2022). Charge severity and aggression during competence restoration. *Journal of the American Academy of Psychiatry Law*, 50(3), 388–395. https://doi.org/10.29158/JAAPL.210096-21.

PATIENT FILE

11. Morrissey, J. P., Burton, N. M., & Steadman, H. J. (1979). Developing an empirical base for psycho-legal policy analyses of ECT: a New York State survey. *International Journal of Law and Psychiatry*, 2(1), 99–111. https://doi.org/10.1016/0160-2527(79)90033-5.
12. Moulier, V., Krir, M. W., Dalmont, M., Group, S., Guillin, O., & Rotharmel, M. (2021). A prospective multicenter assessor-blinded randomized controlled study to compare the efficacy of short versus long protocols of electroconvulsive therapy as an augmentation strategy to clozapine in patients with ultra-resistant schizophrenia (SURECT study). *Trials*, April, 22(1), 284. https://doi.org/10.1186/s13063-021-05227-3.
13. Oltedal, L., Bartsch, H., Sorhaug, O., et al. (2017). The Global ECT–MRI Research Collaboration (GEMRIC): establishing a multi-site investigation of the neural mechanisms underlying response to electroconvulsive therapy. *NeuroImage: Clinical*, Feb., 14, 422–432. https://doi.org/10.1016/j.nicl.2017.02.009.
14. Rojas, M., Ariza, D., Ortega, A., et al. (2022). Electroconvulsive therapy in psychiatric disorders: a narrative review exploring neuroendocrine–immune therapeutic mechanisms and clinical implications. *International Journal of Molecular Sciences*, 23(13), 6918. https://doi.org/10.3390/ijims23136918.
15. Seamon, A., Groth, C. M., Surya, S., & Rosenquist, P. B. (2022). Role of electroconvulsive therapy in treatment-resistant schizophrenia in forensic psychiatry: review. *Journal of ECT*, Sept., 38(3), 156–158. https://doi.org/10.1097/YCT.0000000000000843.
16. Secarea, C. M., Cleary, S. D., & Candilis, P. J. (2021). Factors influencing adjudicative competence and length of time to restoration. *Journal of Forensic Sciences*, 66(3), 982–991. https://doi.org/10.1111/1556-4029.14669.
17. Simpson, J. R. (2016). When restoration fails: one state's answer to the dilemma of permanent incompetence. *Journal of the American Academy of Psychiatry Law*, June, 44(2), 171–179. PMID: 27236171.
18. Stahl, S. M. (2014). *Stahl's Essential Psychopharmacology: Prescriber's Guide*, 5th ed. New York: Cambridge University Press.
19. Witzel, J., Held, E., & Bogerts, B. (2009). Electroconvulsive therapy in forensic psychiatry – ethical problems in daily practice: case report. *Journal of ECT*, June, 25(2):,129–132. https://doi.org/10.1097/YCT.0b013e318185fa55.

23

Sexually violent predators (SVPs): Interrupting the circuit

The Psychopharmocological Dilemma: Psychopharmacological interventions with adult sexual offenders

Rachel Powers and Carolina A. Klein

Pretest self-assessment question

What are the hormonal interventions for managing sexual offending behaviors?

A. Testosterone
B. Gonadotropin releasing hormone agonist
C. Lithium
D. Fluoxetine

Patient evaluation on intake

Patient is a 60-year-old male diagnosed with pedophilic disorder, nonexclusive type, sexually attracted to males, and cocaine use disorder – moderate. He was readmitted to the state hospital under his sexually violent predator (SVP) commitment after he tested positive for amphetamines while on conditional release. He is inquiring about restarting leuprolide acetate in preparation for discharge from the hospital.

Psychiatric history

- Pedophilic disorder, nonexclusive type, sexually attracted to males
- Cocaine use disorder – moderate

Social and personal history

- Only child
- Normal development
- Raised by mother and father in low-income housing
- No history of abuse or neglect
- Mother was disciplinarian, spanking and grounding
- Excellent grades throughout school. Graduated with a diploma
- Attended university for 4 years. Left prior to degree to enter the military
- Entered the military at age 22 and honorably discharged at age 25
- Worked as a journeyman

- Volunteered as an athletic director
  - Patient enjoyed the company of minors and considered them "friends"
  - Was strategic and predatory in his sexual offending, utilizing his role as an athletic director to groom and socially manipulate his victims and their parents
- Established relationships with students and their parents
  - Spent time outside sanctioned activities with students and their families to build trust
  - Identified students who had psychosocial stressors that may increase vulnerability for sexual activity (e.g., family discord, social isolation, etc.)
  - Used his relationships with his victims to gain access to and groom their siblings and other acquaintances
- Used drugs and alcohol in his sexual offending and sexual behaviors
  - To identify "risk takers" whom he believed would also be more vulnerable to sexual abuse
  - To disinhibit his victims, making it easier to coerce them into sexual activity
  - To enhance his masturbatory experiences
- His relational and sexual history
  - Patient has no significant history of intimate relationships with age-appropriate partners
  - He has reported casual sexual contact with adult males
  - He has also offended against adult males
  - Reported occasionally dating women without sexual activity
- Patient's primary sexual partners have been prepubescent and pubescent male victims of his sexual offending
  - The patient has three convictions for sexual offending
  - He has self-reported sexually offending against approximately 125 males throughout his lifetime, the majority of whom were prepubescent and pubescent minors between 10 and 14 years old
  - He estimates the number of individual instances of sexual offending to be approximately 600
  - Non-minor victims included adults who were "passed out" due to intoxication or sleeping at the time of the offense

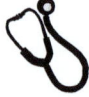

Medical history

- Total left hip replacement in 2017
- Essential hypertension – controlled with lisinopril
- Suspected glaucoma – no indication for treatment at present
- Paternal history of kidney disease

PATIENT FILE

Medication history
- 7.5 mg leuprolide acetate monthly from 2010 to 2014. Discontinued without consultation. Reported it was in preparation for hip surgery
- Declined to restart leuprolide acetate after surgery

Current history
A 60-year-old male diagnosed with pedophilic disorder, nonexclusive type, sexually attracted to males, and cocaine use disorder – moderate, was readmitted to the hospital after testing positive for cocaine and methamphetamines while on conditional release.

Evaluations of risk
- STATIC 99-R: total score = 4; Level Iva: Above Average Risk (5-year recidivism: 10–12%) > Adjusted Risk Level III: Average Risk
- STABLE 2007: total score = 5; Moderate Range (Composite Risk = Level Iva: Above Average; 13–20% 5-year recidivism)

Psychopharmacological interventions
- World Federation of Societies of Biological Psychiatry (WFSBP) algorithm of pharmacological treatment of paraphilic disorders categorizes this patient as a Level 4, which includes: Moderately high risk of sexual violence and severe paraphilic disorders, Pedophilic disorder or sexual sadism fantasies and/or behavior or physical violence; and no compliance or no satisfactory results at level 3
- Treatment at this level of severity should include psychotherapy in the form of sex offender-structured cognitive behavioral therapy (CBT), if indicated and available, and a long-acting gonadotropin-releasing hormone agonist (GnRHa) due to:
  - Diagnosed pedophilic disorder and a prolific sexual offense history with moderate to high risk for reoffending
- No current contraindications for use
- Willingness to re-start leuprolide acetate secondary to guidelines and recommendations for treatment and supervision of individuals with a history of sexual offending
- An SSRI may be associated with the GnRH antagonist, especially if there is comorbidity with anxiety, depression, or obsessive–compulsive symptoms

Psychological interventions: individual, group, and milieu treatment
- Self-management and regulation strategies
- Establishing sufficient social involvement, positive influences, and support persons
- Creating and maintaining healthy and stable sexuality

PATIENT FILE

- Changing distorted attitudes, schemas, and beliefs
- Identification of triggers and early warnings signs for offending

Progress in treatment

- Pharmacological – decreased sex drive, decreased sexual urges, decreased sexual fantasies, and inability to masturbate. Increased voluntary control
- Psychological – increased cooperation with treatment, commitment to sobriety, reduction in criminogenic needs, plan for containment upon release
- Sexual history and maintenance polygraphs – determined to be truthful
- Sexual interest measures – low responsivity

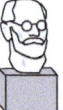

Psychotherapy history

- Saw a therapist in college every 2 weeks for about 1 year, related to "problems with being homosexual"
- Psychiatrically hospitalized for 1.5 months. Diagnosed with acute depression and homosexual pedophilia
- Outpatient treatment for 2 years
- Admission to state hospital as an SVP. Treated for 3 years. Recurrent deviant sexual fantasies
- Discharged to community outpatient treatment. Treated for 8 years. Recurrent use of marijuana and cocaine with positive urinalyses. Undetected alcohol use
- Readmitted to state hospital. Treated for 3 months
- Discharged to community outpatient treatment. Treated for 1.5 years. Repeated use of cocaine; house search found urine samples used to thwart urinalysis; found with a magazine ad of two pre-teen boys with buttocks exposed; described as angry and defiant with treatment and supervision; minimization of sexual offenses
- Readmitted to state hospital. Treated for 2 years
- Discharged to community outpatient treatment. Treated for 3.5 years. Tested positive for methamphetamine and cocaine. Ongoing concerns about compliance and disclosures in treatment, minimization of sexual offending, and indulging deviant sexual fantasies
- Readmitted to state hospital. Returned to inpatient sex offender treatment

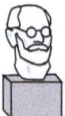

Psychotherapy moment

- Fifteen years after his most recent readmission, the patient received information that one of his victims had died secondary to substance use

PATIENT FILE

- Reflected on his role in introducing the victim to substances, subjecting him to sexual abuse, and how the resulting trauma exacerbated the victim's substance use which ultimately led to his death
- Became less guarded and defensive in treatment and increased his participation.
- Took the initiative to address outstanding recommendations delineated in his individual containment model treatment plan
- Restarted leuprolide acetate to dampen his sexual drive
- Began tracking deviant sexual thoughts and responsivity to derailing them

Mechanism of action moment

Leuprolide acetate is a GnRH receptor agonist, also called a GnRH analog (GnRHa), that decreases the level of testosterone in adult males, with continuous administration, by inhibiting luteinizing hormone (LH) and follicle-stimulating hormone (FSH) production resulting in:

- Decreased sex drive
- Decreased pedophilic sexual urges
- Decreased sexual fantasies
- Decreased masturbation frequency
- Enhanced voluntary control

Attending physician's mental notes

Initial visit

- Requesting to restart leuprolide acetate
- Vocalized concerns regarding long-term side effects
- Recent lab work shows no contraindications
- Significant history of substance use. Last use 15+ years
- Begin monthly injections of leuprolide acetate, 7.5 mg
- Evaluated as moderate–high risk for reoffense

Follow-up visit 30 days

- Recently received second leuprolide acetate injection
- Reduced sexual arousal in response to appropriate sexual fantasies
- Denied inappropriate sexual fantasies
- Continues to attend treatment for sexual offending, substance recovery, and community reintegration

Follow-up visit 60 days

- Reduced sexual arousal
- Difficulties when seeking sexual arousal

PATIENT FILE

- Denied inappropriate sexual fantasies
- No side effects
- Underwent sexual history polygraph – truthful responses

Follow-up visit 90 days

- Disclosed reduction in arousal and sexual fantasies
- Attempts to masturbate are described as "painful" and ineffective
- Penile plethysmography (PPG) testing evidenced "low responsiveness." Supports self-report of reduced arousal

Case outcome

Follow-up visit 120 days

- Inability to attain erection
- Continued reduction in sexual fantasies
- Reduction in effort required to derail inappropriate sexual fantasies
- Is working on relapse prevention plan including supervision and monitoring

Follow-up visit 150 days

- Continued efficacy in reducing arousal
- Discussed role of continued medication adherence in the community
- Shared his relapse prevention plan, including early warning signs and triggers for sexual offending
- Abstained from using, and appropriately reported, cocaine on campus

Case debrief

Background

- 60-year-old male diagnosed with pedophilic disorder, nonexclusive type, sexually attracted to males, and cocaine use disorder – moderate
- Readmitted to the hospital as an SVP after testing positive for cocaine and methamphetamines while on conditional release

Course of hospitalization

- Engaged in and responding to psychotherapeutic interventions
  - Made significant updates to his containment release plan, including warning signs and triggers for sexual offending and substance use
  - In preparation for discharge, the patient is interested in restarting pharmacological treatment for his paraphilic disorder
- Risk assessments and evaluations of paraphilic disorder
  - Above-average risk for reoffending based on composite scores from the Static-99 R and Stable 2007

PATIENT FILE

- Idiographic risk factor – 3 detected sexual offenses involving 2 victims out of 140 individual victims and myriad sexual offenses
- WFSBP Risk Level 4

Pharmacological intervention and outcome

- Restarted GnRH treatment at 7.5 mg leuprolide acetate monthly
  - Reduction in deviant sexual thoughts as detailed in a self-monitoring sheet
  - Faster derailment of deviant sexual thoughts
  - No desire to act on deviant sexual thoughts
  - Impotence
  - Sexual Interest Measure (e.g., PPG) reflected low responsivity
  - Denies any side effects

Take-home points

- Risk evaluation determines type and intensity of treatment interventions regardless of setting, consistent with the Risk–Need–Responsivity (RNR) model.
- Evidence-based treatment interventions include:
  - Pharmacological
  - Psychological
  - Supervision/monitoring
- The aims of pharmacological interventions in the treatment of paraphilic disorders include:
  - Control paraphilic fantasies and behaviors to reduce the risk of sexual offending
  - Control paraphilic sexual urges
  - Decrease distress in persons with paraphilic disorders
  - Increase non-paraphilic sexual interests and behaviors

Performance in practice: confessions of a psychopharmacologist

Medico-legal considerations

- Paraphilic disorders are chronic.
- The presence of a paraphilic disorder is not illegal; however, the behaviors in response to paraphilic urges are frequently associated with sexual offending
- Multimodal treatment is paramount in preventing sexual offending
- Surgical castration and chemical castration laws vary by jurisdiction

PATIENT FILE

Ethical considerations of hormonal treatment, as laid out by the World Federation of Societies of Biological Psychiatry Guidelines for the biological treatment of paraphilias

- The person has a paraphilic disorder diagnosed by a psychiatrist after a careful psychiatric examination
- The hormonal treatment addresses specific clinical signs, symptoms and behaviors and is adapted to the person's state of health
- The person's condition represents a significant risk of serious harm to his health or to the physical or moral integrity of other persons
- No less intrusive treatment means of providing care are available. However, the availability of "less restrictive" alternatives should not preclude the option of choosing to initiate treatment by means of a sex-drive-lowering hormonal intervention
- The psychiatrist in charge of the patient agrees to inform the patient and receive his or her consent, to take responsibility for the indication of the treatment and for the follow-up, including somatic aspects, with the help of a consultant endocrinologist, if necessary
- The hormonal treatment is part of a written treatment plan to be reviewed at appropriate intervals and, if necessary, revised
- "When properly administered, with appropriate protocol in place to detect and treat side effects should they develop, GnRHa treatments constitute no more or less of a risk than most other forms of frequently prescribed psychopharmacological agents"
- "For paraphilias characterized by intense and frequent deviant sexual desire and arousal, which highly predispose the patient to severe abnormal behaviors (such as pedophilia or rape), a hormonal intervention using GnRHa may be needed"

Treatment considerations

- Risk of sexual offending
  - Static – factors that cannot change, except for age, unless additional crimes are committed (e.g., convictions for sexual offenses)
  - Dynamic – factors that have the potential to change with treatment (e.g., poor problem-solving skills, negative emotionality)
  - Idiographic – factors that are unique to the individual and not measurable (e.g., assertions: "I don't know if I can control myself when I see a group of kids")
- Intensity and frequency of deviant sexual fantasies
- Level of engagement and adherence to treatment recommendations
- Previous medical and psychiatric history
- Current medical and psychiatric functioning

- Long-acting GnRH agonists, i.e., triptorelin (3.75 mg IM every 4 weeks) or leuprolide (7.5 mg IM every 4 weeks)
  - Efficacy > 90%
  - Onset of efficacy: 1–3 months
  - Testosterone level measurements may be easily used to control GnRH agonist treatment compliance if necessary
- Cyproterone acetate (CPA) must be associated with GnRHa (one week before and during the first month of GnRHa) to prevent a flare-up effect and to control the relapse risk of paraphilic sexual behavior associated with this flare-up effect.

Tips and pearls

- Pre-initiation of treatment, *rule out contraindications*
  - Active pituitary pathology
  - Thromboembolic disorders
  - Osteoporosis
  - Specific allergies (test dose 1 mg SC)
- Pre-initiation of treatment, *obtain*
  - Informed consent
  - Serum testosterone, LH, FSH, prolactin
  - Urea nitrogen and blood creatinine
  - Complete blood count (CBC) and comprehensive metabolic panel (CMP) including renal and hepatic function, fasting blood glucose, Ca and P levels
  - Bone density scan (if possible)
  - Cardiovascular status and BP, EKG
- *Monitor* during treatment
  - Depression or excessive emotionality q 3 months
  - CBC q 4 months, then q 6 months
  - Testosterone q 4 months, then q 6 months
  - Blood glucose, weight, BP, Ca and P q 6 months
  - LH, FSH, urea nitrogen, creatinine q 6 months
  - Bone density scan yearly
  - Possible side effects: osteoporosis, bone pain, hypogonadism, "flare-up" effect, nausea, vomiting, constipation, weight gain, hot flashes, cold sweats, mood swings (depression), sleep disturbances, hair loss, gynecomastia, headaches, dizziness
- Special considerations in treatment
  - "Flare-up" is a common side effect that occurs upon initiation of luteinizing hormone-releasing hormone (LHRH) agonists and occurs due to sudden increase in testosterone. Management: pair with antiandrogen flutamide for 30 days or CPA 300 mg for 2 weeks

- Osteoporosis: in patients at high risk for osteoporosis, with bone pain, or evidence of demineralization on bone scans, couple with testosterone 25–50 mg every month, to prevent bone mineral loss and erectile dysfunction. Osteoporosis may also be reversible with etidronate and vitamin D therapy.

Two-minute tutorial

Paraphilia

Any intense and persistent sexual interests, urges, fantasies, or behaviors involving objects, activities, and/or situations that are atypical. Paraphilias are not in and of themselves illegal nor constitute a disorder.

Paraphilic disorder

A paraphilia that is causing distress or impairment to the individual *or* a paraphilia that has involved personal harm or risk of harm to others.

Pedophilic disorder

A sexual preference for prepubescent children. It is one of eight delineated paraphilias within the DSM-5-TR; the others are subsumed by a diagnosis of other specified paraphilic disorder.

DSM-5-TR diagnostic criteria for pedophilic disorder

A. Over a period of at least 6 months, recurrent, intense sexually arousing fantasies, sexual urges, or behaviors involving sexual activity with a prepubescent child or children (generally 13 years and younger)
B. The individual has acted on these sexual urges, **or** the sexual urges or fantasies cause marked distress or interpersonal difficulty
C. The individual is at least age 16 years and at least 5 years older than the child or children in Criterion A

Specify whether:

- Exclusive type (attracted only to children)
- Nonexclusive type (attracted to children and adults)

Specify if:

- Sexually attracted to males
- Sexually attracted to females
- Sexually attracted to both

Specify if:

- Limited to incest

PATIENT FILE

WFSBP algorithm of psychopharmacological treatment of paraphilic disorders

- LEVEL 1
  - Aim: control of paraphiliac sexual fantasies, compulsions, and behaviors without impact on conventional sexual activity and on sexual desire
  - May be used in cases of voyeurism, fetishism, frotteurism disorders without any risk of rape or child abuse
  - Treatment: psychotherapy – preferentially cognitive behavioral therapy [CBT], if indicated and available – no level of evidence for other forms of psychotherapy
- LEVEL 2
  - Aim: control of paraphiliac sexual fantasies, compulsions, and behaviors with minor impact on conventional sexual activity and on sexual desire
  - May be used in all mild cases of hands-off paraphilic disorders, with low risk of sexual violence, i.e., exhibitionism without any risk of rape or child abuse
  - No satisfactory results at level 1
  - Treatment:
    - CBT, if indicated and available, as above, *plus*:
    - SSRIs: use fluoxetine $\geq$ 80 mg p.o. daily, or sertraline $\geq$ 100 mg p.o. daily and titrated higher as necessary
      - Onset of efficacy: 1–3 months
      - Efficacy: 70% if no sexual violence
    - Naltrexone: use standard dose 380 mg IM q 4 weeks
- LEVEL 3
  - Aim: control of paraphiliac sexual fantasies, compulsions, and behaviors with a substantial reduction of conventional sexual activity and sexual desire
  - Moderate risk of sexual violence (intellectual disability, neurological comorbid disorders such as dementia)
  - No sexual sadism fantasies and/or behavior (if present: go to level 4)
  - No satisfactory results at level 2
  - Treatment:
    - CBT, if indicated and available, as above, *plus*:
    - CPA: oral, 50–200 mg total daily dose (maximum 300), or 200–400 mg IM once weekly and then every 2–4 weeks (maximum 500 mg every 1–2 weeks), *or*:

- MPA: oral, 50–400 mg/d (maximum 600 mg/d) or IM 400 mg weekly (up to 1000 mg per week) and then monthly, if CPA is not available
  - No markers of compliance if oral form
  - Efficacy 80–90%
  - Onset of efficacy: 1–3 months
- SSRIs may be associated with CPA, especially if there is comorbidity with anxiety, depression, or obsessive–compulsive symptoms
- LEVEL 4
  - Aim: control of paraphiliac sexual fantasies, compulsions, and behaviors with almost complete suppression of sexual activity and desire
  - Moderately high risk of sexual violence and severe paraphilic disorders
  - Pedophilic disorder or sexual sadism fantasies and/or behavior or physical violence
  - No compliance or no satisfactory results at level 3
  - Treatment:
    - CBT, if indicated and available, as above, *plus*:
    - Long-acting GnRH agonists, i.e., triptorelin (3.75 mg IM every 4 weeks) or leuprolide (7.5 mg IM every 4 weeks)
      - Efficacy > 90%
      - Onset of efficacy: 1–3 months
      - Testosterone level measurements may be easily used to control GnRH agonist treatment compliance if necessary
    - CPA must be associated with GnRH agonists (1 week before and during the first month of GnRH agonists) to prevent a flare-up effect and to control the relapse risk of paraphilic sexual behavior associated with this flare-up effect
- LEVEL 5 (Retained)
  - Aim: control of paraphilic sexual fantasies (including sexual sadism and/or behavior or physical violence), high risk of sexual violence, compulsions and behaviors with complete suppression of sexual desire and activity
  - Most severe paraphilic disorders (catastrophic cases)
  - No satisfactory results at level 4
  - Treatment:
    - CBT, if indicated and available, as above, *plus*:
    - In addition to GnRH agonists:

- Use antiandrogen treatment, i.e., CPA oral, 50–200 mg/d (maximum 300) or IM 200–400 mg once weekly and then every 2–4 weeks (maximum 500 mg every 1–2 weeks); or MPA 50–400 mg/d or 400 mg IM weekly (up to 1000 mg per week) and then monthly, if CPA is not available
- SSRIs may also be added

Post-test question

Which of the following options is NOT a necessary component of treatment for a patient with a severe paraphilic disorder with high risk fo sexual violence and a severe personality disorder?

A. Antiandrogen treatment
B. Fluoxetine
C. CBT
D. Group sex offender treatment

Answer: D

References

1. Brankley, A., Helmus, L. M., & Hanson, R. (2017). STABLE-2007 evaluator workbook: updated recidivism rates (includes combinations with Static-99 R, Static-2002 R, and Risk Matrix 2000).
2. Franke, I., Streb, J., Leichauer, K., Handke, S., Dudeck, M., & Tippelt, S. (2021). Efficacy of outpatient treatment of sex offenders. *International Journal of Law and Psychiatry*, Nov.–Dec., 79, 101738. https://doi.org/10.1016/j.ijlp.2021.101738. Epub Sept. 28, 2021. PMID: 34597889.
3. Hanson, R. K., et al. (2017). Reductions in risk based on time offense-free in the community: once a sexual offender, not always a sexual offender. *Psychology, Public Policy, and Law*, 24, 48–63.
4. Helmus, L., Kelley, S., Frazier, A., et al. (2022). Static-99 R: strengths, limitations, predictive accuracy meta-analysis, and legal admissibility review. *Psychology, Public Policy, and Law*, 28(3), 307–331. https://doi.org/10.1037/law0000351.
5. Helmus, L. M., Lee, S. C., Phenix, A., Hanson, R. K., & Thornton, D. (2021). Static-99 R & Static-2002 R evaluators' workbook. Available from www.saarna.org.
6. Paraphilic Disorders. (2024). *Diagnostic and Statistical Manual of Mental Disorders*. https://doi.org/10.1176/appi.books.9780890425787.x19_Paraphilic_Disorders.

PATIENT FILE

7. Schober, J. (2008). Aspects of behavior in pedophilic sex offenders treated with leuprolide acetate. In D. Pfaff, C. Kordon, P. Chanson, & Y. Christen (eds.), *Hormones and Social Behaviour. Research and Perspectives in Endocrine Interactions*. Berlin: Springer. https://doi.org/10.1007/978-3-540-79288-8_11.
8. Thibaut, F., Cosyns, P., Fedoroff, J. P., et al. (2020). The World Federation of Societies of Biological Psychiatry (WFSBP) 2020 guidelines for the pharmacological treatment of paraphilic disorders. *World Journal of Biological Psychiatry*, 21(6), 412–490. https://doi.org/10.1080/15622975.2020.1744723.
9. Thornton, D., Hanson, R. K., Kelley, S. M., & Mundt, J. C. (2021). Estimating lifetime and residual risk for individuals who remain sexual offense free in the community: practical applications. *Sexual Abuse*, 33(1), 3–33. https://doi.org/10.1177/1079063219871573.

PATIENT FILE

24

Pregnancy: Treating for two

The Psychopharmocological Dilemma: Should antipsychotics be continued in the third trimester of pregnancy?

Imran Hassan and Gillian Friedman

Pretest self-assessment question
What is the most common diagnosis that leads to post-partum psychosis?
A. Major depression
B. Medication-induced psychosis
C. Bipolar disorder
D. Methamphetamine
E. Schizophrenia

Answer: C

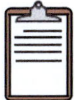

Patient evaluation on intake
- 33-year-old
- 29 weeks pregnant (early third trimester)
- Admitted to state hospital as incompetent to stand trial (IST), secondary to severe mental illness, on charges of assault with great bodily injury
- Presenting symptoms
  - Overt bizarre behaviors indicating active auditory hallucinations: self-laughing, self-talking, gesturing (slapped self on hands at one point, stating she was hitting a person who was disrespecting her). Endorsed hearing voices ("like conservations")
  - Bizarre delusions of thought broadcasting
  - Paranoid ideations
  - Grandiose delusions
  - Pressured speech
  - Elevated affect
  - Disorganized thought process – tangentiality; thought blocking
  - Impaired insight

Psychiatric history
- Psychiatric hospitalizations – reported twice in the past; possibly the first one in mid-adolescence, with a diagnosis of bipolar disorder or schizophrenia
- History of suicide attempts – reported once (drowning in bathtub, age 24)

PATIENT FILE

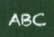
Social and personal history
- Born/raised: California
- Raised by mother and stepfather
- Siblings: "3 brothers and a bunch of sisters"
- Education: dropped out in tenth grade
- Marital: "engaged"
- Children: two

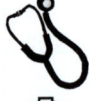
Medical history
None.

Family history
None.

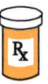
Medication history
- Haloperidol
- Olanzapine
- Paliperidone
- Risperidone
- Quetiapine
- Aripiprazole
- Ziprasidone
- Valproic acid
- Fluoxetine
- Clonazepam
- Trazodone

Current history

<u>Presentation prior to state hospitalization</u>

During incarceration (4–29 weeks of pregnancy), patient continued to exhibit:
- Disorganized behavior
- Thought disorganization and blocking
- Auditory hallucinations
- Pressured speech
- Mood lability, irritability, verbal hostility
- Poor self-care

"She stood in the corner for several minutes alternating between running her fingers through her hair and then staring at the ceiling ... alternated between having an emotionless facial expression and laughing inappropriately throughout the interview."

PATIENT FILE

- Was prescribed risperidone 1 mg p.o. BID and paliperidone palmitate 234 mg IM monthly
- Medication adherence was poor
- Involuntary medication order (IMO) was obtained in jail. Patient became adherent with her medications and remained so even after the expiration of the IMO
- She had limited improvement in her manic and psychotic symptoms
- During a second trimester Obstetrics and Gynecology (OBGYN) visit, she was informed regarding the risks involved with her psychotropic medications, specifically the harm it could cause the fetus
- From then on, she completely refused her oral risperidone
- She decompensated severely. She was defecating in the shower, lying naked in her dorm room, and voicing suicidal ideations (SIs)
- She did accept the monthly injection of paliperidone palmitate
- She continued to be acutely manic and psychotic, with on-and-off SIs
- She was transferred to state hospital for competency restoration

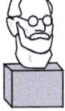

Psychotherapy history

None.

Patient was educated in detail on the importance of medication adherence post-discharge including the postpartum period (the very high-risk time) to decrease the risks of worsening of symptoms, postpartum psychosis/mania, postpartum depression.

Mechanism of action moment

- Dopamine-2 receptor (D_2) blockade

Attending physician's mental notes (at intervals)

When patient first evaluated at 30 weeks pregnancy

- She continues to exhibit overt manic and psychotic symptoms
- Psychiatric symptoms
  - Auditory hallucinations
  - Bizarre delusions
  - Persecutory delusions
  - Disorganized thought process
  - Disorganized behaviors
  - Manic symptoms
  - Very poor insight
  - History of self-injurious ideations and behaviors

Case outcome

- Jail psychiatry records reviewed

PATIENT FILE

- At least on a few occasions, was administered haloperidol, olanzapine, trazodone, risperidone, and patient was last given paliperidone palmitate a week before her transfer to state hospital
- Upon admission to state hospital, serum risperidone < 1.0 + serum 9-OH risperidone 18.4 = total serum risperidone level: 18.4 (quite low)
- Risperidone p.o. was restarted. The dose was given as 2 mg p.o. BID
- Within 2 weeks of taking this dose, patient started showing significant improvement in her mood and psychotic symptoms
- The dose was further increased and consolidated to all in the evening: risperidone p.o. scheduled 6 mg at bedtime (qHS). No side effects reported or observed
- Patient responded well to risperidone, and her manic symptoms, mood lability, and psychotic symptoms showed significant improvement

Psychopharmacology expert recommendations

1. Since she is tolerating risperidone and showing improvement in her psychosis and trial competency efforts, recommend continuing use of risperidone. Generally, antipsychotics have been found to be very safe for use in pregnancy and the risks of undertreated psychosis far outweigh the small-to-undetectable risks to a fetus of antipsychotic use in pregnancy
2. Given the probable bipolar diathesis, avoid using antidepressants to avoid promoting mood destabilization
   - Forensic evaluator assessed the patient and reported that her competency to stand trial had been restored

Reproductive psychiatry expert recommendations

- Continue the monthly paliperidone palmitate injection 234 mg IM in addition to the p.o. risperidone 6 mg qHS
- Rationale: this would potentially help in case the patient had impaired adherence or non-adherence to her p.o. risperidone post-discharge

Treating psychiatrist went ahead and prescribed the medication. Patient had the right to refuse it. She took the paliperidone palmitate 234 mg IM monthly dose. There were no side effects.

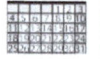

Case outcome

In sum, the patient is a woman with a diagnosis of schizoaffective disorder, bipolar type, in her third trimester of pregnancy. While she did not improve with paliperidone palmitate 234 mg IM monthly alone, she showed improvement on the combination of paliperidone palmitate with an additional dose of risperidone 6 mg p.o. qHS, suggesting insufficient dosing with the paliperidone alone, even at maximum dose formulation.

PATIENT FILE

Take-home points
- Antipsychotics, overall, are quite safe for use in pregnancy, posing little teratogenic risk. There are questions about whether the antipsychotics may contribute to low birthweight, and some studies show neurodevelopmental delay for the first 2 months of an infant's development, although no lasting problems. Some atypical antipsychotics may promote hyperglycemia in the mother
- Risperidone has been found to present a small increase in teratogenic effects compared to other atypical antipsychotics, although this risk is imparted based on first-trimester exposure and no additional risk has been detected for later use in pregnancy

Performance in practice: confessions of a psychopharmacologist
- If poor medication adherence in the community is likely, may consider continuing the paliperidone palmitate long-acting injection (LAI) in addition to the oral risperidone

Tips and pearls
- Paliperidone palmitate maximum dose by itself tends to fall short in improving manic and/or psychotic symptoms in state hospital-level severely ill patients
- Risperidone oral frequently proves far more superior due to the availability of higher doses to achieve a higher dopamine-2 receptor (D_2) blockade
- In third trimester, volume of distribution is increased, so while the first thought may be to give a tiny dose to a pregnant patient, it is better to give a dose that the patient's condition warrants

Two-minute tutorial
- Started refusing psychiatric medications in second trimester due to believing they would harm fetus. This resulted in severe decompensation in an already severely manic episode
- Patient responded well to risperidone and her manic symptoms, mood lability, and psychotic symptoms showed significant improvement
- Recommended to continue the monthly paliperidone palmitate injection 234 mg IM in addition to the p.o. risperidone 6 mg qHS

PATIENT FILE

Post-test question

You receive a patient in her third trimester of pregnancy. She has been acutely manic and psychotic for several months. She is already on paliperidone palmitate 234 mg intramuscular (IM) monthly and risperidone 1 mg oral (po) twice a day (BID). She refuses to continue the paliperidone palmitate but is agreeable to taking an oral antipsychotic. What's the most appropriate course of action?

A. Discontinue the antipsychotics and keep her antipsychotic-free until after the delivery
B. Try getting the patient to agree to a lower dose of paliperidone palmitate
C. Discontinue the paliperidone palmitate and start a different oral antipsychotic
D. Switch to low-dose oral risperidone
E. Increase the risperidone dose

Answer: E

References

1. Betcher, H. K. & Wisner, K. L. (2020). Psychotropic treatment during pregnancy: research synthesis and clinical care principles. *Journal of Women's Health*, 29(3), 310–318.
2. Cohen, L. S., et al. (2016). Reproductive safety of second-generation antipsychotics: current data from the Massachusetts General Hospital National Pregnancy Registry for Atypical Antipsychotics. *American Journal of Psychiatry*, 173(3), 263–270.
3. Wang, Z., et al. (2021) Association between prenatal exposure to antipsychotics and attention-deficit/hyperactivity disorder, autism spectrum disorder, preterm birth, and small for gestational age. *JAMA Internal Medicine*, 181(10), 1332–1340.

PATIENT FILE

25

Schizo-obsessive compulsive disorder (SCZ-OCD), addictions, paraphilia: The collision

The Psychopharmacological Dilemma: Analyzing the various treatment options for comorbid treatment-resistant schizophrenia and obsessive–compulsive disorder (a.k.a. schizo-obsessive disorder)

Hunter Neely

Pretest self-assessment question

What is the first-line treatment for a patient with comorbid treatment-resistant schizophrenia and obsessive–compulsive disorder (OCD) (schizo-obsessive disorder)?

A. Sertraline + olanzapine
B. Haloperidol
C. Clozapine
D. Electroconvulsive therapy (ECT)

Patient evaluation on intake

- 31-year-old male is admitted to the state hospital with the chief complaint of auditory hallucinations, delusions, and obsessive thoughts followed by compulsive behaviors
- I met the patient for the initial evaluation at the state hospital, where he reported experiencing auditory hallucinations, delusions, and disturbing obsessive thoughts and compulsive behaviors
- He was disheveled and his thought process was disjointed at times
- Prior to his instant offense, the patient became increasingly paranoid, as he used increasing amounts of methamphetamine. He began to think that the "demons were out to get [him]"
- The voices from the "demons" commanded him to execute certain behaviors or actions that often involved him engaging in sexually inappropriate behavior with pre-pubescent female children. Of note, the delusions and command auditory hallucinations (CAHs) were also present during periods of sobriety from all substances
- Over time, he became increasingly sexually aroused by watching videos containing non-sexually explicit content of pre-pubescent female children. The videos were benign in nature, such as fully clothed young girls playing with toys, riding their bicycles, or running outside

PATIENT FILE

- He developed the obsessive thought that his genitals were not able to sustain erection or were unexpectedly removed from his body. This resulted in him compulsively masturbating in an effort to alleviate the discomfort the thoughts caused him. He began to masturbate a specific number of times depending on the specific day of the week, with certain days requiring more sessions of masturbation than others. Auditory hallucinations did not command the compulsive masturbation behavior
- Further exacerbation of his psychotic symptoms led to his instant offense, which involved him roaming multiple residential neighborhoods in search of a "sign" or indication that a young female child lived there. Under a delusional belief, and in response to CAHs, he illegally entered a stranger's home with the intent to have sexual intercourse with the young girl whom he assumed lived inside
- The voices commanded him to spread his feces over his body after he had a bowel movement and instructed him to lay with his pants off in his young victim's bed while she slept. His delusion involved the pre-pubescent child victim desiring to have sexual intercourse with him only if his genitals were covered in his feces. After the child woke and screamed, the patient dressed himself in a disorganized fashion and left the victim's house
- The patient was subsequently arrested while roaming the neighborhood as he searched for additional houses that may contain pre-pubescent female children that "wanted" to have sexual intercourse with him. After his arrest, he was taken to jail and was eventually found not guilty by reason of insanity (NGRI) at trial. He was transferred to a state hospital where he has received treatment with the goal of restoring him to sanity and stabilizing his mental illnesses. I met him for the initial evaluation at the state hospital
- He denied depressed mood, suicidal ideation (SI), and homicidal ideation. He did not endorse symptoms of mania/hypomania
- He has been compliant with his antipsychotic medication, aripiprazole, for the last few months, since first prescribed in jail for psychosis

Psychiatric history

- The patient has been diagnosed with schizophrenia, cannabis use disorder, and methamphetamine use disorder
- His first memory of experiencing obsessive thoughts and compulsive behaviors was in adolescence. His initial compulsive behaviors included brushing his teeth a specific number of times and washing his hair on each side of his head for a predetermined duration and manner while showering. His anxiety worsens in intensity until he completes the compulsive behavior, resulting in relief

PATIENT FILE

- As he approached 20 years old, he began to hear voices talk to him. At the same age, he first developed paranoid delusions involving persecutory religious themes
- The patient began smoking methamphetamine at 18 years old. Methamphetamine was his "go-to" drug, which he used daily since he was 20 years old and until his most recent incarceration
- At the age of 20, he started to believe the voices talking to him were those of "demons"
- He has been previously hospitalized twice for "psychotic symptoms and depressed mood," after he reportedly overdosed on an unknown medication. Chart review suggests that his family vaguely mentioned this incident as a suicide attempt although the patient described the overdose as accidental
- He recalls first being sexually attracted to pre-pubescent females when he was in high school, although he has never engaged in sexual interaction with anyone younger than him. When asked, he described that he is sexually aroused by young girls with little to no breast tissue, no pubic hair, and without any secondary sexual characteristics
- He has no history of being the victim of sexual, physical, or emotional abuse
- He has no history of sexually assaulting or molesting pre-pubescent children or adolescents. He has never been charged with sexual involvement with a minor prior to his instant offense

Social and personal history

- The patient's mother was diagnosed with schizophrenia and was an unstable caretaker when he was born. He was raised by his aunt from 3 months old to 13 years old due to his mother being unable to care for him because of her severe mental illness
- After his aunt passed away when he was 13 years old, he went to live with his grandmother. Reportedly, she "kicked him out" of the house when he was 18 years old due to his cannabis use and staying out past curfew. He then went to live with his uncle for 2 years before moving in with his cousin, until he was arrested for his instant offense
- The patient describes himself as a "loner," as he always felt that he did not fit in with his peers. He was bullied throughout middle school and high school. He received many failing grades in various classes due to worsening motivation, interest, and isolation
- The patient did not finish high school. After he overdosed on unknown medications during his senior year in a questionable suicide attempt, he never returned to finish school

PATIENT FILE

- He has never been employed, nor has he provided for himself financially. He has depended on a trust fund from his grandmother, which has supported him until his incarceration
- He has never married, has no children, and has no history of long-term friendships
- His sexual encounters have involved female sex workers on four separate occasions. He had never previously met any of the sex workers he engaged in sexual intercourse with. The patient has never been involved in a romantic relationship with anyone

Medical history

- Essential hypertension
- Obesity
- Hyperlipidemia
- Gastroesophageal reflux disease
- Chronic constipation
- Allergic rhinitis
- Chronic pain
- Dysphagia

Family history

- The patient's mother is diagnosed with schizophrenia
- Per the patient, his grandmother "abused alcohol," although there is no known formal diagnosis
- No known suicide attempts in the family

Medication history

- The patient was initially prescribed fluoxetine for depression after he was hospitalized for overdosing in a questionable suicide attempt in high school. He discontinued this medication prematurely as he did not believe that he was depressed
- He was subsequently prescribed aripiprazole in jail after he was incarcerated for his instant offense, which helped to improve his anxiety, but was not effective in treating his psychotic symptoms

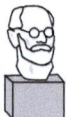

Psychotherapy history

- The patient has received CBT during his current hospitalization, but has been minimally cooperative in attendance and engagement given his undertreated psychotic symptoms. His negative symptoms of schizophrenia significantly impair his motivation, concentration, and ability to engage with others, therefore interfering with the effectiveness of psychotherapy

PATIENT FILE

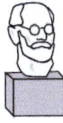

Psychotherapy moment
While the patient remains psychotic, supportive therapy is the most appropriate modality of treatment, with the goal of transitioning to cognitive behavioral work once his psychotic symptoms are fully controlled.

Attending physician's mental notes: initial visit
- This patient's psychotic symptoms and obsessive thoughts / compulsive behaviors have worsened over time, likely exacerbated by methamphetamine use, but this is not likely the sole cause. Despite a history of substance use, which could have led to his acute psychotic episode, he has endorsed a history of psychotic symptoms and obsessive–compulsive symptoms while he has been sober from all substances, making an acute substance-induced psychotic disorder unlikely as the etiology of his clinical presentation
- Given his prominent psychotic symptoms and the lack of evidence to suggest the presence of a comorbid active mood episode currently or previously, this patient's presentation is most consistent with schizophrenia. He experiences persistent perceptual disturbances, paranoid delusions, disorganized thought processes, and impaired self-care and daily functioning which are not attributable to a more likely alternative etiology
- This patient also meets criteria for pedophilia, mucophilia, and coprophilia as supported by at least 6 months of sexual interest in pre-pubescent children, mucus, and feces, respectively. His sexual interests and behaviors have led to impairment in his functioning
- He would initially benefit from discontinuing aripiprazole and starting an alternate antipsychotic medication, such as olanzapine, to target ongoing psychotic symptoms. Olanzapine has a potent dopamine blockade which is more likely to improve his psychotic symptoms in comparison to aripiprazole, which is a partial dopamine receptor antagonist
- Aripiprazole was subsequently discontinued for lack of improvement in his psychotic symptoms. Olanzapine was initiated to target ongoing psychosis due to potent dopamine receptor blockade
- Once his psychosis is well stabilized, cognitive behavioral therapy (CBT) would be an appropriate next step to treat his pedophilic disorder

PATIENT FILE

Case outcome: Interim follow-up visit at 6 months
- His psychotic symptoms have become less distressing, but remain a constant impairment in his daily functioning
- He continues to experience daily auditory hallucinations and delusions regarding "demons" being disguised as female staff in the hospital, whom he believes he should have sex with
- His anxiety remains high as he continues to have obsessive thoughts and compulsive behaviors which cause him stress
- He remains compliant with his medication, and he has not experienced significant side effects
- He remains isolative to his bedroom, not communicating with others or attending any groups

Attending physician's mental notes: first interim follow-up visit at 6 months
- Given the patient's ongoing CAHs and delusions that cause him distress and impair his daily functioning, he would benefit from titrating olanzapine to target ongoing prominent psychotic symptoms
- The patient continues to lack insight into his mental illness and the reality of his delusional thoughts. The patient is agreeable to increasing the dose of his antipsychotic
- He would benefit from initiating a selective serotonin reuptake inhibitor (SSRI) for treatment of anxiety related to obsessive thoughts, in addition to treatment of his paraphilic disorders
- Sertraline is started, with the plan to titrate the dose as indicated based on symptomatic response and tolerability
- Involvement in CBT for his pedophilic disorder is indicated, although the patient remains acutely psychotic, which impairs his ability to engage, concentrate, and benefit from treatment at this time. Will plan to revisit this approach once symptoms are further stabilized

Case outcome: interim follow-up visit at 2 years
- Sertraline was titrated to 200 mg daily due to minimal improvement in his anxiety surrounding the obsessive thoughts / compulsive behaviors. He continued to masturbate excessively, experience intrusive obsessive thoughts, and responded with compulsive behaviors to relieve the internal tension
- Olanzapine was titrated to a total of 60 mg daily, given ongoing auditory hallucinations and delusions of "demons." He continued to hold a false perception of reality and questioned female staff on the unit, paranoid that they were "demons"
- No side effects appreciated

PATIENT FILE

Attending physician's mental notes: interim follow-up visit at 2 years

- The patient has shown minimal treatment response in terms of his ongoing auditory hallucinations, delusions, and preoccupation with "demons." Will add haloperidol to olanzapine in attempts to further target undertreated psychotic symptoms
- The risks of prescribing dual antipsychotics are weighed against the benefits. Given the suboptimal treatment response thus far and no indication of the presence of side effects, will add haloperidol for further symptomatic control
- Will monitor for the development of side effects with regular blood and cardiac monitoring
- He exhibits minimal response to sertraline. Will cross-titrate this medication with an alternative SSRI, as it is standard to begin a trial with a different SSRI if an individual is not responsive or minimally responsive to the first SSRI that was initially tried

Case outcome: interim follow-up at 3 years

- The patient's psychotic symptoms have improved with the maximum dose of both dual antipsychotic medications, although not fully. Improvement has been observed in his ability to communicate his needs, and care for his hygiene, and he is socializing with others
- He continually experiences ongoing auditory hallucinations and delusions of sexual themes involving "demons" dressed as female staff. Psychosis is not fully treated with the dual antipsychotics
- Sertraline was cross-titrated to paroxetine due to poor tolerance of sertraline's side-effect profile and minimal symptomatic improvement. Paroxetine was eventually switched back to sertraline due to risk of ileus and his ongoing subjective complaint of anxiety in the context of the recurrent, intrusive thoughts
- He continues to have frequent sexual fantasies of pre-pubescent female children involving excitement in regard to mucus and feces
- Patient has not been able to fully participate in individualized therapy informed by sexual offender treatment guidelines due to his poor motivation and ongoing hallucinations

Attending physician's mental notes: interim follow-up visit at 3 years

- Patient's psychosis and obsessive/compulsive symptoms remain undertreated and resistant to multiple medications. Will need to consider specific therapies for treatment-resistant schizophrenia

PATIENT FILE

- Given the nature of the obsessive thoughts and compulsive behaviors that result in significant anxiety that has not fully improved, plan to closely observe pattern of symptomatic presentation of symptoms consistent with OCD in relation to his psychotic disorder. Consider adjusting medications at next visit

Case outcome: current presentation

- He continues to find it sexually arousing to fantasize about smearing feces on his genitals prior to sexual intercourse
- The patient continues to become sexually aroused at the thought of pre-pubescent girls gagging on his penis during oral sex and the thought of them sexually desiring him if his genitals are covered in feces
- He continues to hear voices, including those telling him to have sex with "the demons" that he believes are disguised as female staff at the hospital. Although the frequency of the auditory hallucinations has improved, they continue to occur daily and are impairing his functioning
- The patient denies visual, tactile, or gustatory hallucinations
- He continues to experience compulsive behaviors involving masturbating a certain number of times a day based on the specific day of the week. This is in an effort to relieve the internal tension caused by the obsessive thought of his genitals not functioning or being removed
- The patient continues to engage in compulsory behaviors such as brushing his teeth a specific number of times on each side of his mouth, due to the intrusive and obsessive thought that if he does not, his teeth will fall out
- He continues to compulsively wash his hair on each side of his head a specific number of times and in a certain fashion in response to the intrusive thought that his hair will fall out if he does not
- The obsessive thoughts and compulsive behaviors remain unprompted by CAHs
- He is aware of his obsessive thoughts and compulsive behaviors but feels that he is "unable to control them." He believes that if he cannot execute the compulsive behavior in response to the various intruding obsessive thoughts, his anxiety becomes unbearable, and nothing will alleviate the internal tension
- He denies depressive and manic/hypomanic symptoms. He has no current suicidal or homicidal ideations
- Despite being on the maximum dose of two antipsychotics, such as haloperidol and olanzapine, the patient continues to suffer from ongoing psychotic symptoms

PATIENT FILE

- He is compliant with 200 mg of daily sertraline, intended to treat his paraphilias and obsessive thoughts / compulsive behaviors. His treatment response has been minimal at best, with his symptoms continuing to cause him distress and interfere with his functioning

Attending physician's mental notes: current presentation

Diagnostic clarification of co-occurring psychosis and obsessive–compulsive symptoms

- Just as obsessions and compulsions are the main criteria for the diagnosis of OCD, the diagnosis itself or its symptoms are often co-occurring in primary psychotic disorders such as schizophrenia. Literature suggests that there is a "clinical entity proposed for those who show the dual diagnosis: the schizo-obsessive disorder." Although this is not an official diagnosis that is captured in the current DSM-5-TR, it provides a constructive way of thinking about the co-emergence of diagnoses that are distinct yet similar. The pharmacological treatment of these patients is challenging
- The patient's clinical presentation is significant for obsessive thoughts and compulsive behaviors dating back to his childhood and preceding his development of psychotic symptoms per documentation. Although his obsessions and compulsions can be described as related to his psychosis, he also meets the criteria for a diagnosis of OCD independently from his psychotic illness
- In these patients, obsessive–compulsive symptoms are commonly severe and tend to appear during the prodromal stages of psychosis; moreover, patients' insight into their obsessive–compulsive symptoms varies from mild to good, as it does in OCD alone. Compared to their schizophrenia counterparts, schizo-obsessive patients show earlier onset of psychosis, particularly in men; more depressive symptoms and suicide attempts; increased rates of hospitalization; greater dysfunction; higher impairment in social behavior; smaller social networks; and poorer quality of life. Furthermore, these patients tend to be more socially hostile and more anxious, as evidenced by their greater number of panic attacks
- Given that this patient meets criteria for the dual clinical diagnoses of OCD and schizophrenia, his presentation is consistent with the diagnosis of schizo-obsessive disorder

Case debrief

Although this patient's obsessions and compulsions can be described as related to his psychosis, he also meets the diagnostic criteria for a diagnosis of OCD independently from his psychotic illness.

PATIENT FILE

Neither his psychotic nor obsessive–compulsive symptoms have fully remitted despite multiple trials of different antipsychotic and SSRI medications, preventing his progression to remission. Full symptomatic control of the psychotic and obsessive–compulsive symptoms is an appropriate goal to strive for and will require medication adjustments over time.

Given his treatment-resistant psychosis and OCD, clozapine is considered the first-line treatment option if he can tolerate regular blood monitoring. It is appropriate to consider neurosurgical intervention as a potential treatment option if he continues to fail to show significant symptomatic improvement despite initiation of clozapine.

Take-home points

- One must consider the similarities and differences in symptoms and presentations of schizophrenia and OCD, as this can inform treatment for co-occurring disorders
- Contemporary studies have documented a much higher prevalence of obsessive–compulsive symptoms (OCS) in schizophrenia than previously thought, with rates reaching 25% for OCS and 12% for comorbid OCD
- First-line treatment for both psychotic and obsessive/compulsive symptoms (related to themes of sexuality, theft, arson, etc.) is clozapine in patients suffering with schizo-obessesive disorder. Clozapine is indicated until full symptom control is achieved, or the patient reaches optimal plasma levels
- It is appropriate to consider neurosurgical intervention as a potential treatment option if a patient continues to fail to show significant symptomatic improvement despite initiation of clozapine. Notably, DBS for treatment of OCD is highly successful. Patients with OCD treated by DBS typically report that not only compulsions, but the obsessions underlying them, resolve. Given the close association of OCD symptoms with psychosis in schizo-obsessive disorder, treating OCD symptoms by neurosurgical intervention may address treatment-resistant psychosis

Performance in practice: confessions of a psychopharmacologist

What could have been done better here?

- As mentioned previously, a thorough evaluation that allows for timely and accurate diagnoses helps inform clinical treatment
- Assessing for symptoms of obsessive thought and compulsive behaviors in a co-occurring psychotic illness will prevent diagnostic

PATIENT FILE

delay of schizo-obsessive disorder. Given that the first-line treatment for this disorder is clozapine, the provider can avoid prescribing less effective alternatives and dual antipsychotics and treat the patient with a medication which could provide faster and more effective results

Tips and pearls
- Provisional diagnostic criteria for diagnosing schizo-obsessive disorder
  - Symptoms of OCS are present that meet Criterion A for OCD at some time point during the course of the schizophrenia
  - If the content of the obsessions and/or compulsions is interrelated with the content of delusions and/or hallucinations (e.g., compulsive hand washing due to CAHs), additional typical OCD symptoms that are recognized by the person as unreasonable and excessive are required
  - Symptoms of OCD are present for a substantial portion of the total duration of the prodromal, active, and/or residual period of schizophrenia
  - The obsessions and compulsions are time-consuming (more than 1 hour per day), cause distress, or significantly interfere with the person's normal routine, in addition to the functional impairment associated with schizophrenia
  - The obsessions and compulsions in the patient with schizophrenia are not due to the direct effect of antipsychotic agents, substance abuse, or organic factors
  - Although his anxiety has minimally improved, this patient is experiencing ongoing severe psychotic symptoms that have not improved with aripiprazole, an antipsychotic medication. This was the first antipsychotic medication known to be prescribed to treat his psychotic symptoms, which has been ineffective after months of medication compliance
- If clozapine is initiated for the treatment of schizo-obsessive disorder, a slow titration is necessary initially due to significant anticholinergic effects. Given the significant anticholinergic effects of antipsychotic medications the patient is prescribed, a robust and progressive constipation protocol must be initiated and maintained
- Standard monitoring of the patient's clozapine plasma level, as well as the absolute neutrophil count (ANC), will be required regularly and documented in the online REMS database, unless this monitoring system is eventually discontinued
- If clozapine does not result in clinical improvement or shows subtherapeutic results, it is appropriate to consider neurosurgical intervention for treatment-resistant schizo-obsessive disorder

PATIENT FILE

Two-minute Tutorial

Psychopharmacological treatment options for co-occurring disorders, such as schizo-obsessive disorder

Clozapine has been established as the first-line treatment for both psychotic and obsessive–compulsive symptoms in patients suffering with schizo-obessessive disorder. The literature suggests that clozapine may paradoxically heighten anxious and obsessive–compulsive symptoms, although this is dose related.

- Clozapine is indicated until full symptom control is achieved, or he reaches optimal plasma levels
- Given the patient's resistance to pharmacological treatment thus far, it is appropriate to consider neurosurgical intervention as a potential treatment option if he continues to fail to show significant symptomatic improvement despite initiation of clozapine
- Recent scientific literature points to neurosurgical interventions for the management of treatment-resistant schizo-obsessive disorder. In a recent publication authored in 2019, Howard notes:

Notably, deep brain stimulation (DBS) for treatment of OCD is highly successful. OCD patients treated by DBS typically report that not only compulsions but the obsessions underlying them resolve. Given the intertwined nature of OCD symptoms with psychosis in schizo-obsessive disorder, treating OCD symptoms may address psychosis. This interrelated treatment of symptomatology relies on the neuroanatomy of schizo-obsessive disorder combining neuroanatomy of OCD and schizophrenia. This is supported by functional neuroimaging demonstrating hallucinations and delusions share a network with obsessions in schizo-obsessive disorder. To determine if OCD DBS may be adapted to schizo-obsessive disorder, further research is necessary. The similarity between OCD and schizophrenia DBS targets in schizo-obsessive disorder must be assessed.

Post-test question

What is the first-line treatment for a patient with comorbid treatment-resistant schizophrenia and obsessive–compulsive disorder (OCD) (schizo-obsessive disorder)?

A. Sertraline + olanzapine
B. Haloperidol
C. Clozapine
D. Electroconvulsive therapy (ECT)

Answer: C

PATIENT FILE

References

1. Howard, C. (2019). Schizo-obsessive disorder and neurosurgery for schizophrenia. *BMJ Case Reports*, 12(11), e232462. https://doi.org/10.1136/bcr-2019-232462.
2. Poyurovsky, M., Zohar, J., Glick, I., et al. (2012). Obsessive–compulsive symptoms in schizophrenia: implications for future psychiatric classifications. *Comprehensive Psychiatry*, 53(5), 480–483.
3. Reznik, I., Yavin, I., Stryjer, R., et al. (2004). Clozapine in the treatment of obsessive–compulsive symptoms in schizophrenia patients: a case series study. *Pharmacopsychiatry*, 37(2), 52–56. https://doi.org/10.1055/s-2004-815525.
4. Scotti-Muzzi, E. & Saide, O. (2017). Schizo-obsessive spectrum disorders: an update. *CNS Spectrums*, 22(3), 258–272. https://doi.org/10.1017/S1092852916000390.

Case Studies: Index

addiction *see* alcohol use disorder; substance use disorders
ADHD *see* attention deficit/hyperactivity disorder
adjunctive therapy, psychotic aggression 7–8, 11, 13
affective aggression *see* impulsive affective aggression
affective arousal, self-injurious behavior 58
aggression, definition 22, 34; *see also* impulsive affective aggression; psychotic aggression; self-injurious behavior and aggression; violence
alcohol use disorder
    post-psychotic depression 145–146
    primary polydipsia 97, 101
    psychotic aggression 3–4
    treatment planning and options 213, 214
alogia 134, 176, 177, 180, 181, 206, 312; *see also* negative symptoms
amygdala, impulsive affective aggression 24
anhedonia 132, 134, 148, 176, 177, 206; *see also* negative symptoms
anorexia *see* fasting (prolonged)
antidepressants; *see also* drug index
    obsessive–compulsive disorder 240
    post-psychotic depression 155
    sex offending 331, 339, 341
antipsychotics; *see also* drug index
    catatonia 168
    mechanisms of action 238
    mortality rates 94, 167, 225, 277
    neuroleptic malignant syndrome 163, 165–166
    pregnancy 343, 344, 347
    side-effects *see* myocarditis *and see below*
    trimester of pregnancy 343
antipsychotics, side effects of treatment in treatment-resistant schizophrenia 171–172
    case debrief 179–180
    case outcomes 175, 176, 178

constipation 176
further investigations 174, 176, 177, 179
initial evaluation 171–172
medical history 172
medication history and current 173
mechanisms of action 173–174
negative symptoms 177, 182
physician's notes 174, 175, 177, 178
psychiatric history 172
psychopharmacology dilemmas 171
psychotherapy history 173
reflections on clinical practice 181
self-assessment questions 171, 183
social and personal history 172
take-home points 180
tips and pearls 181–182
two-minute tutorial 182–183
antisocial personality disorder (ASPD)
    primary polydipsia 97, 108
    substance use disorders 202
antisocial traits
    non-suicidal self-injury 51, 56
    predatory violence 33, 34
anxiety disorders and comorbidities 259–260
    case debrief 253–254
    case outcomes 253
    comorbidity 258–260, 261–263, 264–265, 266
    current presentation 250
    etiology 255–258
    family history 249
    further investigations 253
    incidence and prevalence 265
    initial evaluation 247
    medical history 249
    medication mechanisms of action 253
    physician's notes 252
    prognosis 260
    psychiatric history 248
    psychopharmacology dilemmas 247
    psychotherapy history 253
    reflections on clinical practice 261–263

anxiety disorders and comorbidities (cont.)
  self-assessment questions 247, 268
  social and personal history 249
  substance use 248
  take-home points 255–261
  tips and pearls 263–265
  treatment planning and options 266
  two-minute tutorial 265–268
arson, SCZ–OCD 235
asociality 132; see also negative symptoms
ASPD see antisocial personality disorder
attention deficit/hyperactivity disorder (ADHD)
  anxiety disorders 247
  traumatic brain injury/encephalopathy comorbid with psychosis 192
auditory hallucinations see hearing voices
autonomic instability
  antipsychotics 163, 165–166
  differential diagnoses 161
  treatment planning and options 164
avolition 132; see also negative symptoms

basal ganglia, calcification 296, 301–302; see also Fahr's disease
benzodiazepines; see also drug index
  catatonia 120, 121–122, 123, 168
  mechanisms of action 164, 291
  neuroleptic malignant syndrome 166
  psychotic aggression 3–4
BFCRS (Bush-Francis Catatonia Rating Scale) 119, 127–128
blunted affect 134; see also negative symptoms
borderline intellectual functioning, impulsive affective aggression 17; see also cognitive impairment
borderline personality disorder
  non-suicidal self-injury 51, 56
  self-injurious behaviors 44
  suicidality 73, 75–76, 79, 80, 81
  two-minute tutorial 80–81
borderline personality disorder with comorbidities
  case debrief 228
  case outcomes 225, 226, 227
  ECT 222–223, 226–227
  family history 220
  further investigations 224–225, 226, 228
  initial evaluation 219
  medical history 220

  medication history and current 220–221
  medication mechanisms of action 221–222
  physician's notes 223–224, 225–228
  psychiatric history 219–220
  psychopharmacology dilemmas 219
  psychotherapy history 221
  reflections on clinical practice 229–230
  self-assessment questions 219, 232
  social and personal history 220
  take-home points 228–229
  tips and pearls 230
  treatment planning and options 219
  two-minute tutorial 230–231
bottom up aggression 22
Bush-Francis Catatonia Rating Scale (BFCRS) 119, 127–128

calcification, basal ganglia 296, 301–302; see also Fahr's disease
calcium deposits, Fahr's disease 300
cannabis 214
  psychotic aggression 3–4
capacity
  evaluation 180
  and insight 174
  targeting symptoms impacting 171, 174; see also antipsychotics, side effects of treatment
Capgras syndrome 88, 93
catalepsy 120, 167, 168
catatonia
  case debrief 124
  case outcomes 119, 120, 121–122, 123, 124
  current presentation 118
  diagnosis 126, 127–128, 167–168
  differential diagnoses 161, 166
  etiology 166, 168
  family history 118
  further investigations 121, 122
  incidence and prevalence 168
  initial evaluation 117
  medical history 118
  medication history and current 118
  medication mechanisms of action 119
  neurological mechanisms 125
  physician's notes 119, 120, 121, 122
  psychiatric history 117
  psychopharmacology dilemma 117
  question 118

reflections on clinical practice 118–119, 125
risk factors 126
self-assessment questions 117, 129
social and personal history 118
take-home points 124–125
tips and pearls 126
treatment planning and options 119, 120, 123, 127–129, 166, 168
two-minute tutorial 126–127
CBT *see* cognitive behavioral therapy
childhood adverse events, self-injurious behavior 44, 58
chronic traumatic encephalopathy (CTE) *see* traumatic brain injury/encephalopathy comorbid with psychosis
cigarette smoking *see* nicotine use disorder
civil commitment 318, 324, 326
cognitive behavioral therapy (CBT)
    post-psychotic depression 155
    self-injurious behavior 60
    sex offending 331
cognitive impairment
    impulsive affective aggression 24, 25
    psychotic aggression 7
    self-injurious behaviors 45
combination regimens
    non-suicidal self-injury 51
    psychotic aggression 47
comorbidity *see* co-occurring disorders
competence to stand trial
    prolonged fasting case 65, 68, 69
    schizophrenia 271, 277
competency
    definition 316
    legal 318
    restoration to 317
Competency Assessment Instrument-Revised 69
constipation, and antipsychotic use 105, 176, 178, 180, 182
co-occurring disorders *see* mood disorders comorbid with borderline personality disorder; post-traumatic stress disorder comorbid with personality disorder; schizophrenia comorbid with obsessive–compulsive disorder; traumatic brain injury/encephalopathy comorbid with psychosis
coping strategies, and self-injurious behavior 58, 59

COVID-19, as trigger for depression/anxiety 228; *see also* myocarditis
CPK (creatine phosphokinase), neuroleptic malignant syndrome 163, 164–165
criminal offending, anxiety disorders comorbid with substance use 265
critical care, neuroleptic malignant syndrome 163, 165
cutting 44; *see also* self-injurious behavior

dangerousness 318, 319
dangerousness to self (DTS) 46; *see also* self-injurious behavior
DBT *see* dialectical behavior therapy
definitions
    aggression 22, 34
    competency 316
    grave disability 318
    violence 22–23, 34
delirium, catatonia 167
delusional disorder, predatory violence 29
delusions; *see also* hearing voices
    prolonged fasting case 65, 67, 70–71
    self-injurious behavior 43–44, 45, 46
depressive symptoms; *see also* post-psychotic depression
    comorbid with borderline personality disorder 219
    schizoaffective disorder 177
    substance use disorders 202, 214–215
diabetes insipidus, primary polydipsia 110–111
dialectical behavior therapy (DBT)
    borderline personality disorder 221
    primary polydipsia 108
    self-injurious behavior 60
dopaminergic pathways, impulsive affective aggression 24
dorsomedial prefrontal cortex, anxiety disorders 261
Dusky v. U.S. legal case (1960) 316

eating disorders *see* fasting (prolonged)
echolalia/echopraxia, catatonia 124–125
electroconvulsive therapy (ECT)
    borderline personality disorder 220, 222–223, 226–227
    catatonia 119, 122, 123, 168
    incompetence to stand trial 320–326
    mechanisms of action 195, 222–223

electroconvulsive therapy (ECT) (cont.)
  negative symptoms of schizophrenia 136
  post-psychotic depression 139, 145–146, 155
  primary polydipsia 106, 109
  psychotic aggression 8, 9, 10, 13
  schizoaffective disorder 177
  self-injurious behavior 45, 47, 48
  traumatic brain injury/encephalopathy
    comorbid with psychosis 195, 196–197
  treatment-resistant schizophrenia 8, 178
emotional dysregulation
  impulsive affective aggression 17, 20
  personality disorders 224
  self-injurious behavior 52, 58
encephalopathy *see* traumatic brain injury/
  encephalopathy comorbid with psychosis

Fahr's disease, psychiatric manifestations
  case debrief 295–296
  case outcomes 295
  current presentation 291
  etiology 301–302
  further investigations 293–294
  genetics 296–298
  imaging 300
  initial evaluation 289
  medical history 290
  medication history and current 291, 293–294
  medication mechanisms of action 291–292
  physician's notes 291
  psychiatric history 289–290
  psychopharmacology dilemmas 289
  reflections on clinical practice 303
  self-assessment questions 289, 306
  social and personal history 290
  symptoms 298–299
  take-home points 296–303
  tips and pearls 304–305
  treatment planning and options 300–301
  two-minute tutorial 305
fasting, prolonged
  case debrief 69
  case outcomes 68–69
  current presentation 67
  family history 66
  further investigations 67–68
  initial evaluation 65
  medical history 66

medication history and current 66–67
medication mechanisms of action 67
physician's notes 67, 68
psychiatric history 65–66
psychopharmacology dilemma 65
psychotherapy history 67
reflections on clinical practice 70
self-assessment questions 65, 71
social and personal history 66
take-home points 69
tips and pearls 70
treatment planning and options 67–68
two-minute tutorial 70–71
felony charges 145, 247, 253, 309
fetus, effect of antipsychotics 345, 346, 347–348; *see also* pregnancy
flat effect 134; *see also* negative symptoms
forensic criteria, predatory violence 34–35
Fregoli syndrome 88, 93
functional somatic disorders (FSD) 262–263

Georgia Court Competency Test 69
gestation, psychosis in *see* pregnancy
gold standard treatments, impulsive affective aggression 17
grave disability 318

hallucinations, self-injurious behaviors 43–44;
  see also hearing voices
head-banging, self-injurious behaviors 44
hearing voices
  misidentification syndromes 88
  obsessive compulsive disorder 239
  schizoaffective disorder 171–172
  self-injurious behavior 43–44
  suicidality 75–76, 77
heavy metal exposure, primary polydipsia 101
hemodynamic instability, neuroleptic malignant
  syndrome 163, 165–166
Historic Clinical Risk Management 20 (HCR-20) 59
hormonal treatment, sex offending 331
hyponatremia, primary polydipsia 99, 106, 109–110

impulsive affective aggression
  case debrief 22
  case outcomes 21
  current presentation 18–19

further investigations 20–21
initial evaluations 17
medical history 18
medication history and current 18
medication mechanisms of action 19–20
physician's notes 20
psychiatric history 17–18
psychopharmacology dilemma 17
reflections on clinical practice 23
self-assessment questions 17, 26
social and personal history 18
take-home points 22–23
tips and pearls 23–25
two-minute tutorial 25–26
impulsive aggression, neurological disorders 289; see also Fahr's disease
impulsive predatory violence 29
incidence and prevalence
  anxiety disorders 265
  catatonia 168
  myocarditis 279
  post-psychotic depression 153, 155
  predatory violence 34
  self-injurious behavior 57, 58
  suicidality 80
incompetent to stand trial (IST)
  case debrief 316
  case outcomes 314–315
  current presentation 312
  ECT 320–326
  family history 311
  further investigations 313
  initial evaluation 309
  medical history 311
  medication history and current 311
  medication mechanisms of action 313–314
  physician's notes 312
  psychiatric history 309–310
  psychopharmacology dilemmas 309
  reflections on clinical practice 324
  self-assessment questions 309, 326
  social and personal history 310–311
  substance use 311
  take-home points 316–319
  tips and pearls 320–324
  two-minute tutorial 324–326
informed consent 325
insertion of foreign bodies, impulsive affective aggression 18

insight
  and capacity 174
  post-psychotic depression 151, 153
intellectual disability, impulsive affective aggression 24, 25
intermittent explosive disorder 56
IQ score, substance use disorders 202

Jackson v. Indiana legal case (1972) 318

Lanterman–Petris–Short Act (1967) 318
lead exposure, primary polydipsia 101
legal considerations, sex offending 335–336
lenticulostriatal pathway, Fahr's disease 296
lithium-induced primary polydipsia 111
long COVID. see myocarditis, risks from clozapine and COVID-19
lorazepam challenge, catatonia 126

malignant catatonia see catatonia
medication compliance
  borderline personality disorder 224
  pregnancy 345, 347–348
  substance use disorders 206, 208, 211, 214
Mental Status Examination (MSE)
  primary polydipsia 98
  psychotic aggression 3–4, 7
methamphetamines, substance use disorders 205; see also stimulant-methamphetamine type use disorder
mindfulness, post-psychotic depression 152
misidentification syndromes (MID)
  case debrief 91–92
  case outcomes 89–90, 91
  current presentation 88
  family history 87
  further investigations 88, 91
  initial evaluation 85
  medical history 87
  medication history and current 87, 94–95
  medication mechanisms of action 88, 92–93
  monitoring regimes 89
  physician's notes 88, 89, 90–91
  psychiatric history 86
  psychopharmacology dilemma 85
  psychotherapy history 87
  reflections on clinical practice 92–93
  self-assessment questions 85, 95
  social and personal history 87

misidentification syndromes (MID) (cont.)
    take-home points 92
    tips and pearls 93
    treatment planning and options 90
    two-minute tutorial 93–94
mood disorders comorbid with borderline
    personality disorder 223–224
mortality rates
    antipsychotics 94, 167, 225
    myocarditis 280
    schizophrenia 277
Murphy conservatorship (MurCon) 319
mutism 118, 120, 124–125, 167, 168
myocarditis 12
myocarditis, risks from clozapine and
    COVID-19 271, 277–281
    case debrief 276–277
    clozapine-associated 12, 271, 272, 273, 276,
        277–281
    COVID-19 associated 278–280
    current presentation 273–274
    family history 273
    further investigations 275
    incidence and prevalence 279
    initial evaluation 271
    medical history 273
    medication history and current 272, 273, 276
    medication mechanisms of action 274–275
    physician's notes 275, 276
    psychiatric history 272
    psychopharmacology dilemmas 271
    reflections on clinical practice 282
    self-assessment questions 271, 285–286
    social and personal history 272
    substance use 273
    take-home points 277–281
    tips and pearls 283–284
    two-minute tutorial 284–285

negative symptoms; *see also* antipsychotics
    (side-effects of treatment); schizophrenia
    (managing negative symptoms)
    schizoaffective disorder 171, 177, 182
    substance use disorders 214–215
negativism, catatonia 124–125
nephrogenic diabetes insipidus, primary
    polydipsia 110–111
neurocognitive deficits, somatic symptom
    disorder 260–261

neurocognitive disorder, predatory violence 29
neurocognitive disorder due to traumatic brain
    injury 192. *see also* traumatic brain injury/
    encephalopathy comorbid with psychosis
neuroleptic malignant syndrome (NMS)
    case debrief 165
    case outcomes 163, 164–165
    current presentation 162
    differential diagnoses 161, 166
    etiology 166
    family history 162
    further investigations 163–164
    initial evaluation 161
    medical history 162
    medication history and current 162, 166
    medication mechanisms of action 164
    physician's notes 163, 164, 165
    psychiatric history 161–162
    psychopharmacology dilemma 161
    reflections on clinical practice 166
    self-assessment questions 161, 168
    social and personal history 162
    take-home points 165–166
    tips and pearls 166
    treatment planning and options 163–164,
        166
    two-minute tutorial 167–168
neurological disorders *see* Fahr's disease
neutropenia, clozapine 94–95
nicotine use disorder, treatment planning and
    options 213, 214
NMS *see* neuroleptic malignant syndrome
non-suicidal self-injury (NSSI); *see also* self-
    injurious behavior
    borderline personality disorder 219–220
    case debrief 56–57
    case outcome 56
    current presentation 53
    family history 53
    further investigations 55–56
    initial evaluations 51
    medical history 53
    medication history and current 53
    medication mechanisms of action 54
    obsessive compulsive disorder 236
    physician's notes 55
    psychiatric history 52
    psychopharmacology dilemma 51
    reflections on clinical practice 60

self-assessment questions 51, 62
social and personal history 52
substance use history 52
take-home points 57–60
tips and pearls 60
treatment planning and options 59–60
two-minute tutorial 61
Not Guilty By Reason of Insanity (NGBRI/NGRI) 235
  anxiety disorders 247
  post-psychotic depression 139, 145

obsessive–compulsive disorder with schizo-obsessive disorder (two separate cases) 235, 241
  antipsychotics 238, 244
  case debrief 240, 357–358
  case outcomes 239, 240, 354–356
  current presentation 237, 356–357
  diagnosis 357
  differential diagnoses 242–243
  family history 349
  further investigations 239, 240
  initial evaluation 235, 349–350
  medical history 237, 349
  medication history and current 237, 349
  non-suicidal self-injury 236
  physician's notes 238, 240, 353, 357
  psychiatric history 235–236, 349
  psychopharmacology dilemmas 235, 349
  psychotherapy history 238, 357
  reflections on clinical practice 241, 358–359
  self-assessment questions 235, 244, 349, 360
  social and personal history 236–237, 349
  substance use disorders 236
  take-home points 240–241, 358
  tips and pearls 242, 359
  treatment planning and options 241, 358
  two-minute tutorial 242–244, 358
opioid addiction, treatment planning and options 213, 214; see also substance use disorders
opioid receptors 204
overgeneralized memory, post-psychotic depression 151–152
oxytocin, and negative symptoms of schizophrenia 132, 133, 134

paranoia, schizoaffective disorder 171–172
paraphilias 338, 357
PCL-R (Psychopathy Checklist Revised) 35–36
pedophilic disorder, diagnostic criteria 338
perinatal psychiatry see pregnancy
personality disorders; see also borderline personality disorder
  comorbid with anxiety disorders 259–260, 266
  impulsive affective aggression 17
polydipsia see primary polydipsia
polypharmacy, personality disorders 220–221
post-acute recovery phase, psychosis
post-psychotic depression
  case debrief 145–146
  case outcomes 144–145
  current presentation 141
  diagnostic definition 153, 154–155
  differential diagnoses 148–149
  etiology 153–154
  family history 141
  further investigations 144
  incidence and prevalence 153, 155
  initial evaluation 139
  medical history 140–141
  medication history and current 140, 143, 145
  medication mechanisms of action 141–143
  physician's notes 144
  post-acute recovery phase 151
  psychiatric history 140
  psychopharmacology dilemma 139
  reflections on clinical practice 149–150
  self-assessment questions 139, 156
  social and personal history 140
  take-home points 146–149
  tips and pearls 150–154
  treatment planning and options 149, 155
  two-minute tutorial 154–155
post-traumatic stress disorder (PTSD)
  comorbid with personality disorder 219, 224
  symptoms 220
predatory violence 31
  case debrief 34
  case outcomes 34
  classification of types 22–25
  current presentation 32
  forensic criteria 34–35
  further investigations 32–33, 34

predatory violence (cont.)
  incidence and prevalence 34
  medical history 31
  medication history and current 32, 36–37
  medication mechanisms of action 32
  physician's notes 32, 33
  psychiatric history 30–31
  psychopharmacology dilemma 29
  reflections on clinical practice 37–38
  risk assessments 35–37
  self-assessment questions 29, 40
  social and personal history 31
  substance use disorder 29, 31
  take-home points 34–37
  tips and pearls 38–39
  treatment planning and options 35–37
  two-minute tutorial 39–40
prefrontal cortex, impulsive affective aggression 23
pregnancy, mental illness in
  case debrief 346
  case outcomes 345–346
  current presentation 343, 344–345
  further investigations 345–346
  initial evaluation 343
  medication compliance 345, 347–348
  medication history and current 344
  medication mechanisms of action 345
  physician's notes 345
  psychiatric history 343
  psychopharmacology dilemmas 343
  reflections on clinical practice 347
  self-assessment questions 343
  social and personal history 344
  take-home points 347
  tips and pearls 347
  treatment planning and options 346
  two-minute tutorial 347–348
prevalence *see* incidence and prevalence
primary polydipsia
  case debrief 106–107
  case outcomes 101–102, 103, 105
  comorbidities 110–111
  complications 109–110
  family history 99
  further investigations 101, 103, 104–105
  initial evaluation 97–98
  lithium-induced 111
  medical history 99

medication history and current 99–100, 103, 105, 108
medication mechanisms of action 100
Mental status examination 98
physician's notes 100–101, 102–103, 104, 106
psychiatric history 98
psychopharmacology dilemma 97
psychotherapy history 100
reflections on clinical practice 107–108
risk factors 108–109
self-assessment questions 97, 111
social and personal history 98–99
take-home points 107
treatment planning and options 98, 103
treatment planning and options and options 109
two-minute tutorial 109–111
prolonged fasting *see* fasting, prolonged
psychogenic polydipsia *see* primary polydipsia
psychopathy, predatory violence 33, 34
Psychopathy Checklist Revised (PCL-R) 35–36
psychopharmacology dilemmas
  anxiety disorders 247
  borderline personality disorder 219
  catatonia 117
  clozapine-resistant schizoaffective disorder bipolar type 43
  constipation secondary to antipsychotics 171
  Fahr's disease 289
  impulsive affective aggression 17
  incompetence to stand trial 309
  misidentification syndromes 85
  myocarditis, risks from clozapine and COVID-19 271
  negative symptoms of schizophrenia 131
  neuroleptic malignant syndrome 161
  obsessive–compulsive disorder 235
  post-psychotic depression 139
  predatory violence 29
  pregnancy 343
  primary polydipsia 97
  prolonged fasting 65
  SCZ–OCD 349
  self-injurious behaviors 51
  sex offending 329

substance use disorders 201
suicidality, severe 73
traumatic brain injury/encephalopathy comorbid with psychosis 189
psychosis; *see also* post-psychotic depression; psychotic aggression; schizophrenia; traumatic brain injury/encephalopathy comorbid with psychosis
  catatonia 117, 119
  differential diagnoses 242
  misidentification syndromes 86, 88
  myocarditis, risks from clozapine and COVID-19 275
  prolonged fasting case 67, 70–71
  schizo-obsessive disorder 235–236
  side-effects of medication 248
  substance-induced psychoses 205
  substance use disorders 201–202, 214
  trimester of pregnancy 343
psychotic aggression
  case debrief 10
  case outcomes 7, 8–9
  further investigations 7, 8, 10
  initial evaluations 3–4
  medical history 4–5
  medication history and current 5, 6
  medication mechanisms of action 6
  Mental status examination 3–4, 7
  physician's notes 6, 7–8, 9–10
  psychiatric history 4
  psychotherapy 6
  reflections on clinical practice 11
  self-assessment questions 3, 13
  social and personal history 4
  take-home points 10
  tips and pearls 11–12
  two-minute tutorial 13
psychotic violence, classification of types 22–25; *see also* psychotic aggression
PTSD *see* post-traumatic stress disorder

reality testing 31
recovery, psychosis caused by substance use 205
risk assessments
  sex offending 331
  violence 35–36, 37
risk of death *see* mortality rates
rule breaking 103

schizoaffective disorder, non-suicidal self-injury 51
schizo-obsessive disorder *see* obsessive–compulsive disorder with schizo-obsessive disorder
schizophrenia; *see also* treatment-resistant schizophrenia
  competence to stand trial 271
  mortality risks 277
  myocarditis 271
  post-psychotic depression 145–148
  primary polydipsia 97, 101
  psychotic aggression 3–4
  two-minute tutorial 243–244
schizophrenia, managing negative symptoms 133
  case debrief 134
  current presentation 132
  family history 132
  further investigations 134
  initial evaluation 131
  medical history 132
  medication history and current 132, 133–134
  physician's notes 133–134
  psychiatric history 131–132
  psychopharmacology dilemma 131
  psychotherapy history 133
  reflections on clinical practice 135
  self-assessment questions 131
  social and personal history 132
  take-home points 134–135
  tips and pearls 135
  two-minute tutorial 135–136
schizophrenia spectrum disorder, impulsive affective aggression 17
SCZ–OCD *see* obsessive–compulsive disorder with schizo-obsessive disorder
seizures
  clozapine 91
  primary polydipsia 99, 106
selective serotonin reuptake inhibitors (SSRI)
  obsessive–compulsive disorder 240
  primary polydipsia 102, 103
  sex offending 331, 339, 341
self-assessment questions
  anxiety disorders 247
  borderline personality disorder 219, 232
  catatonia 117, 129

self-assessment questions (cont.)
constipation secondary to antipsychotics 171
Fahr's disease 289
Fahr's disease, psychiatric manifestations 306
impulsive affective aggression 17, 26
incompetence to stand trial 309, 326
misidentification syndromes 85, 95
myocarditis, risks from clozapine and COVID-19 271, 285–286
negative symptoms of schizophrenia 131
neuroleptic malignant syndrome 161, 168
non-suicidal self-injury 51, 62
obsessive–compulsive disorder with schizo-obsessive disorder 235, 244, 360
post-psychotic depression 139, 156
predatory violence 29, 40
pregnancy 343
primary polydipsia 97, 111
prolonged fasting case 65, 71
psychotic aggression 3, 13
schizoaffective disorder 183
SCZ–OCD 349
self-injurious behavior 43
sex offending 329
substance use disorders 201, 215
suicidality 73, 81
traumatic brain injury/encephalopathy comorbid with psychosis 189, 199
self-compassion, post-psychotic depression 152
self-injurious behavior (SIB); see also non-suicidal self-injury; suicidality
definition 57
incidence and prevalence 57
substance use disorders 202
types 57
self-injurious behavior and aggression
case debrief 46
case outcomes 46
current presentation 44–45
ECT mechanisms of action 45
family history 44
further investigations 46
initial evaluations 43
medical history 44
medication history and current 44
physician's notes 45–46

psychiatric history 43–44
psychopharmacology dilemma 43
psychotherapy 45
reflections on clinical practice 47
self-assessment questions 43
social and personal history 44
take-home points 47
tips and pearls 47
two-minute tutorial 48
self starvation see fasting, prolonged
serotoninergic pathways, impulsive affective aggression 24
sex offending see sexually violent predators
sexual violence risk assessment (SVRA) 331
sexually violent predators (SVPs)
case debrief 334–335
case outcomes 332–333, 334, 335
current presentation 331
family history 330
initial evaluation 329
medication history and current 331, 335
medication mechanisms of action 333
physician's notes 333–334
psychiatric history 329
psychological interventions 331–332
psychopharmacology dilemmas 329
psychotherapy history 332–333
reflections on clinical practice 335–337
relational and sexual history 330
risk assessments 331
self-assessment questions 329
social and personal history 329–330
take-home points 335
tips and pearls 337–338
treatment planning and options 331, 336–337
two-minute tutorial 338–341
SIADH see syndrome of inappropriate antidiuretic hormone secretion
sialorrhea, primary polydipsia 105
SIB see self-injurious behavior
smoking see nicotine use disorder
sodium imbalance, primary polydipsia 99, 106, 109–110
somatic symptom disorder 260–261
specific gravity, primary polydipsia 98
SSRIs see selective serotonin reuptake inhibitors
starvation see fasting, prolonged

stimulant-methamphetamine type use disorder
  impulsive affective aggression 17
  non-suicidal self-injury 51, 56
subjective doubles, misidentification
  syndromes 93
substance use
  and anxiety disorders 248, 264–265
  incompetence to stand trial 311
  myocarditis 273
  non-suicidal self-injury 52
  self-injurious behavior 57
substance use disorders (SUD)
  case debrief 210
  case outcomes 206, 207–208, 209
  comorbid with borderline personality
    disorder 220
  family history 203
  further investigations 206, 207, 208–209,
    210
  initial evaluation 201
  medical history 203
  medication compliance 206, 208, 211, 214
  medication dosing conventions 211–212
  medication history and current 203–204, 205
  medication mechanisms of action 212
  obsessive compulsive disorder 236
  opioid receptors 204
  physician's notes 205, 206–207, 208, 209
  predatory violence 29, 31
  psychiatric history 201–203
  psychopharmacology dilemmas 201
  psychotherapy history 204
  reflections on clinical practice 211–212
  self-assessment questions 201, 215
  social and personal history 203
  substance-induced psychoses 205
  take-home points 210–211
  tips and pearls 213–214
  treatment planning and options 201, 213, 214
  two-minute tutorial 214–215
substance-induced anxiety enhancement
  theory 263
suicidality
  case debrief 79
  case outcomes 77–79
  current presentation 75–76
  family history 74
  further investigations 77
  initial evaluation 73

medical history 74
medication history and current 75, 76, 78
medication mechanisms of action 76
physician's notes 76, 78
psychiatric history 73–74
psychopharmacology dilemma 73
psychotherapy history 76
reflections on clinical practice 78
role of medication 80
self-assessment questions 73, 81
social and personal history 74
substance use disorders 202
take-home points 79
tips and pearls 80
treatment planning and options 77
two-minute tutorial 80–81
surrogacy, incompetence to stand trial 325
SVPs *see* sexually violent predators
syndrome of inappropriate antidiuretic
  hormone secretion (SIADH), primary
  polydipsia 102, 103

temporal lobe, impulsive affective aggression
  24
thirst *see* primary polydipsia
thromboembolism 271
tobacco use *see* nicotine use disorder
top down aggression 22
transcranial magnetic stimulation,
  schizophrenia 136
trauma, and personality disorders 224; *see also*
  post-traumatic stress disorder
traumatic brain injury, predatory violence 29
traumatic brain injury/encephalopathy
  comorbid with psychosis
  case debrief 195–196
  case outcomes 192, 193, 194–195
  current presentation 189
  ECT 195, 196–197
  ECT mechanisms of action 195
  medical history 191
  medication history and current 191
  patient evaluations 191
  physician's notes 191–192, 193, 194
  psychiatric history 190
  psychopharmacology dilemmas 189
  reflections on clinical practice 198
  self-assessment questions 189, 199
  social and personal history 190

traumatic brain injury (cont.)
 take-home points 197
 two-minute tutorial 198
treatment-resistant schizophrenia (TRS);
  see also antipsychotics (side effects of treatment in TRS)
 antipsychotics 175
 ECT 178
 misidentification syndromes 85, 88
 two-minute tutorial 93–94
trimester of pregnancy
 antipsychotics 347
 psychosis 343
TRS *see* treatment-resistant schizophrenia

vasopressin, primary polydipsia 110–111
violence; *see also* aggression; predatory violence; psychotic violence; self-injurious behavior and aggression; sexually violent predators
 classification of types 22–25
 clozapine 12
 coinciding with ECT treatment 10
 definition 22–23, 34
 and impulsivity 11, 18, 22–25
 risk assessments 35–36, 37
 urge to inflict 6
viral infection *see* COVID-19
voices, hearing *see* hearing voices

water intoxication 97; *see also* primary polydipsia
women's mental health in pregnancy *see* pregnancy
World Federation of Societies of Biological Psychiatry (WFSMP), sex offending 331, 339–341

Index of drug names

acamprosate 213, 214
amantadine 315
amisulpride 135–136, 171, 183, 207
amitriptyline 220–221
amphotericin B 109, 110
aripiprazole 5, 25, 132, 173, 193, 203–204, 210, 211–212, 220–221, 226, 229, 231, 237, 272, 344, 349, 353
armodafinil 132
atropine 105

benztropine 66–67, 99–100, 117, 203–204, 272, 273, 291, 293–294
botulinum toxin 105
bromocriptine 164, 166
buprenorphine 213
bupropion 5, 203–204, 210, 213, 214, 220–221
buspirone 98, 107, 252, 253, 254

carbamazepine 75, 120, 229–230, 237
cariprazine 135–136, 179, 180, 181, 183, 207, 210–211
chlorpromazine 78, 79, 176, 193, 220–221, 275
cidofovir 109, 110
citalopram 5, 7–8, 193, 203–204, 210, 220–221, 226
clomipramine 240, 241, 242
clonazepam 5, 66–67, 99–100, 203–204, 210, 344
clonidine 30
clozapine 4–5, 6, 7–8, 9, 10, 11, 12, 13, 17, 19, 20, 21, 22, 23, 24, 25, 43, 44, 45, 46, 47, 54, 55–56, 57, 85, 87, 88, 89, 90–91, 92–93, 94–95, 99–100, 103, 104–105, 106, 107, 132, 133–134, 135–136, 140, 145, 149–150, 162, 171, 175, 176, 177, 178, 179–180, 181, 183, 189, 193, 203–204, 207–208, 209, 210, 211, 215, 220–221, 225, 229, 235, 244, 271, 274, 277, 280–281, 284–285, 290, 292, 293–294, 295, 303, 306, 312, 313–314, 315, 316, 321, 324, 358, 359, 360
clozaril 37, 38, 39, 349
COVID-19 vaccine 271, 277, 279, 284–285

dantrolene 164, 165, 166, 167
demeclocycline 109, 110
dextroamphetamine 237
diazepam 163
digoxin 12
diphenhydramine 105, 203–204, 210, 273, 274, 275, 276
disulfiram 213, 214
divalproex 5, 19, 21, 22, 47, 48, 54, 55–56, 57, 79, 107, 142, 144, 145, 192, 193, 220–221, 237, 248, 291, 292, 293–294, 295, 313, 314, 315, 316
doxepin 173, 210
duloxetine 78, 79, 132, 142–143, 145, 173, 203–204, 210, 220–221, 229, 263

escitalopram 5
etomidate 8, 9, 13

famotidine 11, 87
ferrous sulfate 6
fludrocortisone 315
fluoxetine 5, 75, 76, 78, 97, 99–100, 102, 103, 105, 107, 108, 111, 135–136, 203–204, 210, 220–222, 225, 229, 242, 339, 344, 349
fluphenazine 5, 54, 55–56, 57, 99–100, 107, 193, 203–204, 209, 211–212, 220–221, 225
fluvoxamine 229
foscarnet 109, 110

gabapentin 132, 145, 210–211, 212–213, 229–230
glycopyrrolate 105
guanfacine 75, 294, 295, 306

Index of drug names

haloperidol 4, 5, 6, 7, 17, 20, 21, 22, 32, 33, 66–67, 86, 99–100, 104, 107, 143, 144, 145, 162, 173, 193, 203–204, 207–208, 209, 210, 211–212, 220–221, 225, 229, 235, 244, 271, 272, 273, 274, 275, 276, 292, 293–294, 295, 312, 313, 314, 315, 316, 344, 345–346, 349, 355, 360
hydroxyzine 6, 32, 33, 99–100, 103, 105, 142, 145, 203–204, 210

ifosfamide 109, 110
imipramine 132
indomethacin 148
isoniazid 294

ketamine 8, 9, 13, 226, 228

lactulose 6
lamotrigine 5, 7–8, 132, 229–230
leuprolide acetate 331, 333–334, 335
levetiracetam 120, 290, 306
levodopa 301, 303, 306
levothryroxine 6
lithium 5, 17, 20, 21, 22, 44, 47, 48, 54, 55–56, 57, 78, 79, 85, 90–91, 97, 99–100, 102, 107, 109, 110, 111, 120, 132, 142, 144, 145, 149–150, 156, 173, 175, 178, 193, 203–204, 207–208, 209, 210, 220–221, 225, 226, 290, 292, 293–294, 295, 300, 313, 314, 315
lofexidine 213, 214
lorazepam 5, 99–100, 117, 118, 119, 120, 121, 122, 123, 124, 125, 126, 168, 203–204, 210, 220–221, 248, 252, 253, 272, 273
loxapine 99–100, 107, 173, 175, 193, 235, 244
lurasidone 88, 89, 175, 176, 178, 220–221

melatonin 220–221
memantine 11
metformin 6, 132, 231
methadone 213, 214
methohexital 8, 9, 13
methylphenidate 237
minocycline 11
mirtazapine 5, 102, 143, 144, 145, 173, 203–204, 210, 220–221

naloxone 213, 214
naltrexone 87, 106, 109, 203–204, 205, 206, 207–208, 210–211, 213, 214, 215, 220–221, 226, 229–230, 231, 339
norclozapine 10, 12

ofloxacin 109, 110
olanzapine 5, 6, 30, 44, 68–69, 86, 88, 89, 98, 99–100, 102, 103, 104, 105, 106, 107, 135–136, 143, 144, 145, 171, 173–174, 175, 176, 180, 183, 189, 192, 193, 203–204, 210, 211–212, 220–221, 225, 229, 252, 253, 254, 271, 272, 273, 312, 344, 345–346, 353, 354, 355
omeprazole 290
ondansetron 135–136
oxcarbazepine 132
oxytocin 132, 133–134

paliperidone 118, 203–204, 209, 210, 211–212, 229, 291–292, 293–294, 343, 344, 345–346, 347
pantoprazole 290
paroxetine 99–100, 107, 173, 220–221, 242, 248, 252, 253, 254, 355
perphenazine 210, 235, 244
polyethylene glycol 6
prazosin 76, 78, 79, 220–221, 225
propranolol 5, 192, 193, 203–204
pyridoxine 294

quetiapine 5, 66–67, 68, 99–100, 107, 132, 173, 193, 203–204, 210, 220–221, 229, 237, 271, 272, 273, 344

rifampin 294
risperidone 5, 7–8, 44, 76, 86, 99–100, 107, 143, 145, 171, 172, 173, 175, 183, 193, 203–204, 209, 210, 211–212, 237, 239, 240, 272, 275, 276, 343, 344, 345–346, 347

sertraline 5, 143, 173, 203–204, 209, 210, 220–221, 239, 240, 242, 273, 275, 339, 349, 354, 355, 360

tamsulosin 6
temazepam 220–221
thioridazine 176

thiothixene 173
topiramate 120, 192, 203–204, 206, 207–208, 210–211, 212–213, 220–221, 229–230, 252, 253, 254
trazodone 99–100, 107, 135–136, 173, 203–204, 220–221, 344, 345–346

valproate 25, 145

valproic acid 5, 30, 99–100, 107, 120, 121, 193, 220–221, 229–230, 344
varenicline 213, 214
venlafaxine 203–204, 207–208, 210, 229

ziprasidone 5, 141–142, 144, 145, 203–204, 207–208, 229, 252, 253, 272, 273, 344
zolpidem 220–221